The HOME MEDICAL HANDBOOK

The HOME MEDICAL HANDBOOK

Jack I. Stern, M.D. & David L. Carroll

William Morrow and Company, Inc. New York

Library of Congress Cataloging-in-Publication Data

Carroll, David.
    The home medical handbook.
    Bibliography: p.
    1. Medicine, Popular—Handbooks, manuals, etc.
2. Self-care, Health—Handbooks, manuals, etc.
I. Carroll, David, 1942–   . II. Title.
RC81.S777   1987   616   87-1726
ISBN 0-688-06073-0

Printed in the United States of America

2   3   4   5   6   7   8   9   10

BOOK DESIGN BY BARBARA MARKS

CONTENTS

INTRODUCTION

The What's and the Why's of Medical Self-Care

You know the story well enough: costs of hospitalization rocket daily without foreseeable limits. Health care institutions grow increasingly overpopulated, out-priced, and understaffed. Fees shoot up unchecked. The frenetic world of institutionalized medical services relies more on high-tech machinery and less on loving human care while, sadly, the commercial and government authorities which are in a position to do something about this unfortunate situation, are unable—or unwilling—to act.

Thus, the birth of the medical consumer lobby. If those in charge are not going to help reduce the burden of medical care on the average person, they say, then we will take matters into our own hands. If the medical establishment insists on providing less than adequate services while raising their prices for the privilege, then the line must be drawn and action must be taken. Enter medical self-care.

Medical Self-Care: What Is It?

In a nutshell, it is *patient-applied* medical therapy and rehabilitation. To varying degrees—and always, of course, within the limits of medical safety—the patient self-administers many of the medical tests, procedures, and therapies that thirty years ago fell within the exclusive domain of hospitals and physicians. In some cases these methods are practiced under a doctor's supervision. In others, the patient applies the techniques alone. In both cases, endless return trips to the hospital or to the doctor's office for services just as easily applied at home are rendered unnecessary.

Self-care techniques, with some overlap between areas, fall into three general categories:

1. *Preventive self-care*

A college student with a past history of minor bladder symptoms purchases an over-the-counter urinalysis kit and tests himself each month for ten different potential urinary problems. If and when abnormal test results appear, he immediately visits the doctor.

A health-conscious dress designer anxious to know more about the workings of her own body learns how to perform basic self-examination techniques—blood pressure, pulse, respiration rates, breast check—and now gives herself a regular abbreviated physical checkup every six months.

2. *Therapeutic self-care*

The mother of a child sick with the flu controls the child's temperature with over-the-counter medications, monitors all the vital signs herself, applies appropriate home remedies, stays on top of the ailment from beginning to end—and saves a costly trip to the doctor.

A copywriter who has been suffering from migraine headaches all her life buys a portable biofeedback kit and attempts to relieve the headaches at home.

3. *Convalescent self-care*

An elderly laborer who was hospitalized once for severe hypertension is taught how to use a sphygmomanometer at home, how to control his diet, how to exercise and generally improve the quality of his life style; he now monitors his own blood pressure, and knows when and when not to consult a physician.

An elderly executive who is prone to painful back problems learns a series of helpful back exercises. By following this regime faithfully every morning and night he improves both the strength and flexibility of his entire lower back area.

Self-care works on several levels. It encourages patients to learn the basics of self-diagnosis for minor disorders, and, when necessary, to pass this information on to physicians. It supports preventive medicine of all kinds, from dietary control to exercise to good dental hygiene. It supplements a doctor's diagnosis and care. It gives patients more say in their treatment, therefore allowing them to feel a part of their own healing processes. It helps patients learn, when a disorder may be serious, and when they can be their own physician. It educates laymen in the basics of health care, physiology, and healthful life-style habits. It saves money, time, and energy. And, of course, it keeps the person who practices it healthy, alive, and alert.

The Limits of Self-Care

Of course, not all disorders are self-treatable. Certainly no one in his or her right mind would suggest that you treat yourself for tuberculosis or that you sew on a severed limb at home. Extreme cases, perhaps, but both have been tried. In general, self-care should always be just that—self-*care*—and should be practiced only:

1. For simple acute ailments that can be controlled by over-the-counter medications and/or home remedies, and that are known to respond well to self-treatment. Colds, cold sores, ringworm, constipation, headaches are examples.

2. For chronic ailments that are first diagnosed and treated by a doctor, then monitored at home by the patient in between visits to the physician. Arthritis, back injuries, and hypertension are typical cases.

3. For convalescence from a major disease or serious accident. In this instance self-care must almost always be practiced under a physician's guidance.

4. For certain psychophysical disorders which, though not diseases per se, can have a debilitating effect if left untreated for long periods of time. Stress or sleeping difficulties are examples.

Given these limitations, the question then arises: When should the doctor be consulted? Though advocates will answer this question in many different ways, general rules of thumb are:

1. In *all* emergency situations—call a doctor.

2. When an ailment does not respond to home care within a reasonable amount of time—call a doctor.

3. When symptoms of a disorder recur on a regular basis—call a doctor.

4. When unusual symptoms or pains not ordinarily associated with the ailment appear—call a doctor.

5. When there is a sudden, unpredicted, and potentially harmful turn for the worse—call a doctor.

6. When there is severe pain—call a doctor.

Again, it is difficult to be precise in this matter, as every dis-order comes packaged with its own symptoms and eccentricities. As a help in this direction, the self-care instructions given for specific disorders in this book contain a section describing when a physician's care is required.

The Doctor's Role

Although many physicians continue to resist patient-adminis-tered care, and certain powerful medical associations seem deter-mined to keep patients as far removed from their own medical treatment as possible—even in instances where self-care is clearly both practicable and advisable—there is a growing grass roots recognition among many physicians that patient self-help is a cause whose time has come. Articles on the subject crop up with in-creasing frequency even in the most conservative medical jour-nals. Industries of all kinds are producing almost a billion dollars' worth of home-care medical equipment a year. Popular maga-zines such as *Medical Self-Care* regularly feature lists of health care practitioners around the country who are amenable to these new ideas. Pushed from behind, as it were, by this popular move-ment, the doctor's role is changing along with the patient's, and both are profiting.

What then is the doctor's role in medical self-care? Potentially, he or she has several key roles to play. First, the doctor should be an *adviser*. Consultations over the phone save unnecessary of-fice visits, and in many cases can accomplish as much as actual trips to the doctor, especially if the ailment is minor. The patient saves money, and the doctor saves time and effort better spent on patients requiring immediate medical attention or on patients desiring information concerning risk factors and methods of pre-vention.

The doctor should be an *educator*. By teaching patients to use the blood pressure cuff and the stethoscope to perform home medical tests and self-exams, the health-care professional be-comes both coach and tutor. Certainly a patient who knows the rudiments of medical terminology and tentative self-diagnosis will make the physician's job easier. Such a patient follows directions more clearly, describes symptoms in a more informed way, and generally has a firmer grip on the mechanics of his or her own curative processes. As a result, the doctor spends less time and less guesswork in making a diagnosis. Many doctors responsive to self-care even *insist* that their patients learn basic principles of physiology and self-examination, and some go so far as to print their own booklets on the subject. Most of these doctors are available whenever they are needed as sources of information, counsel, and further treatment.

Finally, the doctor should be a willing *partner* in helping patients take some degree of responsibility in the process of their own healing. A growing number of men and women feel it is not acceptable for a medical practitioner to silence patients with a homily such as: "My job is to cure you, not to educate you." Indeed, they believe that the processes of education and of cure should often be the same.

In short, the era of the impotent patient and the omnipotent doctor is coming to an end. Today's medical consumers are better educated, more sophisticated in medical matters, and a good deal more wary of physician authoritarianism than ever before. And the physician, the new physician who is willing to make patients partners in health care, is already more than halfway toward the goal of regaining a lost trust.

Why Self-Care Today

Forty or fifty years ago a great deal of our health care was administered by close friends or family members—at home. Traditionally, Americans have doctored themselves partly in the bedroom, partly in the physician's office, and partly, as a last resort, in the hospital.

Following World War II, however, medicine became a big business as well as a personal calling. Doctors allied themselves with hospitals and unilaterally abolished the time-honored service of the house call. Both private and government insurance plans *forced* patients to enter hospitals on the slightest provocation, and high-tech testing and therapeutic machinery kept them there. As a result, institutionalized medicine quickly became the norm. The fact remains, however, that in many cases the hospital is the least desirable, most expensive place to get health care; it has been estimated that at least *25 to 30 percent of the patients* now in health care institutions do not need to be there.

There are, as well, other reasons for the self-care revolution. In brief, these are:

• Advances in electronics, chip technology, and medical research are providing consumers with low-cost, home-use medical machinery and self-testing devices that were simply not available even three or four years ago.

• Medical self-care for minor ailments is less expensive and in many cases equally as effective as professional medical care.

• Hospitals and health-care institutions are usually crowded, expensive, confusing places. If home health options are available, many consumers will leap at the chance.

• Home-care programs associated with hospitals or with pri vate nursing agencies, once heavily discouraged by the medical profession, are coming to play an increasingly conspicuous role in American health care.

• Medical consumers are more sophisticated in health-related matters than ever before. Many consumers have already used some type of self-care service or device. Many of them like it; many of them want more.

• A growing number of doctors are dissatisfied with the present patient-physician relationship. They are seeking new approaches to health care that are more suitable to both parties.

SELF-CARE: GETTING STARTED

Most ailments treated in a physician's office could as easily be dealt with at home by patients who know the self-care ropes. In some cases these ailments are acute problems for which standard home remedies and over-the-counter medications are available; all the doctor can do in such situations is suggest simple therapeutic measures which an informed medical consumer would know about already. In other instances the ailment may be a chronic one; and here again, after the preliminary diagnosis is made by the physician, self-maintenance, supported by phone consultations and constant progress updates, will accomplish as much as an office visit—or at least make such visits less frequent.

Although many elements of medical practice are highly technical, the basics can be learned by anyone of average intelligence. Educators have urged that such skills be taught throughout grade school and high school, and that self-care be made a part of every young person's consciousness. In the words of Dr. Jonas Salk: *

---

*Larry Holden, "The Man Who Eradicated Polio—30 Years Later: Jonas Salk," *The Continental* (March 1985), p. 70.

It's for this reason that studying human nature—to see how to help people help themselves to become their own health managers—is the new challenge. Such studying of human nature has to start very early in life. Beyond reading, writing and arithmetic, we have to introduce into the educational system an understanding of biology, especially human biology. That understanding will guide us in becoming skillful in living healthy, constructive, contributing lives.

So far, of course, our educational system has not responded to the call. Yet there is nothing stopping any of us from taking matters into our own hands and beginning the process of medical self-education now, right away, this very day. Indeed, it could be said that, of all the self-help options open to Americans, medical self-care is the most pressing and significant.

This book will get you started. The first section describes methods of self-treatment for most of the common minor ailments you will be likely to encounter. The emphasis is on:

1. Learning to identify specific symptoms.
2. Applying appropriate therapies.
3. Recognizing when an ailment can be self-treated and when it should be seen by a doctor.
4. Locating tools, services, and resources helpful in treating the disorder.

In some instances standard over-the-counter medications are recommended. In others, tried-and-proven natural and home remedies are suggested. In still others, both options are included.

The second section starts with a lengthy chapter teaching you how to perform a medical self-examination. This description takes you through the basics, from performing a respiration count to diagnosing abnormalities in your own urine. Next follows a chapter describing the most useful medical self-tests currently available, and another on the basics of home care. The last chapter tells you how to practice preventive health techniques and how to maintain good health.

The third and final sections provides an exhaustive list of basic and secondary self-care aids and resources. Included are self-care organizations, services, literature, audiovisual materials, telephone aids, and computer software.

Use this book as a reference and as a guide. The reference materials will help you locate information on self-care techniques and show you how to track down the many resources available in this growing area of medicine. The chapters on therapy and treatment will advise you on the best self-applied techniques for getting well. The sections on self-examination, prevention and medical self-testing will teach you how to stay that way. Good luck. Good health. And remember the adage, tried and true: God helps those who help themselves.

MEDICAL SELF-CARE FOR COMMON AILMENTS

CHAPTER 1

INSOMNIA

WHEN YOU CAN'T FALL ASLEEP

Insomnia is an ailment of degrees. It ranges from occasional nights of wakefulness to a chronic and prolonged inability to fall asleep under any circumstances. (There have actually been cases of individuals who never sleep, and who simply rest in a kind of half-waking, half-sleeping state for several minutes at a time.) In a majority of instances the former variety, the occasional sleepless night, is due to one or a combination of traceable causes. Most of these can usually be helped. They include:

- Caffeine stimulation (too much coffee, tea, No-Doz, or soft drinks, especially when taken later in the day).
- Worry, mental excitement, depression, anxiety over personal and work-related problems.
- Lack of exercise.
- Snoring, respiratory problems, chronic coughs.
- Uncomfortable sleeping conditions: noise, light, a new or uncomfortable bed, etc.
- Sleeping too late in the morning.
- Napping for long periods during the day.
- Excessive drinking of alcoholic beverages.
- Side effects of medications (especially diuretics—stay away from them at night).

- Low-level physical discomfort (such as the kind caused by indigestion, leg cramps, skin irritations, etc.).

A couple of "maybes" you can add to this list include excess intake of salt; heavy smoking (cigarettes sometimes act as a stimulant); dieting (some people have a difficult time getting to sleep on an empty stomach); and excess use of sleeping pills.

Interestingly, while one might assume that the items mentioned above are all obvious sleep inhibitors, many people, even insomniacs, fail to recognize them as such, simply because these activities have become so familiar and habitual in their lives. Doctors constantly hear complaints of sleep disorders from patients who, when questioned carefully, admit to drinking two cups of coffee each night after dinner or napping from five to seven every evening. "But Doctor," they protest when this is brought to their attention, "I've *always* done that!"

The first rule of insomnia self-treatment is therefore a simple one: Review your daily activities. Look for ordinary habits and activities that you may take for granted but that may be causing the sleep problems.

The Anatomy of Sleep

Here is a brief description of the sleep process itself. Two phases of sleep activity are most important:

1. Rapid Eye Movement Sleep (REM Sleep) which takes place when we dream.
2. Non-REM Sleep (NREM) which occurs in the non-dream state.

These phases can be differentiated on a polygraph by the facts that during REM sleep:

1. The eyes register a certain number of movements per minute beneath the lids.
2. Brain waves are almost as active as during the waking state.
3. Muscle tone approaches a condition akin to paralysis.

During NREM sleep, on the other hand, brain waves are slower, rapid eye movements cease, and some muscle tone returns.

When the body's normal patterns of REM and NREM sleep are disturbed—when there is too much REM sleep at the expense of the deeper NREM or when NREM itself is not deep enough—problems arise. All the items listed above are potential inhibitors of normal REM and NREM sleep.

SELF-DIAGNOSIS OF INSOMNIA

Self-diagnosis of insomnia is relatively straightforward. The primary symptom is as follows: *If you are regularly spending at least one hour a night or more trying to fall asleep, then you probably have some form of sleep disturbance.* Note, too, that early morning rising with an accompanying inability to fall back to sleep is also a form of insomnia. So is a regular pattern of nocturnal awakenings, especially when it occurs at approximately the same hour each night. Also, a consistent feeling upon awakening that you slept poorly or not at all. Watch out during the day for unreasonable sensations of irritability, restlessness, and malaise—prolonged sleep deprivation will inevitably produce all three. Concentration may become impaired and one's work and social and personal life may suffer accordingly.

PREVENTIVE TECHNIQUES AND SELF-CARE FOR INSOMNIA

The type of self-care used for insomnia depends to a large extent on the specific factors causing it. Although in some cases this means there are things you can do to help the problem, in other cases it means there are things you must *stop doing*.

Eight Ways to Prevent Sleeplessness

1. *Control Caffeine Intake*

The treatment here is obvious: Stop drinking so much caffeine. This is especially true if you are prone to "coffee nerves" or if you tend to drink caffeine later in the day. Remember, while coffee, tea, and soft drinks in the morning often have little effect on sleep patterns, if taken from four P.M. on, their stimulating properties can be felt far into the night. If you have any question as to whether or not caffeinated substances are causing sleep disturbances, abstain from them for a week or two. And keep in mind that caffeine is hidden in certain foods such as cocoa, chocolate, and cola drinks and in medications such as antidepressants, appetite-suppressants, stimulants, aspirin compounds, cold pills (e.g., Excedrin), and decongestants containing pseudoephedrine and phenylpropanolamine.

2. *Get a Handle on Worry, Mental Excitement, Depression, and Anxiety over Personal Problems*

Many sleep disorders are based on the ordinary frustrations

and excitements that build up during the day and take their revenge at bedtime. In fact, it has been estimated that from 50 to 90 percent of all insomnia stems from depression, worry, and stress. If you can identify these problems and isolate them, so much the better. But even if you can't, there are things that can be done. Counting sheep is still a favorite, and it works for some. Another good exercise is to relax your body entirely, then imagine a blackboard with the number ten written on it. Picture a hand entering the frame, erasing the number, and writing a nine in its place. After a moment, the hand erases the nine and draws an eight; and so on down to zero. Then repeat the whole process. This simple exercise can produce wonderful results. The notion behind such methods, of course, is to remove your mind from worrisome subjects, suspend the thoughts of the day, and lull the body into a state conducive to slumber.

Another remedy for nighttime anxiety is the relaxation exercise. This also comes in many forms, of course, though its goal is always to release psychophysical tensions and slow metabolism rates. For effective examples of such exercises, consult the chapters on headache and stress, and see the section below on technology and resources for information on recorded relaxation tapes.

3. *Exercise Regularly*

Many of us have desk jobs that limit daily physical activities. Since our bodies were built to remain intensely active during the day, we pay a higher price for the sedentary way of life. What to do? An obvious antidote is exercise. Many people find that a half hour to forty-five minutes of daily calisthenics or jogging calms the mind and body at night and helps in falling asleep.

Generally speaking, it's advised that you exercise four to six hours before going to bed. As it turns out, one of the most critical factors in getting to sleep is body temperature. If your temperature is going down at bedtime, you will have an easier time falling off; if it's going up, there can be trouble. Exercise tends to raise the metabolic rate for several hours and hence the body temperature as well. After five or six hours have passed, the metabolism slows down again and the temperature drops. People who take scalding baths to relax at night should be warned on this count. Hot baths raise the body temperature and interfere with sleep. Lukewarm baths are almost as relaxing and have a negligible effect on the body's thermostat. Also, since intense exercise raises body temperature, it's better to confine all pre-bed

calisthenics to mild stretching. Jogging at night may be a pleasure, but it is no aid to falling asleep. (Of course, if you do have
problems falling asleep even *without* jogging, then keep on jogging.)

4. *Make Your Sleeping Environment As Comfortable
As Possible*

Seemingly small factors such as a poor mattress, a stuffy room
or too much noise can interfere with sound sleep. Some tricks in
this area include:

• Sleep on a really *good* mattress. The investment may be considerable, but if it buys you a night's sleep, it's worth any price.

• If you share a bed with another person, make sure you are
not too cramped. A king-size bed may help. Occasionally, the
only solution is to sleep in separate beds, or separate rooms if
snoring is part of the problem.

• Keep the room dark, quiet, and well-ventilated. A stuffy
sleeping area can keep you awake and interfere with the quality
of your rest.

• Try falling asleep to soft music or to relaxation tapes. For
some people they work. Studies have found, incidentally, that low
droning noises, such as an air conditioner, may interfere with
REM sleep and disturb sleep patterns. Note, however, that for
some people droning noises actually aid in sleep.

• Try elevating your legs a few inches at bedtime. This simple
trick has helped many people get a sounder rest.

• Make sure you have enough blankets and that all coverings
feel pleasant to the touch. Lamb's wool undersheets are touted
by some as improving the quality of sleep, though nothing has
been proven. Don't use too many covers. Their weight can be
disturbing. Experiment with an electric blanket or down com-
forter if blanket weight is a problem.

• The quality of the pillow is important. Is it too hard or too
soft? Is it stuffed with materials that feel good under your head
and neck? As with a mattress, a good pillow is an expensive but
valuable investment.

• Clutter can be disturbing. Make sure the environment around
your bed is quiet and tidy before you get in. A made bed is some-
how more enjoyable than an unmade bed. Clean sheets are more
comfortable than soiled ones.

• Wear nightclothes that are comfortable and non-binding. If
they scratch or irritate, replace them.

5. Don't Sleep too Late in the Morning or Nap too Late in the Day

The brain is programmed to fall asleep a limited number of times during the day and night. If you use up too many of these opportunities before bedtime, you'll find yourself tossing and turning at night. Naps should be brief and taken at the same hour every day, preferably before three o'clock in the afternoon. Right after lunch, as Europeans understand, is the best time. As for sleeping late, any break in patterns of rising and retiring can disrupt the subtle time clocks and hormonal rhythms that govern our behavior. The best thing to do is to establish regular rising and bedtime hours and *stick to them*. After awhile, the body will become accustomed to its schedule and reward you accordingly.

6. Curtail Excessive Drinking of Alcoholic Beverages

In small amounts alcohol can be relaxing. Too much liquor puts a person into a stupor, interferes with all-important periods of REM sleep, and produces a daze (if not a hangover) the next morning. Alcohol metabolizes quite rapidly and its effects wear off long before the seven or eight hours necessary for a sound sleep have passed, causing people to wake at odd hours of the night and seriously disrupt sleep patterns.

7. Watch Out for the Side Effects of Medication

Many medicinal drugs include stimulants of some kind such as caffeine, or occasionally stronger chemicals like amphetamines. Be sure to read the information on the label of all medications, both prescription and non-prescription, and consult your physician about the possible sleep-inhibiting—and nightmare-producing—effects of whatever medications you may be taking.

8. Be on the Lookout for Hidden Physical Discomforts

Pains such as indigestion, slight joint aches, skin sensitivities, and mild chest or nose congestion all hover on the margins of awareness and can be just distracting enough to keep a person awake. The insidious thing about these annoyances is that they are sometimes so slight that the sufferer does not recognize them as the culprits. Become more aware of your body as you lie sleepless at night. Run a mental searchlight over yourself from head to toe, paying special attention to your stomach, skin, head, and joints. Search for hidden sources of irritation or malaise. An act as simple as taking an aspirin (without caffeine!) or an antacid before bed may be all that is necessary to overcome these problems and get a sound night's sleep.

The Sleeping Pill Question: Should You or Shouldn't You?

One thing to bear in mind about sleeping pills is that their effectiveness—when they *are* effective—often wears off after several weeks. As a rule, ten to fourteen days is the average time it takes for sleeping preparations to lose their sleep-inducing powers.

Add to this that sleeping pills can easily become addictive; that many of them interfere with the natural rhythms of REM and NREM sleep; that some contain chemicals of questionable safety; and that the side effects are often unpleasant and severe—and you have some powerful strikes against the sleeping-pill route to sleep.

Take note, as well, of the following information on popular sedative drugs and their possible side effects:

• *Phenobarbital* (Brand names: Barbipil, Eskabarb, Floramine, Henomint, Luminal) Possible side effects: drowsiness, skin rashes, nausea, unusual bleeding, mental apathy, hepatitis with jaundice, sluggishness

• *Secobarbital* (Brand names: Seconal, Seco-8, Tuinal) Possible side effects: allergic reactions, anemia, delirium, skin rashes, dizziness, nausea, muscle and joint pains

• *Chloral Hydrate* (Brand names: Aquachloral, Cohidrate, Dormal, Felsules, Kessodrate, Oradrate, Somnos) Possible side effects: severe skin reactions, vomiting, nausea, nightmares, hangover effect, delirium, heartburn

• *Glutethimide* (Brand names: Doriden, Dorimide) Possible side effects: hives, skin rashes, confusion, fatigue, sore throat, nausea, blurred vision, addiction, unusual bleeding, fever

• *Methaqualone* (Brand names: Parest, Quaalude, Sopor, Somnafac) Possible side effects: skin rashes, hives, diarrhea, unusual bleeding and bruising, indigestion, fatigue, fever, sore throat, bone marrow depression

• *Methyprylon* (Brand name: Noludar) Possible side effects: dizziness, hangover effect, unusual bleeding, numbness in the arms and legs, indigestion, nausea, diarrhea, hives, sore throat, fever, bone marrow depression

• *Flurazepam* (Brand name: Dalmane) Possible side effects: dizziness, blurred vision, slurred speech, hallucinations, jaundice, excitability, nausea, headache, indigestion, skin rashes, lightheadedness

What About Over-the-Counter Sleeping Pills?

What about over-the-counter sleep remedies such as Nytol, Sominex, Nite Rest, and the others? Many of these depend on antihistamines such as diphenhydramine hydrochloride for their somnambulistic effects, a drug that works for some people and not for others. This family of drugs, moreover, can produce mental torpor, sometimes intense, along with dry mouth, dizziness, and occasionally nausea and blurred vision. According to Goodman and Gilman in *The Pharmacological Basis of Therapeutics*, "About one person in four will experience some bothersome reaction during treatment with a given antihistamine." In other words, nonprescription sleep-inducers will work—but only sometimes and only for certain people.

As of the writing of this book, the FDA has approved only two substances, *Diphenhydramine* (diphenhydramine hydrochloride and diphenhydramine monocitrate) and *Doxylamine succinate* as being both effective and safe nonprescription sleep-inducing chemicals. Look for both on the label when buying an over-the-counter product. *Pyrilamine maleate* has been only conditionally approved, while aspirin, passionflower extract, bromides, salicylamide, all scopolamine compounds, and the vitamin thiamine hydrochloride have been deemed either unsafe or ineffective for insomnia.

Commercial sleep aids that have been recognized as safe and effective include Unisom, Nytol with DPH, Sominex Formula 2, and Compoz Tablets. Of questionable use are Nytol, Quiet World, and Relax-U Caps.

In short, sleeping pills are a chancy and, perhaps, even dangerous route to a good night's sleep. This does not mean, of course, that they are without value. When carefully prescribed by a thoughtful physician they have their place; and over-the-counter sedatives are useful for occasional sleepless nights and for those times when the frustrations of life have us keyed up beyond our control. All in all, however, it is advisable to try other, less volatile alternatives before turning to this problem-ridden option.

Warning: If You Must Take Sleeping Pills, Be Careful. The following list includes important details that your doctor may or may not give you. If you have any questions about a particular sleep medication, be sure to raise them at the time the prescription is written, *not* after you have been taking the drug for a week or so.

FACT ONE:
Sleep-inducing drugs can sometimes lessen the effectiveness of other medications (secobarbital, for instance, can reduce the effects of anticoagulants; phenobarbital can interfere with the pain-killing effects of aspirin). Sedatives can also *increase* another drug's effect, sometimes to an unwanted degree (secobarbital increases the strength of antihistamines and tranquilizers; chloral hydrate may heighten the effects of oral anticoagulants, causing abnormal bleeding and even hemorrhage). Get all the information you can on this subject *before use.*

FACT TWO:
Never mix a sleeping pill, and especially a barbiturate, with alcohol. Together the two can increase both the sedative and depressant action on the brain. In certain instances the combination can be fatal.

FACT THREE:
Women who take oral contraceptives should be aware that phenobarbital, by speeding up the contraceptive's clearance rate from the body, reduces its effectiveness as a pregnancy-inhibitor.

FACT FOUR:
Many forms of sleeping pills, including chloral hydrate, seco-barbital, glutethimide and others, can become psychologically and physically addictive. Be sure to learn the details of this potential problem before starting an extended course of the drug. Be warned, furthermore, that while barbiturates are perhaps the most addicting of sleep drugs, central nervous system depressants (glutethimide, methaqualone, methyprylon), which are touted as being less habit-forming, sometimes produce the same results.

FACT FIVE:
The drug flurazepam (Dalmane) remains in the body for long periods of time. Therefore, it tends to make patients groggy and hampers coordination. To make matters worse, users are often oblivious of the cumulative effects of the drug and serious acci-

dents may result. If you are using Dalmane regularly, be extremely careful when driving, performing dangerous tasks, etc.

FACT SIX:

Pregnant women should *always* be wary of sleeping pills. Sedatives can have a direct effect on the fetus, while the drowsiness they produce can make a pregnant woman more prone to falls, slips, household accidents, and the like.

FACT SEVEN:

It is not uncommon for a person to have an intolerance to certain sedative drugs. If unusual skin, respiratory, or digestive symptoms result from medications, discontinue use and check with your physician.

FACT EIGHT:

When discontinuing sleep-inducing drugs it is sometimes necessary, in order to avoid a "rebound effect," to taper off the medication rather than to stop it abruptly. Each drug is somewhat different in this respect and requires different procedures. Seek professional medical advice.

FACT NINE:

If sleep-inducing drugs are used for extended periods of time, periodic physical examinations may be necessary to check for organ damage. Prolonged use of chloral hydrate, for instance, requires that the kidneys be monitored. Liver function tests and complete blood cell counts may be necessary for persons taking secobarbital.

FACT TEN:

Certain sedatives, such as secobarbital, can produce seasonal problems in patients such as light sensitivity in summer or cold sensitivity in winter, especially in older people. Again, check with a health care professional.

FACT ELEVEN:

If your physician prescribes sleep-inducing drugs, and if any of the following factors are pertinent to your situation, volunteer all information concerning them *even if you are not asked*:

- If you suffer from any allergies or drug intolerances.
- If you have any kidney, liver, or digestive problems.
- If you plan to have surgery or general anesthesia in the near future.
- If you are taking any other type of medication.
- If you use narcotic drugs or excessive amounts of alcohol.
- If you are attempting to become pregnant.
- If you suffer from a specific disease such as epilepsy or porphyria.
- If you are taking birth control pills.
- If you are being treated by any other health-care professional such as a psychiatrist or a psychologist (they may not want you to use sleep medications).

More Helps and Hints on Getting to Sleep

For occasional nights of sleeplessness:

• Try reversing your normal sleeping position, placing your feet where your head goes and vice versa.

• Light a candle and gaze into it for fifteen minutes before retiring. Flame-gazing tends to calm the nervous system—this is a Yogic technique.

• Drink a calming infusion before bed. Camomile tea has a definite sedative effect. Teas made from hops, skullcap, peppermint, and valerian are all proven natural sleep-inducers. Be careful, however, of that cup of hot chocolate before retiring. Cocoa contains caffeine.

• The amino acid L-tryptophan, available in pill form at most natural food stores and at the vitamin counters of many pharmacies, is believed to have sleep-inducing qualities. Tryptophan comes naturally in milk, which is one reason why warm milk with a little honey (also a mild soporific) before retiring acts as a natural sedative.

• If the need to urinate in the middle of the night is waking you up, keep your liquid intake to a minimum after dinner. Also, be careful of taking diuretic drugs at night.

• Attempt to sleep *only* when you are tired. If you get in bed feeling wide awake, the chances are against you. Stay up awhile instead, read a little, listen to some soothing music, have a small carbohydrate snack (not too much and not too heavy; fruit warmed to room temperature is the most easily digested of snacks), keep warm, drink a soothing herbal tea. When you're feeling at ease and a little sleepy, try again.

• Force yourself to stay up late at night and to get up early in the morning. Follow this schedule for several weeks straight and do not deviate from it. This one takes discipline, but it works. Eventually, you will become so tired at night that you will fall asleep without prompting.

• Self-suggestion helps. In the chapter on headaches, a step-by-step self-hypnosis program is outlined that will prove very useful for insomnia. Simply repeating to oneself words such as "relax" or "sleep," and picturing these words spelled out before your mind's eye can be of help.

• Lull yourself to sleep with soothing music. Harp music is particularly effective for this purpose. Consult the technology and resources section below for information on sleep-inducing audio-cassette tapes.

When to Call the Doctor

If you experience an inability to get to sleep for more than two weeks straight, and if all self-applied remedies fail to work, a visit to the physician is appropriate. Chronic sleep disorders can be the result of many possible problems, most of them minor, a few of them major. Sleep apnea (temporary cessation of breathing), depression, muscle spasms, respiratory ailments, stomach problems, anxiety, hysteria, prostate disease, and many more factors can cause chronic insomnia. A careful checkup should reveal the origin of your particular problem.

Technology, Resources, Aids, and Services

1. Many sleep problems result from uncomfortable head support. *Propillow,* engineered to support the head and spine at just the right angle, was designed by a doctor and eliminates the need to support the head with the hands. Purchase it from *The Self-Care Catalog,* P.O. Box 999, Pt. Reyes, CA 94956, for $25.00. The catalog is free and is published as a service of *Medical Self-Care Magazine.* You might also consider Hammacher Schlemmer's *goosedown travel pillow,* a 12 x 17-inch travel pillow filled with European white goosedown, incredibly soft yet tightly packed and all natural. It costs $39.95 from Hammacher Schlemmer, 147 East 57th Street, New York, NY 10022, (800) 543-3366. More information on pillows is available in the technology and resources section in the back and neck chapter.

2. *Inflatable sleep incliners are wedge-shaped shoulder and head supports* designed both to reduce tension in the back and neck and to make breathing at night easier. Available from CLEO, Inc., 3957 Mayfield Road, Cleveland, OH 44121, for $8.00

3. *Sheepskin sheets,* soft, springy, natural, eight to nine feet square, are believed by some to improve the quality of sleep. Available for $45.00 from CLEO (address in number 2 above).

4. *Electric home beds* adjust via a button to any desired inclination. They are an excellent solution for the person who has trouble getting comfortable in bed. Also a good idea for bedridden patients. Available for $666.85, and must be ordered through a health-care professional from Abbey Medical, 13782 Crenshaw Blvd., Gardena, CA 90249, (800) 421-5126; in California call (800) 262-1294.

5. *Electronic massaging devices* come in many shapes and sizes and can be ordered from a number of different sources. They are useful for relaxing troubled sleepers before bedtime. *Cushion massages, twin head massagers, variable speed hand massagers, and deep heat massagers* are all available through a health-care professional from Abbey Medical (address in number 4 above). *Hand vibrators* (from $2.50), *home massage kits* ($19.00), *vibra massage kits* ($16.95) are available from CLEO (address in number 2 above). *A flexible hand-held adjustable neck massager* is available for $49.50 from Hammacher Schlemmer (address in number 1 above). *A professional oscillating motion deep-penetration variable-speed massager* is available from the same source for $107.50. For more suggestions, see the technology and resources section in the back and neck chapter.

6. Listening to *sleep-inducing self-hypnosis tapes* before bed has helped many insomniacs sleep better. These can be obtained directly from B. K. Enterprises, 9478 Olympic Boulevard, P.O. Box 6248, Beverly Hills, CA 90212. Write for their complete catalog. Another source is Applied Subliminals, P.O. Box 135, Cresskill, NJ 07626. For more information on relaxation tapes, see the technology and resources sections in the chapters on stress and headache.

7. *Relaxation tapes—guided imagery and music on 30-minute cassette tape engineered for relaxation at bedtime*—are available for $9.95 from Inner Guidance System, Gwynedd Plaza II, Suite 301, Spring House, PA 19477. Another tape, "Letting Go of Stress," is available from *The Self-Care Catalog* (address in number 1 above) for $10.95. Other available tapes include "Re-

laxation and Stress Reduction" and "The Relaxation & Stress Reduction Workbook." Write for details to New Harbinger Publications, 2200 Adeline, Suite 305, Oakland, CA 94607. Finally, you can order sample relaxation tapes from a selection of ten different antistress cassettes for $2.00 from Emmett Miller Tapes, P.O. Box W, Stanford, CA 94305 (ask for their catalog).

8. *Electronic sleep sound generators are solid-state bedside machines that generate soothing sounds* of surf, waterfalls, and rain. The manufacturers' claim tests show "sound conditioned" sleepers receive about 50 percent more Delta (deep stage NREM) sleep, which may or may not be true. Available from *The Sharper Image Catalog,* 406 Jackson Street, San Francisco, CA 94111 for $129 plus postage. Call (800) 344-4444 for further details.

9. *Electronic mattress massager—A vibrating bedboard* that fits under the mattress and provides relaxing massage to feet, back, neck at bedtime. It costs $69.00 from *The Sharper Image Catalog* (address in number 8 above).

10. *Books and periodicals on sleep and insomnia:*

- *A Guide to Better Sleep,* for $1.00 from The Better Sleep Council, 1270 Avenue of the Americas, New York, NY 10020.
- *A Doctor Discusses Learning How to Live with Nervous Tension,* for $2.00. Contains a lot of information on stress and sleep. Order from Milex Products, 5915 Northwest Highway, Chicago, IL 60631.
- *Consumer Fact Sheet: Insomnia,* is free from Consumer Information Center, Pueblo, CO 81009.
- *Night Time and Your Handicapped Child.* For handicapped children with insomnia; from The Association for Retarded Children, National Headquarters, P.O. Box 6109, Avenue 'E' East, Arlington, TX 76011.
- *The Complete Book of Sleep* by Dianne Hales (Reading, MA: Addison-Wesley, 1981).
- *Morpheus and Me* by Phyllis Rosenteur (New York: Funk and Wagnalls, 1957).

CHAPTER 2

INSECT BITES AND STINGS

First a word of clarification. A *biting* insect such as an ant or beetle has mandibles and literally takes a nip out of its victim. This attack produces a momentarily painful experience but almost never a serious one. A stinging insect *injects* its stinger into the skin of its victim and either removes blood (such as a tick or mosquito) or puts poison in (such as a bee or wasp). Here is where potential trouble lies.

Be Careful: Stings Can Be Serious

Medically speaking, there are two types of insect sting reactions. The first, known as a *local reaction,* consists of a sharp burning sensation at the sting site caused by poisonous substances in the insect's venom. At times this reaction can involve a large area of the body such as the whole hand or face, but the swelling will *always* be contiguous with the sting site itself. Such stings occasionally become infected. If they do, the condition becomes evident one or two days after the sting when the wound takes on a raised, red, and swollen appearance and feels tender and warm to the touch. Treat such reactions immediately or they may worsen and require antibiotic therapy.

The second reaction, known as a *generalized multisystem response,* is triggered by an *allergy* to the insect venom. This response can be identified by the fact that the reaction usually takes place *on a part of the body separate from the sting site.* For example, a person is stung on the back of the hand. Within several minutes his face swells up, his throat starts to close, and breathing becomes labored. Such a response, known medically as an *anaphylactic reaction,* can sometimes become extremely severe, involving a change in blood pressure, impaired breathing, nausea, vomiting, loss of bowel and bladder control, and rarely, death. Obviously, such a condition requires immediate medical aid.

Most of the potentially dangerous stinging creatures come from the *hymenoptera* order of insects, containing bees, wasps, yellow jackets, hornets, and fire ants. With the exception of the fire ant, which lives mostly in the Southern states, these creatures are found everywhere in America and can be identified immediately after the attack has occurred. Although bees have a barbed stinger that stays lodged in the wound and remains behind, the stingers on wasps, hornets, and yellow jackets are straight and removable—which means these creatures can sting a person many times in a row and come back to sting some more. The presence of a stinger in the wound is a sign that you have been stung by a bee; the absence suggests a hornet, yellow jacket, or wasp. In either case, the attackers will deposit a small but virulent drop of venom into your blood, which will cause the site to redden and swell within five to fifteen minutes after the event. Pain usually accompanies the swelling, and if the recipient is particularly sensitive, the wound may throb. Note that bumblebees *do* sting, but only if thoroughly provoked. Treat their stings as you would any other bee sting.

SELF-CARE FOR ORDINARY, NONALLERGIC BEE, WASP, OR HORNET STINGS

There are many simple self-care remedies you can apply when treating a localized reaction from a bee, wasp, or hornet sting. Most of these remedies aim to keep the swelling down and reduce pain. Here's what to do:

1. Wash the sting site thoroughly.

2. If you have been stung by a bee, do not attempt to pull the stinger out directly (grabbing it will cause you to squeeze more venom into the wound). Rather, flick it off with the thumb and forefinger as quickly and as smoothly as possible.

3. Place ice on the sensitive area for a few minutes to keep the swelling down. Then try any of the following remedies:
- Witch hazel
- Calamine lotion
- Alcohol
- Meat tenderizer (monosodium glutamate)
- Baking soda
- A slice of raw onion
- A cut potato
- A mixture of vinegar and lemon juice
- A piece of raw meat
- A drop of honey (for bee stings only)
- Submerge in ice water
- Other substances that have been used on stings include castor oil, detergent, wheat germ oil, hot salt water, and shreds of tobacco.

SELF-CARE FOR OTHER TYPES OF INSECT STINGS AND BITES

Mosquitoes

Try placing a poultice combining lemon juice, cornstarch, and witch hazel on the bite. Lime juice, wet soap, salt, cobwebs, ice cubes, or your own saliva will all help curtail the itching and reduce the swelling. To repel mosquitoes in general, there is some evidence that taking 100 milligrams of thiamine about an hour before exposure will reduce the chance of being bitten. Note also that mosquitoes prefer the color blue, so avoid wearing it if you are going into mosquito country.

Fire Ant

Fire ants arrived in the United States in the last century and since then have migrated into thirteen southern and south central states. Extremely aggressive, their bite produces a pustule that develops within twenty-four hours after the attack and then slowly subsides. Wash the sting site, treat it with a steroid cream and perhaps an antihistamine, and allow it to run its natural course.

Gypsy Moths

Besides ravaging the countryside, these unpleasant pests are also capable of producing a skin rash upon contact. Wash the rash, dab a little wet baking soda on it, and make sure it gets plenty of air and light while it heals.

Chiggers

Chiggers are bloodsuckers that work their way under the skin and remain embedded, producing small, round, itchy, red spots. Wash the sores frequently and apply any good over-the-counter anti-itch cream such as Chiggerex. Refrain from scratching the spots; they easily become infected.

Ticks

Ticks bore into the skin and suck their victim's blood, but mercifully take a few minutes to sink their pinchers into the skin. During this time they may be plucked off by gripping the insect's body firmly with fingers or tweezers and pulling with a quick, unscrewing motion. If, however, you pull at the tick and it has bored too deeply into the skin for easy removal, *by no means rip it out forcefully.* The head may break off inside the skin and cause an infection. (On rare occasions ticks can also transmit Rocky Mountain Spotted Fever, whose symptoms include chills, high fever, muscle pains, and a rash that starts, characteristically, on the wrists and ankles.) Instead, take a lit cigarette and hold it slightly behind the tick's abdomen, just far enough away so that the ash doesn't sear your skin. This method usually causes the creature to release its grip and back out posthaste. If, for some reason, the cigarette trick fails to work, cover the tick with Vaseline, alcohol, or kerosene and remove it carefully with tweezers, making sure that the head is not left behind in the skin. Then wash the wound with soap and water and keep a close eye on it for several days. If there is any sign of infection—red streaks, tenderness, immediate pus emissions—or if a fever and swollen glands appear within ten days after the bite—see a physician immediately.

A Quick Guide to Dealing with Insect Itch

Some hints: Hot water dabbed onto a bite will often stop the itching. So will your own spittle.

When going into mosquito territory, take along some thiamine pills. Approximately 300 milligrams a day seems to have a strong deterrent effect against many biting insects.

Try a dab of ammonia on a mosquito, flea, or chigger bite.

Also, a wet cloth compress made with cold milk or a solution of water and cornstarch.

For chigger bites, a combination of 1 percent phenol and 10 percent benzocaine (your pharmacist can provide both) applied twice a day to the irritation with a plastic toothpick will speed the healing.

Eau de cologne will help when applied to spider bites.

Some over-the-counter anti-itch preparations deemed safe and effective by the FDA include Nupercainal ointment and cream, Quotane ointment, Cortaid cream, Xylocaine ointment, Pro-Cort cream, Caladryl cream and lotion, and Dermoplast spray.

SELF-CARE FOR A GENERALIZED REACTION TO AN INSECT BITE

1. *Get immediate medical help!*

If you (or anyone near you) is stung by an insect and develops a generalized multi-organ response, go *immediately* to the nearest medical facility. This condition is, or often can be, a medical emergency, possibly life-threatening. There are only a limited number of things you can do on your own until help is found.

2. Take an oral antihistamine, if one is available.

3. Use an Epi-Pen or Ana-Kit, both of which are often kept on the person of those susceptible to insect sting allergies. The contents of an Ana-Kit include ample portions of the drug epinephrine (Adrenalin) in a pre-filled syringe, along with several antihistamine tablets. An Epi-Pen is an injection device containing a pre-loaded dose of epinephrine that automatically discharges when pressed firmly against the skin. Both items can be procured only by prescription; your physician will show you how to self-administer these useful aids (also, see the technology and resources section below).

4. If you are the victim of severe insect sting reactions, it is wise to keep a Medic-Alert tag or bracelet on your person at all times. This handy device identifies your allergic susceptibilities in writing and provides appropriate instructions for treatment should you be found unconscious. It can be purchased at most pharmacies.

TECHNOLOGY, RESOURCES, AIDS, AND SERVICES

1. If you are allergic to any type of insect bite, acquiring a prescription for an ANA-KIT will present no problem. You can purchase the kit from a pharmacy or directly from Hollister-Stier

Laboratories, P.O. Box 3145, Terminal Annex, Spokane, Washington 99220. Contact them for recent prices and ordering details.

2. *Medical alert necklaces, bracelets and cards* can be purchased directly from Medic-Alert Foundation International, 1000 N. Palm, Turlock, CA. For a small lifetime fee, the Medic-Alert organization will put your name and medical history on file, key it to your Medic-Alert serial number, and make this information available to any doctor or health care professional on a twenty-four-hour-a-day basis.

3. Booklets that may be of help for insect allergies include:

Insect Allergy
Booklet #NIH 78-1046
National Institute of Allergy and Infectious Diseases
Information Office
Room 7A-32, Bldg. 31
9000 Rockville Pike
Bethesda, MD 20014
Free

Prevention of Stings by Hymenoptera:
Bees, Wasps, Hornets, and Yellowjackets
American Academy of Allergy
1444 Sixteenth Street, N.W.
Washington, DC 20009
Free

CHAPTER 3

SIMPLE HEADACHES

There is a saying among Japanese physicians: "One headache, a hundred and ten causes." This is not an exaggeration. A headache can be a symptom of an amazingly wide span of ailments ranging from simple tension to a brain tumor. Happily, approximately 90 percent of headaches are the result of muscular tension in the neck and scalp, and even the remaining 10 percent rarely signal a serious disorder.

There are two basic types of headaches: *vascular* and *psychogenic*.

1. *Vascular (Pathologic Headaches)*

These begin when the blood vessels in the brain expand, exert pressure on the vessel walls, and create sensations of pain in various locations throughout the head, along with blurred or double vision. Migraine headaches and hypertensive headaches both fall under this category. Ordinarily such headaches should be handled by a physician, at least in the preliminary stages when diagnosis and prescription medications are required.

2. *Psychogenic Headaches*

These headaches arise from daily psychological and physiological ups and downs: depression, pollution, stress, eye strain, etc.

All fall into the category of "simple headache," and fortunately all are among the easiest of maladies to self-medicate, even without the option of the aspirin tablet.

THEY ARE NOT ALWAYS EASY TO DIAGNOSE

Most simple headaches go undiagnosed. It is not, after all, entirely essential for you to know why your head is splitting—whether it is because your eyes are tired, your blood sugar level is off, your neck is tense, or whatever. The important thing is to get relief. On the other hand, the reasons for simple headaches are sometimes obvious, and they can be traced to one or more of the following common factors:

- Tension in the back, shoulders, neck, scalp, or jaw
- Depression
- Eyestrain
- Caffeine withdrawal
- Sinus pressures
- Pollution
- Poor room ventilation
- Stress
- Lack of proper or adequate sleep
- Colds or flu
- Premenstrual condition
- Reactions to certain foods or medications

Self-Diagnosis of Simple Headaches

Simple tension headaches become chronic for many people. They can be recognized by their dull, throbbing pain, as if a metal band is slowly being tightened around the temples. Sometimes tension headaches are accompanied by nausea and even vomiting, though this is rather unusual. Loss of appetite, dizziness, and a general lassitude may also occur from time to time.

SELF-CARE FOR SIMPLE HEADACHES

The Aspirin Route

1. The most simple and accessible antiheadache remedy is to take two aspirin (or an aspirin substitute such as acetaminophen) every four hours until the headache goes away. If your stomach is sensitive to aspirin, take aspirin with a meal or coat your stomach beforehand by drinking a glass of milk.

2. While waiting for the headache to disappear, relax as much as possible.

3. Stay away from television, reading, bright lights, and loud noises.

4. Take a few deep breaths and settle into a comfortable position. Lying down is the best posture for most people.

5. Although aspirin comes as close as anything we have to an over-the-counter wonder drug, it is not without its drawbacks. If you use aspirin on a regular basis, here are a few important and little-known facts to bear in mind:

• According to most knowledgeable opinion, all aspirin is the same. This means that one commercial brand is no better than another, and that it is pointless to believe commercial hype and to purchase the most expensive varieties. Generic aspirin is probably just as good as any of the more expensive brands.

• For some people aspirin has a mild sedative effect. This is good if you want to relax, bad if you want to get work done or if you are driving. Be careful.

• If an aspirin is crumbly or smells like vinegar, throw it away. It is decomposing.

• Due to aspirin's blood-thinning qualities, it is recommended that a person not take this drug for at least two weeks before undergoing surgery.

• Too much aspirin can kill children. In 1976, twenty-five youngsters died from aspirin overdose. We also see many nonfatal aspirin O.D.'s in the emergency room every year. Keep bottles sealed and away from little fingers at all times.

• Aspirin is not without its possible side effects. For some people it causes stomach upset or gastrointestinal bleeding. For others, it produces ringing in the ears. Aspirin may interact unfavorably with prescription medications such as anticoagulants, insulin, probenecid (for gout), and certain corticosteroid drugs. It can also trigger an allergic reaction in some people. Excessive long-term use (which means more than two straight weeks) can produce a psychological dependency, and on certain rare occasions it leads to stomach ulcers and/or kidney damage. People who drink alcohol on a daily basis must be extremely careful of aspirin since *both* agents—alcohol and aspirin—are gastric irritants.

Do not, furthermore, take aspirin without a doctor's guidance if:

1. You have a history of peptic ulcers or hiatal hernia.
2. You have had a previous allergic reaction to it.
3. You are taking anticoagulant drugs.
4. You are a hemophiliac.
5. You are pregnant.

• With aspirin, familiarity often breeds contempt. The most popular drug in the world and surely one of the most useful, aspirin is also perhaps the most misused and overused. Take no more than two tablets at a time, and keep dosage periods spaced at least four hours apart. Unless your doctor puts you on a regular course of aspirin (its anticoagulant effects are apparently proving effective when used on a daily basis for some victims of coronary disease), do not use it unnecessarily. For instance, some people take two aspirin with every meal as "insurance" against a cold. This is nonsense. Aspirin has no proven prophylactic capabilities against viruses, and besides, excessive use can lead to side effects. A moderate overdose of the drug, for instance, may cause impaired hearing, nausea and vomiting, dizziness, and a ringing in the ears. Massive overdose can produce rapid pulse, hallucinations, fever, rapid breathing, delirium, errosive gastritis, hemmorhage, and even death.

Profile of Over-the-Counter Aspirin Substitutes

Acetaminophen—The most popular aspirin substitute and probably the best. It comes in brands such as Tylenol, Datril, Dolanex (elixir form), Valadol, Febrinol; its generic name is acetaminophen or APAP. Dosage recommended by the FDA is between 325 to 650 milligrams every four hours. If you take this drug for more than ten days without relief, see a doctor. Acetaminophen is quite safe and produces few if any side effects, but note that overdose can cause severe liver and kidney damage.

Codeine—Though a powerful pain reliever in large doses, the small amounts allowed by the government in nonprescription brands (it comes mixed in cold and cough remedies) makes it largely ineffective for headache relief. This means that you shouldn't count on a codeine cough syrup or cold remedy to relieve head pain.

Magnesium salicylate—Comes in Doan's Pills. Generally considered safe and effective when taken as directed. Can be used by persons allergic to aspirin.

Choline salicylate—Comes in a liquid called Anthropan. Generally considered safe and effective for headaches.

Eliminating Headaches Without Aspirin

Massage. Simply rubbing your head front and back will often bring relief from headache pain, but there are more interesting and systematic methods to follow. One of these, based on the Oriental technique of acupressure, can be done in five minutes and often brings surprisingly effective results. Here's how it works:

STEP ONE:

Sit up straight in a comfortable chair and take a moment to relax your mind and body. Take ten deep breaths, wait several moments, then take ten more. (Deep breathing alone can often have a beneficial effect on headaches, especially if the headache is due to insufficient oxygen intake or stress.) Start by rubbing the back of your neck, making small circles and working your way up to the top of the head, applying firm, kneading pressure. Next, bunch the fingers till they come to a point, place the points in the hollows of the neck directly behind and adjacent to the earlobes, and press for thirty seconds. Massage these hollows in small, firm circles with pointed fingers for approximately thirty seconds.

STEP TWO:

Draw an imaginary line from the bridge of the nose, up the center of the forehead, directly over the top of the skull, down to the hollow at the base of the neck. With bunched fingers (as above) start at the bridge of the nose and massage upward, moving carefully along this imaginary line, making small circles with the fingers as they move slowly up the forehead, over the top of the head and down to the base of the skull. Take about two minutes to complete this maneuver. There should be some relief already. Now repeat, this time drawing two lines, one starting above the center of the left eye, one above the right and extending up and over the skull to the hollows of the neck behind and adjacent to the ears. Massage slowly along these lines in small circles, taking about a minute to complete the movement.

STEP THREE:

Place your palms on either side of your temples and press firmly inward for thirty seconds. Next, take your head in your hands, tuck your thumbs beneath the chin, and gently pull the head upward so that the neck gets a good stretch for twenty or thirty seconds. Massage the entire top and back area of the head. Take a fistful of hair and firmly tug and twist it, to stimulate the scalp. End the session by placing the thumbs along the jaw at the base of the earlobes, massaging upward in small circles to the temples.

A *word of warning:* Since the carotid arteries are located just below the hollows described above, and since too much accidental pressing of these arteries can reduce blood flow to the brain, these exercises are not recommended for older people, especially those who have suffered from atherosclerosis or stroke.

Breathing imagery. This technique is also unexpectedly effective and is especially useful for headaches caused by stress, depression, and overwork. For some years the healing power of mental imagery has been recognized by an increasing number of physicians, and "imaging" techniques of various kinds are being used for a wide range of therapeutic purposes, from stress reduction to cancer therapy.

To practice breathing imagery, find a quiet, well-ventilated space (outdoors is ideal) and sit in a comfortable, upright position—spine straight, feet planted solidly. Take ten slow, deep breaths through your mouth, and with each inhalation visualize a stream of silver light pouring in with the breath and flowing up through your head, to the exact spot where the pain is located. Hold the inhalation, along with the image of the light, for five seconds. Then exhale, visualizing the pain moving with the breath down through your head and out your mouth. Each individual will have a different picture of what his or her pain looks like. One person will envision a black vapor; another, little demonlike figures; a third, jackhammers pounding cement. Conjure up whatever image is most evocative. Do three sets of breaths, ten deep breaths each, pausing a minute between sets.

Self-suggestion. Here's another natural healing method that takes a few minutes to perform and that, when combined with any of the remedies mentioned above, will get to the heart of tension, eyestrain, sleep deprivation, and depression headaches. As with breathing imagery, you'll need a quiet room and about ten minutes alone to practice it. If you've never tried self-hypnosis you are in for an interesting experience.

STEP ONE:

Settle into a comfortable chair, take several deep breaths, then begin preparation for self-hypnosis by entirely relaxing your whole body. There are, of course, innumerable methods for attaining this state of relaxation. Here is one that works particularly well:

Pre-hypnosis relaxation exercise

- Tense the muscles of your face for ten seconds, then relax them. Start with the muscles at the top of your head. Tighten your scalp for ten seconds, then release. Move down to the forehead: tense, relax. Then the eyes and eyebrows; the ears; the nose and mouth; the cheeks and chin.
- When your face feels loose and relaxed, move to the neck. Tighten and release.
- Now down to your chest, your arms, hands, stomach, hips, thighs, calves, and feet.
- After detensing your whole body—the process should take three or four minutes—sit quietly and reduce the flow of thoughts through your mind. A minute of mental silence and you are ready to begin.

STEP TWO:

Silently repeat to yourself trance-inducing suggestions more or less to this effect:

"My eyes are growing heavy, they are starting to close, starting to feel as if lead weights were attached to them. I am becoming more and more tired, relaxed, so relaxed. I am feeling drowsy. It's getting harder and harder to keep my eyes open. The lids are getting heavier and heavier, and now my eyes are beginning to blink. I will let them blink. This is a sign that they are getting ready to close. They want to close. I will let them close. They *are* closing. Slowly and steadily. I am becoming more and more relaxed. I am sinking into a blissful, relaxed state. It's so hard to keep my eyes open as I become more relaxed, more at ease, more deeply relaxed. Harder and harder to keep them open. I'm sinking into a deep, relaxed state."

The first time you perform this exercise you may be surprised to see that your eyes *are* closing. It is always something of a shock to learn how responsive we are to self-suggestion. Repeat this self-hypnotic litany until your eyes close firmly. The process shouldn't take more than a few minutes. Once your eyes are shut, go on to Step Three.

STEP THREE:

You are going to deepen what has already become a light trance:

"Now that my eyes are closed, I am sinking more and more into a deep, quiet state where nothing in the world can hurt me or bother me. I am totally at peace. I am sinking deeper and deeper, totally relaxed and absorbed. Outside noises and disturbances do not affect me in the slightest way. I feel so drowsy, so comfortable, so happy. I am relaxing more and more, sinking more and more with every breath I take. My whole body feels as if it has turned to stone. The outside world is disappearing. Every part of my body is relaxed now; my arms . . . my hands . . . my neck . . . the back of my head . . . my eyebrows . . . my elbows . . . my chest . . . my stomach . . . my knees . . . my feet . . . everything. I feel I am sinking into the chair, getting heavier and heavier. So relaxed now. I could move if I wanted to, but I don't because I am too comfortable and relaxed. My arms are so pleasantly heavy. My legs. My head. All so comfortably relaxed. Nothing bothers me now. My problems have gone far, far away. Nothing can bother me now, nothing can touch me, nothing can affect me or worry me. The deeper I go, the more pleasant it feels." And so on.

This step should require about five to ten minutes to take effect, or as long as it takes to feel a measurable increase in relaxation and well-being. By no means will self-suggestion turn you into a zombie, and you must not look for unconsciousness or rigidity as signs that the suggestion is taking. On the contrary, you will feel a strange sense of alertness, but it will be coupled with a floating sensation and a feeling of detachment from the world.

STEP FOUR:

Now imagine yourself standing at the top of a long flight of stairs. Peer down these stairs. See how they lead down, down, down into a deep but not unpleasant darkness. Tell yourself that you will now walk down these stairs, and that each step you take into the darkness will bring you deeper into hypnosis, deeper into relaxation and your own unconscious.

Now start down, slowly, step by step. At each step, sink a little deeper into trance. One slow step at a time until you reach the tenth step. Here you will come to a landing. Pause at this landing in a state of relaxation. Look back up the stairs and see how far you have come. Feel how deep your trance is becoming. Now walk down another ten stairs, pause at the landing, and then down another, letting yourself sink deeper and deeper into trance with every step down. At the bottom of the third landing, tell yourself that you have arrived. Your mind is relaxed and open enough to start the process of self-suggestion.

Now, for the most crucial step.

STEP FIVE:

While in a state of trance, all the suggestions you give yourself should be simple, gentle, direct, totally positive, and not overly directive. They are literally suggestions, not commands. Tell yourself: "My headache is feeling better and better all the time," not "My headache will immediately cease." Gentle and polite advice to your unconscious is the key. Something like: "I am feeling better now. Better and better. I like feeling better; I like not having a headache. When I come out of trance, my head will feel just fine and will stay that way for the rest of the day."

While in trance, repeat all your messages at least five times. No need to say them over and over again indefinitely, however; your unconscious is more open than usual now and more receptive. A few hints will usually do the trick.

To give more strength to the suggestions, accompany them with compelling mental images. Imagine yourself walking along a sunny street feeling wonderful. The sky is blue, flowers are blooming, your headache is gone. Or visualize yourself with a golden band of light revolving around your head. You are smiling and feeling better. This combination of verbal guidance and visual imagery is a powerful weapon against tension.

Do not tell your mind how to go about the actual healing process. Procedural instructions are unnecessary. State your suggestions, repeat them several times, visualize, and leave the rest up to the unconscious.

Stay in this state for three or four minutes, then end the session in the following way.

STEP SIX:

Start the return to wakefulness by imagining yourself standing at the landing of the dark staircase, looking up. Imagine that you are about to ascend, and that with each step you are bringing yourself closer and closer to normal consciousness. Then start slowly up the thirty stairs, step by step. When your reach the top, tell yourself that you are now out of the trance, perfectly normal, and ready to go about your business feeling terrific.

Practice this exercise daily, preferably at the same time each day. A very good method is to prerecord your monologue on a cassette tape, complete with whatever suggestions you wish to give yourself and then play it back during the self-hypnosis sessions. This method allows you to stay entirely relaxed during the process without having to make the mental effort of talking to yourself.

Finally, it should be mentioned that the program for self-suggestion outlined above is useful not only for headaches, but also for a number of daily disorders such as simple insomnia, stress, depression, fatigue, and even (for some people) such problems as bad backs, sore necks, and the malaise of a cold or flu. Also for addictions to food, alcohol, or cigarettes.

BIOFEEDBACK FOR HEADACHES

Many of the body's functions such as circulation, pulse, skin temperature, and blood pressure work without our conscious knowledge or participation. We are their passive recipients, if not their prisoners. Recent developments in biological electronics, however, have made it clear that the mind can exert greater command of these functions than was previously supposed, and that if certain unconscious functions like blood pressure or involuntary muscle movements are monitored electronically, the mind can both modify and control these processes.

The device best suited for this task is *the biofeedback machine,* both the sophisticated apparatus used in professional clinics and the commercial varieties designed for home use. Clinical biofeedback is ordinarily done on an electromyograph (EMG) machine using electrodes attached to the patient's forehead to monitor tension changes in the muscle system. These changes are registered by a series of high-pitched sounds (or sometimes flashes of light, beeps, etc.) that rise and fall in synchronization with shifting tensions. This method of sensitive, continuous measurement creates a precise graph of the patient's muscular activity as the muscles grow alternately more and less relaxed.

While monitoring the sounds of the machine, the patient and the biofeedback therapist work together on a set of visualization and relaxation exercises. As relaxation increases, the machine emits sounds at an increasingly lower frequency. This information reinforces the patient's determination along with his or her sensitivity to the body's subtle physiological processes. The procedure is a kind of benevolent Pavlovian interface between man and machine, where effort to relax is rewarded by signal, which in turn inspires more effort.

Eventually, by regular use of biofeedback, patients learn to relax many physiological functions ordinarily considered involuntary. The final goal is to become free of the machine entirely and to manipulate these bodily functions by the power of one's mind alone.

Is treating headaches with biofeedback a realistic self-care alternative? In most cases, yes, especially now that home biofeedback machinery is available. As a rule, of course, the machines used in a clinic are more elaborate and sensitive than the home-care varieties, and anyone seriously interested in using biofeedback is encouraged by professionals to take the clinic route first. This is especially true if you plan to use biofeedback to control symptoms of serious diseases such as cerebral palsy, heart problems, epilepsy, or rheumatoid arthritis. On the other hand, home machines definitely have their place, especially for use with simple headaches, hypertension, and tensions. The section on technology and resources below lists sources where biofeedback equipment can be purchased.

OTHER SELF-APPLIED HEADACHE REMEDIES

There are, it seems, as many headache cures in this world as there are headache sufferers, and all of us have our pet remedies. The following methods are among the most popular and are culled from traditional cures. They work for some people—sometimes. They usually heal quickly, when they heal at all, and as a rule they take little effort. If there is no improvement soon after you have tried one of these techniques, it probably isn't going to do the trick. If your headache persists, try another, then another, until you find one that works for you.

Herbal Teas

Any of the following teas are useful for headaches:

basil	peppermint	catnip
fennel	camomile	hops
rosemary	sage	ginger

Boil a cup of water, steep the herb in the hot water for five to ten minutes, and drink. Add honey to make sour-tasting brews such as sage or fennel more palatable.

Meditation

Linked in many ways to both self-hypnosis and biofeedback techniques, the practice of meditation has helped many chronic headache sufferers to relax and reduce the physical tensions that cause headaches. Today there are meditation groups just about everywhere, both secular and spiritually oriented. Look for advertisements and announcements in the newspaper and on bulletin boards or ask around.

Exercise

When suffering from a throbbing headache, exercise is the last thing in the world anyone wishes to think about. While a little stretching and some simple eye exercises can help the circulation and hence the headache, we are not suggesting strenuous calisthenics as a remedy. The best plan for chronic headache sufferers is to engage in at least fifteen minutes of daily exercise, such as aerobics or yoga. Many tension headache sufferers have found that establishing a regular calisthenics or jogging schedule is a painless, natural way of eliminating a problem that might otherwise require frequent medication.

Acupressure

Acupressure is acupuncture without needles. The same vital points along the body are stimulated as in acupuncture, but the stimulation is applied with the fingers and thumbs. To treat headaches:

• Make a fist. With the thumb of one hand apply steady pressure to the center of the mound of flesh formed at the base between the thumb and index finger on the other hand for ten to fifteen seconds. Repeat with the other hand.

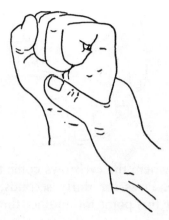

• Turn the hand palm up with the wrist exposed. Press the point on the wrist directly below, and in line with, the pinky. Press for ten to fifteen seconds on each wrist.

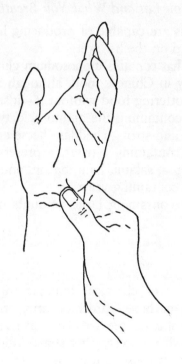

• Press the point on the top of the foot approximately a finger's width below the intersection of the big toe and a second toe for fifteen to twenty seconds on each foot.

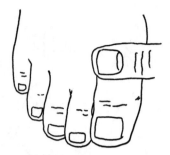

• Press the spot where the eyebrows come together, above the bridge of the nose. Press for thirty seconds, then squeeze and knead the skin over this point for another thirty seconds. Repeat several times.

• Rub and massage the outer shell of both ears, the outer corners of both eyes (very carefully), and the hollow of the back of the neck. Rub and knead for thirty seconds. Repeat several times.

Watch What You Eat and What You Breathe

Certain foods are capable of producing headaches in sensitive people. Included on the list are:

• Any food that contains monosodium glutamate (MSG). (MSG is found mostly in Chinese food, although some Chinese restaurants are now offering food without it—just tell the waiter.)

• Any food containing the amino acid tyramine: pickled herring, red wine, and strong cheddar cheese are some examples.

• Any food containing nitrites, a preservative. These include hot dogs, bologna, salami, ham, bacon, and lunch meats.

• Any foods containing yeast.

• Any foods containing large amounts of chemical preservatives.

• Liquor

• Cigarettes

• Chocolate

Also, be wary of chemical fumes from photographic dark-rooms, copying machines, garden or farm sprays, auto repair shops, factories, etc. Some people are also sensitive to the odors of hair spray, nail polish remover, after-shave lotion, smoke, soap, etc. Heavy smoking can also cause headaches, especially in a poorly ventilated room.

For some people, blood sugar fluctuations may be the problem behind the headache. In such instances, it's best to avoid candy bars, ice cream, soft drinks, cakes, and cookies, and to eat six small meals daily consisting of high fiber and complex carbohydrates such as potatoes, legumes, pasta, breads, and green leafy vegetables.

Finally, there's salt. According to Dr. John B. Brainard, author of *Control of Migraine,* salt can be responsible for triggering a hormonal response that leads to serious headaches—particularly migraines. Try reducing salt intake and observing the results. In general, overuse of salt should be avoided by everyone. It can raise blood pressure and increase fluid retention.

Simple Rest

Lie down in a darkened room. Relax. (You can use the relaxation exercises mentioned above; also, the tapes described in the technology and resources section below.) Take several deep breaths. Sleep is often the best remedy, but if this is not possible, simply lie as still and quiet as you can for fifteen minutes.

And a Few Last Resorts

• Take a medium-sized paper bag, place it over your nose and mouth, and inhale and exhale into it for about a minute. This simple technique seems to be helpful, especially for migraine sufferers.

• Place cold washcloths on the top of your head and the back of your neck. For some people, cold water poured over the head helps, as does a two-minute cold bath or shower. For others, taking hot and cold showers in sequence is helpful. Those with heart or blood pressure problems who are not constitutionally fit for the shock of the hot and cold treatment can place a piece of ice in the back of the mouth when headache pain begins, and suck on it until the ice melts. This method was developed by Augustus Rose at the University of California Center for Health Sciences in Los Angeles.

• Place hot towels on the back of your neck. Freshen the towel with a new application of hot water every three or four minutes.

• Breathe deeply ten times in a row, rest for a minute, then repeat.

• Drink three tablespoonsful of apple cider vinegar mixed with a teaspoonful of honey.

• Open a jar of vinegar and sniff the fumes.

• Drink a cup of black coffee.

When to Call the Doctor

As a rule, headaches are common and harmless. Occasionally they can be signs of a more serious underlying condition. How to tell the difference? If any of the following symptoms accompany the headache, you must seek a physician's advice immediately:

- The headache continues for longer than four days.
- The pain is unusually severe and comes on with unexpected speed. This should be given special attention if the pain center is situated in a part of the head not usually involved in ordinary tension headaches (tension headaches are usually located in the back of the head, and over the temples).
- The headache is accompanied by unusual and disturbing symptoms such as nausea, vomiting, dizziness, loss of equilibrium, double vision, weakness, numbness of the extremities, or blurred vision.
- If you feel unusually drowsy and listless during the headache. Losing consciousness may be an indication of a serious condition—get medical help immediately.
- If the headache is accompanied by motor difficulties such as slurred speech or faulty coordination.
- If you have recently experienced a head injury of any kind.
- If you feel an explosion in your head followed by any of the above symptoms.

How to Treat Sinus Headaches

These can be caused by colds, inflammation of the ears or nose, nasal polyps, infection, nasal congestion, and allergies. Treatment consists of applying hot compresses to the sinus areas, though any source of heat will help, including a heating pad on the neck, warm saltwater gargles and, in a pinch, an electric light bulb placed directly over the sinus areas (naturally, you shouldn't bring the hot bulb too close to your skin). Stay away from irritants such as alcohol and cigarettes, and carefully avoid mucous-producing foods, especially dairy products. Keep your environment as dust-free as possible; sometimes a humidifer will help, or even steam from a bowl of boiling water. Promote sinus drainage by remaining upright. Accompanying symptoms such as a stiff neck or sore throat can be relieved with aspirin. Antihistamines may also help, although you should avoid using decongestants for more than three or four days in a row. They can end up producing a "rebound effect" whereby they cause the very symptoms they are supposed to prevent.

TECHNOLOGY, RESOURCES, AIDS, AND SERVICES

1. Some reliable sources for *home biofeedback equipment* include: The GSR 2 is a small, hand-sized piece of *biofeedback apparatus* that comes with an earphone, battery, instruction book, and clinically designed learning system on cassette. The price is around $50.00. For information write:

Thought Technology Ltd.
2180 Belgrave Avenue
Dept. #485
Montreal, P.Q.,
Canada H4A 2L8

A *liquid crystal thermometer ring* that works on somewhat the same principle as biofeedback, by monitoring skin temperature, is available from:

Futurehealth, Inc.
P.O. Box 947
Bensalem, PA 19020

Home biofeedback equipment can be purchased from the following:

Echo, Inc.
P.O. Box 87
Springfield, OH 45501

Conscious Living Foundation
P.O. Box 513
Manhattan, KS 66502

Abbey Medical Catalog Sales Department
13782 Crenshaw Blvd.
Gardena, CA 90249

(Must be ordered through a health care professional. Abbey sells both home and highly sophisticated laboratory biofeedback machinery.)

A *video teaching cassette* on the subject of biofeedback (order

#900050) is available from Medcom Film Library, P.O. Box 16, Garden Grove, CA 92642, (800) 854-2485 (in California call [800] 472-2479).

Relaxation tapes that can be used in conjunction with biofeedback are obtainable from:
William S. Kroger, M.D.
BK Enterprises
P.O. Box 6248
9478 Olympic Blvd.
Beverly Hills, CA 90212

HR & A
830 Terrace 49
Los Angeles, CA 90042

Emmet Miller Tapes
P.O. Box W
Stanford, CA 94305

Self-Control Systems, Inc.
Suite 223
Lake Air National Bank
4901 Bosque Blvd.
Waco, TX 76710

BioMonitoring Applications
Audiocassette Programs
270 Madison Avenue
Suite 1704
New York, NY 10016

Books on biofeedback include:
Biofeedback: Turning on the Power of Your Mind by Marvin Kalins and Lewis Andrews (New York: Lippincott, 1972).

Biofeedback: Potential and Limits by Robert M. Stern and William Ray (University of Nebraska Press, 1980).

New Mind, New Body by Barbara Brown (New York: Harper and Row, 1974).

If you have any general questions on the subject of biofeedback, or if you are searching for a practitioner in your vicinity, get in touch with the following organizations for information and referrals:

The Biofeedback Society of America
4301 Owens Street
Wheat Ridge, CO 80030
(303) 422-8436

American Association of Biofeedback
2424 Dempster Street
Des Plaines, IL 60016
(312) 827-0440

2. Other *relaxation aids* include: *Progressive muscle relaxation exercises conjoined with mental imagery,* a system developed by James Lipton, a psychologist at the University of Texas Health Science Center in Dallas, which has received a good deal of publicity. For information on this system, contact:
James Lipton, Ph.D.
University of Texas Health Science Center
5323 Harry Hines Blvd.
Dallas, TX 75235
The prerecorded cassette tale "Letting Go of Stress" is available from:
The Medical Self-Care Catalog
P.O. Box 999
Pt. Reyes, CA 94956
Video tapes showing tranquil scenes designed to induce relaxation are available from:
CMA Video Productions
P.O. Box 414
Bend, OR 97709
Tapes to aid self-hypnosis are available from:
Creative Dimensions
P.O. Box 1056-N
Aptos, CA 95001

Tapes
P.O. Box 614
Santa Barbara, CA 93160
(write for free catalog)

Lifeworks
24A Ohayo Mountain Road
Woodstock, NY 12498
3. *A sinus mask* designed to fit over the face and use moist (or dry) heat to relieve sinus discomfort is available for around $17.00

from Sears Home Health Care (call [800] 323-3274 for information on ordering, or for the Sears nearest you). For people
who have trouble swallowing pills, *a hand pill-splitter* will prove
exceptionally useful. It costs $4.98 (catalog item B3971) from
Harriet Carter, Dept. 16, North Wales, PA 19555.

4. The National Migraine Foundation offers an eight-page bimonthly newsletter for $4.10 a year that presents the latest infor-
mation and advances in migraine research. Write to the National
Migraine Foundation, 5214 North Western Avenue, Chicago, IL
60625.

5. *A home use self-help program for migraine sufferers,* complete with workbook and biofeedback device, is available for
$21.95 from Biofeedback Clinic, Lakeview Medical Bldg., 3216
N.E. Place, Seattle, WA 98105.

6. Some helpful books on the subject of headaches include:
Freedom from Headaches by Joel Saper, M.D., and Kenneth
Magee, M.D.
New York: Simon & Schuster, 1981

Dealing with Headaches by Wendy Murphy and the Editors of
Time-Life
Alexandria, VA: Time-Life Books, 1982).

Headaches: The Kinds and the Cures by Arthur Freese
New York: Doubleday, 1973

*Then Two Aspirin: A Complete Guide to Identifying, Under-
standing and Solving Your Headache Problem* by Seymour and
Ferling Diamond and William B. More
Chicago: Follett, 1976

No More Headaches by Alan C. Turin, M.D.
Boston: Houghton Mifflin, 1981

7. *Related problems.* See sections on Stress, Ringing in the Ears,
Colds and Flu, Eyestrain.

CHAPTER 4

MOTION SICKNESS

For people in the grip of motion sickness it is difficult to believe that life will continue past the present hour, or that it makes much difference if it does. For those prone to this unpleasant malady, the most comforting thing we can say is: No matter how bad the condition feels right now, it *will* get better when the movement stops. Furthermore, it practically never causes lasting damage.

SELF-DIAGNOSIS OF MOTION SICKNESS

Motion sickness is triggered by abrupt shiftings of fluid in the inner ear, which in turn are caused by sudden changes in direction and acceleration of a moving vehicle.

What are the symptoms? Nausea, of course, possibly accompanied by dizziness, sweating, fatigue, breathing difficulties, pallor, excessive salivation, headache, vomiting, and general malaise and lassitude. If the situation drags on for hours or even days, a person may become exhausted, dehydrated, limp, and deeply depressed. What can be done to help?

SELF-CARE FOR MOTION SICKNESS

In most cases the symptoms of motion sickness disappear when the trip is over. The obvious and best remedy is to get off the boat, bus, or helicopter, and go home. This is not always possible, of course, so other alternatives must be tried. Here are some of the better ones:

1. If possible, lie down. This is an especially effective position for seasickness. Wear a warm coat or blanket. Breathe deeply and evenly. Don't focus on any object that is too busy or too close; this means no reading, no knitting, etc. Fast, jerky motions or sudden rotations of the head, shifting the eyes, or bouncing up and down will all trigger or intensify motion sickness. Find a place where you can remain still, and stay there, preferably with your eyes closed.

2. The symptoms of motion sickness can be heightened by food or chemical odors. Stay away from kitchens, bars, factories, and exhaust fumes.

3. Children and dancers are taught that keeping their eyes fixed on a certain spot while turning circles can prevent dizziness. The same principle holds true for motion sickness: Focusing your eyes on a *fixed, distant* point can reduce symptoms. If you are on a boat, concentrate on a cloud or an object on deck. Do *not* look at the rolling waves or the tilting horizon.

4. Motion sickness is most likely to develop in an enclosed, claustrophobic environment such as the cabin of a ship. If it is possible, go outside where you can breathe deeply and fix your attention on a distant object.

5. *Crème de menthe* poured over ice is an effective home remedy. Plain ice can also be useful. Also, cola or ginger ale in small sips is good for upset stomachs and nausea.

6. If circumstances allow, try stimulating the following acupressure points:

- Measure one hand's width distance up from the bony protrusion on the inside part of the ankle. Massage this point along the bone, fifteen seconds on each leg. Repeat.
- Massage the solar plexus for thirty seconds. Repeat twice.
- Massage a point on the center of the inside wrist approximately two inches above (i.e., toward the elbow) the main crease on the wrist for fifteen seconds. Repeat twice on each wrist.
- Push on the mastoid process, which is located on the bony protrusion directly below and behind the bottom of the earlobe.
- Massage the hollow in the center of the neck directly at the base of the skull.

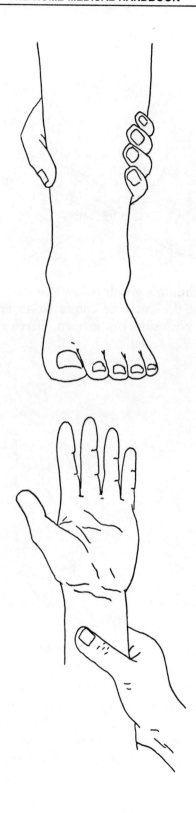

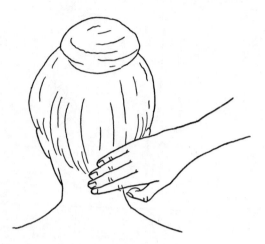

- Measure one thumb's width below the base of the earlobe to the spot where the jawbone comes to an end. Stimulate this point twice on both sides of the head, fifteen seconds each time.

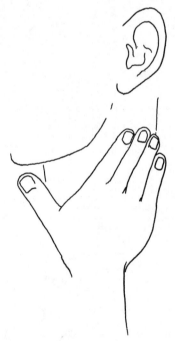

7. People who have travel phobias or panic in planes, cars, etc., are more prone to motion sickness than those who travel easily. If you are among the former, it is best to prepare by taking medications ahead of time. More on this below.

8. Proper ventilation is extremely important, both as a preven-

tion and as a cure. Keep the car windows open. Sit near an open window on a bus or train. Stay on deck when traveling by boat. Point the air conditioning nozzle directly toward you on an airplane.

9. For those prone to motion sickness, the best seating position on a plane is directly over the wing. Be sure you get a seat in the nonsmoking section; if you smoke, try to abstain while traveling. On a bus, forward seats are best, away from the bouncing rear. Sit toward the front on a train as well, as close to the engine as possible. On a ship, remain in the middle of the vessel. Avoid facing backward in all vehicles; you should see the scenery coming toward you, not moving away. When driving, stop the car frequently, walk around, breathe deeply, rest your eyes, and relax.

10. Restrict eating before a trip, and beware of rich bon voyage feasts. Bland foods are good, and plain soups and hot teas are better. Stay away from chewing gum; it will make you swallow too much air. Whatever you do, don't overeat before setting out on your journey.

11. In Japan, fresh-brewed green tea is taken to ward off motion sickness before the trip begins.

12. Nibble at a root of fresh ginger before departing. In several laboratory tests, this substance has proven more effective against motion sickness than Dramamine. Powdered ginger is okay if the fresh variety is not available.

What About Medication for Motion Sickness?

There are three antiemetics (i.e., anti-nausea medicines) that the FDA has deemed safe and effective for use in over-the-counter motion sickness drugs. These are:
1. cyclizine
2. dimenhydrinate
3. meclizine

Medications containing twenty-five to fifty milligrams of meclizine will last most of the day. Cyclizine in fifty milligrams is good for about half a day, and the same is true of dimenhydrinate. All three seem to be about equally effective in controlling motion sickness, although some experimentation may be necessary to find which is best for you. Take the drugs a half hour to an hour before starting out; later on, nausea may make it a good deal harder to get the medications down. Children's doses are smaller than adult doses. Ask your pharmacist for instructions on this, and read the directions. Cyclizine, dimenhydrinate, and meclizine are found in the following commerical medications:

Drug	Brand
Cyclizine	Marezine (tablet)
Dimenhydrinate	dimenhydrinate (generic name) Dramamine (tablet, liquid, and children's formula) Eldodram (tablet) Marmine (tablet) Dipendrate (tablet) Travel Aids (tablet) Traveltabs (tablet)
Meclizine	meclizine hydrochloride (generic name) Bonine (tablet) Vertrol (tablet) Antivert (tablet) Lamine (tablet) Motion Cure (capsule, chewable tablet)

When Not to Use Antiemetics for Motion Sickness
- If you are pregnant.
- If you must drive (they make you drowsy).
- If you are performing intricate or dangerous work.
- If the nausea results from something other than the motion sickness.
- If you are drinking alcohol or taking tranquilizers.

Note: Do not give over-the-counter antiemetics to pets before a journey. In some cases these drugs can prove fatal to animals.

WHEN TO CALL THE DOCTOR

As a rule, motion sickness is not dangerous, but if other problems accompany it, a doctor may be necessary. Consult a doctor if:
- Intense vomiting occurs continuously for more than several hours
- There are signs of blood in the vomit.
- There are indications of dehydration (decrease in urination, sunken eyeballs, rapid breathing, drowsiness, fever, refusal to take liquids).
- The symptoms continue for several days after the journey is over.

CHAPTER 5

NOSEBLEEDS

An ordinary nosebleed stems from injury to the soft tissue of the nose, especially from ruptures of the surface blood vessels in the lower parts of the nostrils. A common childhood ailment, it can be caused by cold symptoms, dried mucous membranes, or nose picking, and is rarely reason for alarm. In adults, it may occasionally signal an underlying pathology, and it is necessary to be able to distinguish serious forms from harmless ones.

SELF-DIAGNOSIS OF NOSEBLEEDS

As a rule, the origin of the nosebleed will be evident (if it is not, this fact in itself may be reason for concern). Common causes to look for include:

- Sneezing and runny nose.
- Any type of self-inflicted trauma to the delicate veins of the nostril such as picking, continuous nose blowing, rubbing, etc.
- Direct injury to the nose.
- Exposure to high altitudes.
- Dried out nasal membranes, especially those caused by forced hot-air household heating units.

Self-Care for Nosebleeds

1. The best way to treat a bloody nose is to pinch the wings of the nostrils together until the bleeding stops. Squeeze firmly but not to the point of pain. Grip the entire nose, not just the tip. Occasionally pressure applied to the upper lip (as if stopping a sneeze) will also help.

2. Do not lie down while the bleeding continues. Lean forward whenever possible. After the bleeding has stopped, do not pick, blow, rub, or otherwise disturb the clotting process inside the nose.

3. If the bleeding is stubborn, an ice pack or cold compress placed over the forehead and the bridge of the nose will prove useful. Also, try raising both arms over your head.

4. If the bleeding is profuse and you can't stop it with any of the above measures, pack the nostrils with a clean gauze pad (not with cotton) and continue to apply pressure to the nostrils as described above. Be sure a corner of the pad is left protruding from the nostrils so that the gauze can be easily removed. Use this method only if the others described do not work.

Nosebleed Prevention: Some Quick How-To Advice

• Cracked and dried nasal mucous membranes are one of the chief causes of recurrent nosebleeds. These are often produced by low household humidity caused by indoor heating. The person who wakes up every morning suffering from what seems to be a sore throat may not be suffering from a virus or bacteria but from a simple lack of moisture in the air.

A humidifier placed in several rooms of the house will help solve this problem by bringing the household humidity up to 35 or 45 percent (anything below 25 percent can cause nasal irritation). Although simple methods such as placing bowls of water on top of radiators will raise the moisture content of the air, electric humidifiers are far better. The best of these is the *ultrasonic cool mist humidifier*. This space-age mechanism uses sound waves to produce a superfine vapor that remains suspended in the air for long periods of time. The water droplets are so small they easily penetrate the mouth and nose. For information on procuring cool mist humidifiers, see the technology and resources section below.

- Avoid abusing your nose when you have a head cold. When you blow your nose, do it gently. Be especially careful of the blood vessels in the lower part. After several days of a runny nose, they become particularly vulnerable.
- Avoid the use of over-the-counter nasal sprays and drops. Their continued use will not only aggravate the bleeding, but also may cause eventual injury to the nasal membranes.
- In a dry environment, rub petroleum jelly on the nasal membranes in the morning and at night. This will keep the membranes from cracking and is especially appropriate during the winter.

CAN NOSEBLEEDS EVER BE SERIOUS?

Yes, but only when they are symptoms of a more severe disorder. Rarely, nosebleeds can be a sign of rheumatic fever (in children), typhoid fever, internal head injuries, heart problems, high blood pressure, allergies, foreign bodies in the nose, anemia, or malignant nasal growths (in adults). You should consult a physician if:

- The bouts of mild bleeding continue for more than several days. This is especially true if you are not ordinarily prone to bloody noses.
- You have recently experienced an accident of some kind, especially a head injury.
- If the nosebleed persists for more than a half hour without abating and without responding to any of the above self-care methods.
- If you are having difficulty breathing.
- If you are taking anticoagulant drugs.
- If you have a medical history of blood problems, heart, kidney or liver ailments, or high blood pressure.*

TECHNOLOGY, RESOURCES, AIDS, AND SERVICES

1. Many drugstores and appliance stores carry room *humidifiers* and *air filters*. Sears sells a *dehumidifier* that is sometimes needed by people whose allergies are worsened by dampness and high humidity. HSA, P.O. Box 288, Farmville, NC 27828, (800)

---

*Although the relationship between nosebleeds and hypertension has not been proved, it would be wise in this instance to opt for the more conservative attitude and see a physician.

334-1187 (in North Carolina call [800] 672-4214), offers a good line of *vaporizers, cool mist humidifiers,* and *HEPA-type air purifiers* (see p. 188 for a description).

2. For a *free pamphlet on using humidifiers,* send a stamped, self-addressed envelope to ARI, Dept. HB, 1501 Wilson Blvd., Arlington, VA 22209.

CHAPTER 6

ACUTE BRONCHITIS

Bronchitis is an inflammation of the inner lining of the bronchial tubes. It often develops as a complication from a cold or respiratory infection, although it may also be triggered by the inhalation of irritating fumes and chemicals, gases, dust, tobacco smoke, or other airborne pollutants. Whatever the reason, the resultant mucous buildup in the bronchial passageways, coupled with the body's attempts to rid itself of this mucous, produces the persistent bouts of coughing that are characteristic of this ailment. Although many other maladies have symptoms similar to those of bronchitis, self-diagnosis is possible with careful observation.

SELF-DIAGNOSIS OF ACUTE BRONCHITIS

Bronchitis is typified by the following symptoms:

• A persistent, congested cough. The cough tends to be worse at night and is often accompanied by much spitting up of mucous.

• Chest pains, especially a tightness toward the center of the chest. Prolonged coughing causes pain throughout the rib area due to repeated muscular trauma caused by stretching the muscles that hold the ribs together.

• A rattling wheeze and sometimes shortness of breath (but

usually without the sense of suffocation that characterizes more serious respiratory problems such as asthma).

• If caused by a bacterial or viral infection, the coughing can be accompanied by a low-grade fever, hoarseness, and general malaise. The mucous will be thick and yellowish green.

SELF-CARE FOR ACUTE BRONCHITIS

If you are suffering from bronchitis, the following steps will help keep it under control:

1. Avoid inhaling irritating particles or fumes. If your bronchitis is caused by airborne pollutants such as dust or chemical fumes, the first thing you must do is avoid such irritants or at least wear a mask when you are near them. Needless to say, you should stop smoking. If you don't, the smoke will irritate the bronchial tubes, damaging the cilia (little hairs) in the mucosal linings that keep mucous flowing *out* of the lungs. Coughing and congestion could continue for months if the irritating source is not removed.

2. Increase fluid intake. Juices, herb teas, chicken soup, and plain water are all good for thinning the mucous and preventing dehydration. Self-treatment in this case is designed to break up congestion and get it out of the body.

3. Watch what you eat. Although some controversy surrounds this question, it is believed by many professionals that dairy foods produce mucous, and that when suffering from respiratory congestion of any kind, it is best to steer clear of milk, cheese, cream, butter, and yogurt. Also on the possible mucous-producing list are chocolate, coffee, and nuts. Eat plenty of fresh vegetables and stay away from sweets.

4. Inhale steam. Bring a pot of water to a boil. Being careful not to get too close to the scalding steam, bend over and inhale the vapors. A towel or sheet placed over the head while you breath will keep the steam concentrated. Do this several times a day. It should help break up the mucous. (Some doctors advise patients not to put the face directly over the boiling water but to keep it to the side of the pot, "whiffing" the steam toward the nose and mouth with the hands.) Humidifiers, steam baths, steamy showers, and moist warmed air are generally helpful for loose bronchial coughs.

5. Be careful of cough suppressants. They tend to dry up the mucous membranes, not a helpful service in this case. Remember,

coughing is the body's way of cleansing the lungs. If you must use a cough suppressant, here are some guidelines:

- If your cough is *dry* and *hacking* without mucous or sputum discharge (this is known as an irritative cough), a cough suppressant is advisable.
- If your cough is *thick* and *wet* with much chest rattling, spitting up of phlegm, and general mucous build-up (this is called a congestive cough), it is probably best not to use a cough suppressant. An expectorant *may* be of use here, though there are no guarantees.

Over-the-counter cough suppressants are all much the same. A majority use dextromethorpan as the primary ingredient, and a minority contain codeine. The latter is said to be harmless in small doses, but it pays to be careful, and drugs containing this chemical should always be kept well away from children. Be wary of spending your money on commercial expectorants. Most doctors agree that they don't work very well. Cough drops sold at candy counters are almost useless for controlling a bronchitis cough, but they can help soothe "cougher's throat."

6. Massage the chest. This will increase blood circulation, improve muscle tone, and produce a general feeling of well-being. Have a friend or family member rub your chest twice a day, using a soothing mentholated salve such as Vicks. Hot mustard plasters placed over the chest may also loosen congestion. If there is much mucous in the chest, hanging over the edge of the bed sometimes helps bring it up. Pounding the person's back with cupped hands produces vibrations that also seem to loosen mucous secretions.

7. Try home remedies. Some people have luck with simple homemade cough syrups such as lemon and honey mixed with hot water. The oils from eucalyptus, peppermint, clove, and wintergreen, when added to a vaporizer, are believed to help dissolve

---

Be on the Alert

When suffering from acute bronchitis, children tend to swallow their mucous rather than spit it out. Too much of this swallowing can cause an upset stomach, nausea, and eventual vomiting. Encourage spitting up.

---

mucous. Two tablespoons of apple cider vinegar mixed with a teaspoonful of honey taken three times a day is a popular New England remedy. So is plain honey.

8. *Remember, acute bronchitis is highly contagious,* most particularly in the early stages. Expose as few people as possible, especially children.

WHEN TO SEE A DOCTOR

A doctor's advice should be sought if:
- The cough does not go away after two weeks.
- The condition seems to be getting worse after four or five days with thickening and darkening of the mucous.
- The condition returns regularly every few months.
- The person appears to be having progressive difficulties breathing.
- There are signs of blood in the mucous.
- There is persistent pain in the chest.
- The fever goes above 101° F several times daily accompanied by chills and sweating.

WHAT ABOUT CHRONIC BRONCHITIS?

Chronic bronchitis is a serious ailment that is a long time coming and a long time staying, if it goes away at all. Lung function must deteriorate as much as 30 percent before this disease manifests itself as wheezing and shortness of breath—which is surely a testament to the lung's reserve capacity. Chronic bronchitis is characterized by an unpleasant and persistent cough caused by the swelling of the mucosal lining of the lungs and by copious amounts of sputum that clog and narrow the bronchial tubes. The condition is usually worse in the morning and is accompanied by much spitting up of secretions plus regular shortness of breath. Although there is not a great deal to be done once chronic bronchitis has appeared, measures *can* be taken to prevent it:

• Stop smoking now. Smoking is the number one cause of chronic bronchitis *and* emphysema (the two usually come together). If you smoke, your chances of developing both ailments are high. The good news is that if the chronic bronchitis is due to smoking, and if emphysema has not yet developed, then quitting can ultimately cause a return to almost normal lung function. But quit *now*.

• Stay away from chemical pollutants and toxic fumes (long-term inhalation is a primary cause of chronic bronchitis). If your job requires exposure to fumes, a mask should always be worn.

• At the first sign of a cough that does not go away, see your physician.

• Get plenty of rest and exercise. Running, deep breathing, good diet, and sound sleep are all specifics against this ailment.

TECHNOLOGY, RESOURCES, AIDS, AND SERVICES

1. *Portable oxygen units* for use in respiratory emergencies, both the single cylinder units and the twin-pac, are available from Sears Health Care Catalog (call [800] 323-3274 to order by mail or to get the address of the nearest Sears store).

2. A variety of *respiratory and lung care supplies*—Oxygen analyzer, oxygen mask, mouth-to-mouth breather, oral airways kit, humidifier, nebulizer, filters, respiratory exerciser, etc., are available from Health Supplies of America, P.O. Box 288, Farmville, NC 27828, (800) 334-1187 (in North Carolina call [800] 672-4214).

3. The following pamphlets on the subjects of bronchitis and chronic respiratory disease are available free:

The Lungs: Medicine for the Layman
Office of Clinical Reports and Inquiries
Building 10, Room 1A05
National Institutes of Health
Bethesda, MD 20014

Breathing . . . What You Should Know
American Lung Association
1740 Broadway
New York, NY 10019

Take a Look at the Facts: Your Lungs
American Lung Association (address above)

The Facts About Your Lungs
American Lung Association (address above)

The Facts About Your Lungs: Chronic Bronchitis
American Lung Association (address above)

If You Have Emphysema or Chronic Bronchitis, This Booklet Is for You
Emphysema Anonymous
P.O. Box 66
1364 Palmetto Avenue
Ft. Meyers, FL 33902

Chronic Obstructive Lung Diseases: Emphysema and Chronic Bronchitis
National Heart, Lung and Blood Institute
Public Inquiries and Reports Branch
9000 Rockville Pike
Bethesda, MD 20014

CHAPTER 7

COLD SORES

Cold sores are a mild skin condition caused by a virus known as *herpes simplex type 1*. Generally speaking, the virus tends to form on the area of the lips and mouth. Once contracted, the herpes simplex virus tends to remain dormant in the body for a long period of time, recurring periodically, especially after a cold or flu (they are not called "fever blisters" for nothing), exposure to intense sun, or in times of stress. Though not harmful or dangerous (do not mistake herpes simplex with *genital herpes (herpes simplex type 2)* or *herpes zoster [shingles]*), cold sores are highly contagious, especially in the early stages, and activities such as kissing or sharing common eating utensils should be discouraged.

SELF-DIAGNOSIS OF COLD SORES

The sores take the form of small, red, shiny blisters that come in clusters and eventually dry out, scab, and fall off in one to three weeks. If rubbed too violently they will weep a clear, colorless fluid that is highly contagious. The scab tends to be a yellowish-brown color. In most cases, cold sores form on the mouth, especially on the upper lip and the corners of the mouth, although they may also appear on the inside of the cheeks, on the tongue, and on the eyeballs, where they can cause considerable trouble. The blisters are mildly painful, especially if irritated.

SELF-CARE FOR COLD SORES

Basically, there is no cure for cold sores other than time. As with many ailments, however, certain remedies and approaches tend to work for *some* people *some* of the time. Although there are no guarantees here, it doesn't hurt to try. For certain individuals they seem to speed up the healing process, and for others they relieve pain and irritation.

1. Dab rubbing alcohol over the sores. This method tends to speed up drying and healing.

2. As soon as the cold sore begins to appear—veterans of this ailment come to recognize the early symptoms by a special kind of itching and tingling sensitivity—apply ice for at least an hour or, preferably, two. Although this method can be bothersome, especially since the ice pack must be shifted every few minutes, many people report that careful application causes sores to disappear before they erupt.

3. Somewhat the reverse of the above, another method calls for placing a hot washcloth over the sores before they erupt and continuing the treatment for at least an hour, periodically changing the cloth.

4. During the time that the sores are active, remain on a bland diet, avoiding hot or spicy foods and favoring those containing yeast, like yogurt (yeast may have a good effect on the healing rate of herpes). Stay away from chocolate, nuts, and seeds, all of which contain high amounts of the amino acid arginine, which is suspected of increasing the activities of the herpes simplex virus.

5. Although the definitive word is not yet in on the effectiveness of the many over-the-counter topical salves and balms presently on the market for cold sores, many people report that preparations made with menthol, camphor, peppermint oil, beeswax, sesame oil, white petrolatum, and benzoin all tend to speed up the healing process. Topical ointments containing tannic acid, allantoin, and phenolphthalein are all considered either unsafe or ineffective by the FDA.

Caution

Cold sore balms containing hydrocortisone and hydrocortisone acetate will spread the herpes virus and must be avoided.

6. Recently, several nonprescription preparations for cold sores have come on the market, two of which are derived from entirely natural ingredients. The first, marketed in tablet form as *DoFUS* and *Lactinex*, contains *lactobacillus acidophilus* or *lactobacillus bulgaricus*. Both ingredients are extracted directly from yogurt and both are considered promising by the FDA for cold sore relief. The amino acid *lysine*, sold in tablet form as *Enisyl* and *L-Lysine*, has also proved effective in suppressing the virus when taken in doses of from three hundred to one thousand milligrams a day. Other oral remedies, especially cold tablets containing acetaminophen, caffeine, phenolphthalein, and phenylephrine hydrochloride are not generally considered effective.

WHEN TO CALL THE DOCTOR

Although cold sores are not in themselves serious, they may on occasion be symptoms of an underlying pathology. Consult a physician if:
- The sores do not clear up within a month.
- The sores spread to the eyes.
- Other skin problems appear along with the herpes lesions.
- The sores become infected—as evidenced by reddening, profuse pus secretions, swelling, and rapid spreading.

CHAPTER 8

MINOR
EAR PROBLEMS

Connected by a series of intersecting tubes and tissue, the ears, nose, and throat are part of a mutually interacting system that is as sensitive as it is effective. The disorders that arise in these areas are sometimes serious, especially in the delicate inner mechanisms of the ear and nose. More commonly, they are minor and can be easily controlled at home. Here are some of the most frequent ailments that occur specifically in the ears, along with methods for self-help therapy. Problems of nose and throat will be treated in subsequent chapters.

Excess Wax in the Ears

Happily, the most common problem of the ear, wax accumulations, is also the most remediable. Many seemingly serious ailments such as deafness, earaches, running ear, ringing in the ear, dizziness, and lightheadedness may be due to the simple fact that wax secretions, while performing their function as lubricator of the auditory canal, become compacted into semi-hard plugs. These plugs block the auditory canal, interfere with hearing, and serve as a potential culturing media for infections. Occasionally the condition can cause pain. More commonly, it produces a sense of low-level pressure in the head. The condition should be attended to quickly before complications arise.

Some people have a tendency to form large amounts of excess earwax. Such accumulations do not mean that the person is dirty or that his or her hygiene is remiss. It is simply a quirk, perhaps inherited, of the person's auditory apparatus.

SELF-DIAGNOSIS OF EAR WAX PROBLEMS

Suspect wax buildup if:

• Your hearing seems impaired, but there is no serious pain or suspicious symptoms accompanying the condition. This condition can become acute if the wax accumulation "flips" over to cover the eardrum or block the ear canal, at which point patients usually complain of sudden onset of deafness.

• There is a constant sense of pressure in the ear, usually without pain.

• Large wax accumulations are apparent when looking into the ear.

SELF-CARE FOR EAR WAX PROBLEMS

1. Do *not* go after the wax with a pointed instrument. This includes cotton swabs, cotton balls on the end of matchsticks, nail files, toothpicks, etc. Such methods, besides being ineffective, may cause damage to the delicate ear canal and can end up packing the wax tighter or even puncturing the eardrum.

2. The best method of cleaning out ear wax is as follows:

• Lie on your side.

• With a medicine dropper or syringe, *carefully* squeeze (or have someone squeeze) lukewarm water into your ear. Let the water remain there for ten to fifteen minutes, then shake it out. Repeat, this time using hydrogen peroxide. Wait ten minutes, then rinse the hydrogen peroxide out with water.

• Wait several minutes, then lie down again. This time, place several drops of warm (not hot) olive or mineral oil into your ear and allow it to remain for approximately fifteen minutes. The oil will soften the wax and allow it to exit the ear naturally. Repeat again in three hours if the ear is still not clear.

Caution

Do not use the water and oil method if there is any suspicion of a perforated eardrum.

---

3. Even if you suffer from excess wax deposits, cleaning should be done only occasionally. Excessive cleaning removes the ear's natural lubricating and protective substance and leaves the ears especially vulnerable to infection.

WHEN TO CALL THE DOCTOR

A visit to the physician in is order if:
- The above cleaning method does not work and wax continues to build up regularly in the ear.
- There is any suspicion of a perforated eardrum.
- The ear becomes painful.

Ringing in the Ears (Tinnitus)

Ringing in the ears, or *tinnitus* as it is technically called, is a common affliction that takes different forms for different people, from a kind of muffled thumping sound to a dull buzz to a hum, pop, flutter, or even a roar. Basically a response of the auditory nerve to any type of irritation or stimulation, ringing in the ears can arise from many causes ranging from allergies to high blood pressure to side effects from medication.

SELF-DIAGNOSIS OF RINGING IN THE EARS

Ringing in the ears is self-evident. Although it can take the forms mentioned above, it decidedly does *not* take the form of voices in the ears or strange noises, both of which belong in the category of auditory hallucinations. Be aware, moreover, that after a haircut small hairs are sometimes swept into the ear where they get trapped in the canals and rub against the eardrum, causing a deep thundering sound. A special instrument known as an *otoscope* can be used to examine the external ear canal for such renegade hairs and for other foreign particles as well. The otoscope is, in fact, a good tool for everyone to keep as part of their home medical kit. Information on obtaining one is provided at the end of this section, along with instructions for its use.

SELF-CARE FOR RINGING IN THE EARS

1. Occasional ringing in the ears is nothing to be alarmed about. There are so many possible causes, including exposure to loud noises, drug side effects (aspirin and aspirin compounds are the most common offenders here), toxins in the food, and, some believe, stress, that a bit of it now and then will cause no harm.

2. On the other hand, after checking for wax buildup and other problems in the external ear canal, there is not a great deal that can be done to make it stop.

3. Keep the ear passages as clean as possible, avoid harsh sounds and stress, and let time do the healing.

WHEN TO SEE A DOCTOR

See a physician if:
- Severe ringing continues for more than several hours.
- The ringing occurs when you are taking drugs and medications.
- You suffer from arthritis, high blood pressure, or any chronic disease.
- The ringing is associated with hearing diminution, dizziness, loss of coordination, or intense headache.

Foreign Objects in the Ear

Do not assume that the presence of foreign particles in the ear will necessarily be obvious. A hair, a piece of grass, a tiny insect all can enter and lodge without causing obvious discomfort. The trouble will come later, when infection sets in.

SELF-DIAGNOSIS OF FOREIGN OBJECTS IN THE EAR

Consider the possibility of foreign objects lodged in the ear if you suffer from:
- A constant itching or draining from the ear.
- A sense of pushing against the eardrum; a feeling of pressure, bursting, or swelling.
- A sense that something is "moving inside the ear."
- Pain deep in the ear canal.

SELF-CARE FOR FOREIGN OBJECTS IN THE EAR

Removing foreign objects from the ear is a tricky matter. Probing into the ear with a pointed object and "fishing" for the lodged particle on your own is not a wise idea. Physicians have special instruments for such jobs, and even then it is not always easy to remove the offender without damaging surrounding ear tissue.

1. The one self-care option you have is the warm oil method described on page 79.

2. If this technique does not work, go directly to a physician.

3. Do *not* attempt to probe for the foreign object yourself.

A Trick for Removing Live Insects from the Ear

As everyone knows, insects are attracted to light. If a gnat, fly, or other winged creature flies into your ear, place a flashlight against your ear and turn the light on. Nine times out of ten the insect will move toward the light and out of your ear. If a live insect becomes trapped and the light method does not work, don't panic. Though it makes a good deal of noise fluttering around, it will rarely do damage. Get yourself to a medical professional as quickly as possible and have the insect extracted. Do not try to drown it by irrigating your ear, as the body of the insect may become lodged and cause infection.

Bleeding from the Ear

Bleeding from the ear is due to two things—an injury to the lining of the ear canal or a more serious injury within the eardrum or head.

Rule: Unless you are absolutely positive that the bleeding is due to a minor cut or tear to the ear lining, see a doctor. Bleeding from the ear can be a serious symptom. It's best to let a professional evaluate the situation before home treatment is considered.

Running Ear

Occasionally, ears will "leak" a clear or greenish-yellow fluid. Such discharges often have a foul smell and may be a sign of several possible ailments:
• Chronic infection of the external ear canal or middle ear (with perforated ear drum).
• A boil in the ear canal.
• A skull fracture.
• Damage to the ear drum.
• A trapped object in the ear.
• Tumor of the middle ear.
All of the above are serious enough to warrant an immediate trip to the doctor. While waiting for help, you can loosely pack a little cotton in your ear to absorb the drippings. Take aspirin

or acetaminophen if there is pain. By no means should you wash a dripping ear or probe it with a cotton swab.

Pierced Ear Infections

So many people, male and female, young and old, have pierced their ears that infections of the earlobe are becoming epidemic. Problems can occur both at the time of piercing—usually due to unsterilized instruments—or later, from infection. As a rule, problems are minor and can be dealt with without a doctor's help. Occasionally, they become chronic and should be treated professionally.

SELF-DIAGNOSIS OF EARLOBE INFECTIONS

Note the following symptoms:
• The earring hole becomes red and raw, warm, tender, and may produce discharge.
• The earlobe is swollen and sensitive to the touch.
• There is indication of eczema or other scaly, itchy skin conditions.

SELF-CARE FOR EARLOBE INFECTIONS

1. Part of the treatment is simple prevention. When the ear is pierced, be *absolutely certain* that the piercing instrument is sterilized and that all procedures are sanitary.

2. Once the training earring is in place, keep the lobe especially clean and shift the earring's position frequently to avoid chafing. Note, too, that problems in the lobe sometimes stem from allergic skin reactions to the metallic alloys used in earrings and studs. Treatment in this case is simply to stop wearing jewelry made from these materials.

3. When an infection does occur, remove the earring immediately and do not replace it until all signs of the infection are gone.

4. Keep the infected area scrupulously clean with several daily washings, make sure the wound is exposed to the air, and allow it to heal on its own.

5. If there is no improvement after a week, consider applying an antibiotic skin cream such as Neosporin, Tri-Salve or Bacimycin. As a rule, the problem will heal by itself with proper hygiene.

Consult a physician if:
- The pierce shows no signs of healing after a week, or if the infection seems to be getting worse.
- Lumps form in the pierced area.
- There is any unusual discharge from the infected earring hole.

Earache

Quite frequently, especially among children, a cold or flu causes blockage in the Eustachian tube, the channel that connects the back of the nose to the middle ear, home of that most delicate and important organ, the eardrum. Unrelieved, this blockage can become infected, producing what is commonly called an earache, and what is medically termed *otitis media*. If the ailment is not given immediate attention, pressure builds up within the middle ear and damage to the eardrum can occur. Serious complications such as facial paralysis, permanent hearing loss, and meningitis are possible effects. Generally speaking, an earache is nothing to ignore or leave untreated.

SELF-DIAGNOSIS OF EARACHE

Because most of us have at one time or another suffered from earaches, the early symptoms are relatively familiar: clogging of one or both ears with slight but recurrent pain. As the condition worsens, a fever appears—sometimes a fever as high as 102°F or 103°F (up to 105°F in children)—accompanied by a boring pain, severe throbbing, dizziness, stomach upset, and a sensitivity of the ear to external pressure. Sore throat, vomiting, ringing in the ear, and diminished hearing are all possible effects. If the disorder does not receive adequate attention, the eardrum may bulge and eventually burst, with an accompanying outpouring of pus, mucous, and blood. You will recognize this condition not only by sight, but also by the fact that all pain ceases immediately; it is to be hoped that you will never allow an earache to reach this extreme point.

What causes earache? Although the aftermath of colds and flu often cause fluid accumulations in the middle ear, a foreign object lodged in the ear or an overabundance of ear wax can also be the culprit. So can a boil in the ear. For young children who

are not articulate enough to identify clearly the cause of their distress, earaches can be recognized by these signs:
- The child cries constantly.
- Fever is high.
- The ear may be hot and sensitive to the touch.
- The child's hearing seems affected.
- The child constantly touches, cups, and pulls at his or her ear.
- The child has recently had a cold or flu, gone swimming, flown in an airplane, suffered from a stuffy nose, or has had a history of ear problems.

SELF-CARE FOR EARACHE

In many cases, an earache will require antibiotics and a doctor's care. In some cases, home care may be all that is required. If you are going to take the latter route, be aware of a few important DON'TS":
1. Don't allow the ear to be exposed to drafts or cold.
2. Don't attempt to probe the ear with any type of instrument or cotton swab.
3. Don't allow the pain to become too intense. This may be a sign that the eardrum is under pressure and is about to rupture.
4. Don't place warm oil, water, hydrogen peroxide, or any other liquids into the ear without first consulting a doctor.
5. Don't blow your nose with too much vigor. It will increase the pressure already built up in the middle ear.
   And some DO'S:
1. Give simple aspirin or acetaminophen for pain.
2. Keep the ear warm at all times. Use a hot water bottle or an electric heating pad. Lie on your side and place the heating apparatus directly under the ear. Keep it in place as long as possible.
3. A humidifier by the bed will keep the ear canal moistened and the waxy mucous thinned.
4. In some cases, an antihistamine will control mucous in the nasal areas. The use of nasal decongestants to shrink the membranes of the nose and open the Eustachian tube for drainage can sometimes help, too.
5. Remain relaxed and quiet. Get plenty of rest. Keep your diet simple and bland. Soups and liquids are best. Drink plenty of cool water and do not eat hot, spicy, or mucous-producing foods.

6. A hot compress may help. The best is made of salt. Take a half cupful of salt, warm it in a frying pan, then pack the salt in a clean cloth and hold the cloth against the afflicted ear. Keep the compress in place while you sleep. Reheat the salt periodically.

WHEN TO CALL THE DOCTOR

As mentioned, *otitis media* can develop into a serious ailment. Contact a physician if any of the following symptoms develop:
- The pain continues to increase or becomes too severe.
- There is no sign of healing after two weeks, or if the condition seems to be getting worse after the first two or three days.
- The fever goes above 101° F.
- The ear oozes fluids.
- Hearing becomes progressively impaired.
- Dizziness, lightheadedness, or nausea become especially intense.

Performing an Ear Exam with an Otoscope

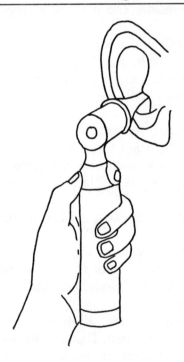

An otoscope is a kind of flashlight cum viewing scope that throws a concentrated beam of light directly into the ear canal and allows for close examination. Insert the ear piece very carefully into the external ear canal, being sure not to force it in. Insertion is facilitated by gently taking hold of the ear shell and pulling it upward, opening a clear view into the canal. Now look through the lens. Any sign of undue redness or infection will be apparent; the ear canal will appear inflamed and raw. Pus, mucous and excess ear wax may be similarly visible. An otoscope can be ordered through a medical supply house with a health professional's help or directly from companies that cater to home care. Addresses are given below in the resource section. Also, check the medical self-examination chapter for more information on using this instrument.

COMMONSENSE METHODS FOR PREVENTING EAR PROBLEMS

Earaches and related ear problems are by no means inevitable, and there are many simple things you can do to discourage them. As always, prevention is the best medicine.

1. Some people tend naturally to produce large accumulations of wax. If you are among this group, a periodic ear cleaning with hydrogen peroxide or warm oils (see self-treatment for ear wax) will discourage bacteria formation, wax buildup, and possible infection.

2. If you are prone to ear infections, avoid immersing your head in water, and do not use a diving board when swimming. This is especially true for children. Although it seems a bit cruel to make a child give up water sports entirely, the amount of time spent in the water should be curtailed (no longer than twenty minutes at a time), and only in chlorinated pools (swimming in the ocean, rivers, ponds, and lakes can lead to infections). Some people wear earplugs in the water for added protection, but this is a double-edged sword, as earplugs may cause impaction of earwax.

3. Again, for children, if a child has a recurring history of ear ailments, have his or her adenoids and tonsils checked. Trouble in either of these areas can lead to chronic ear infections.

4. Treat all head colds with decongestants early, especially if you or a child has a history of ear problems. Shrinking the nasal membranes can help avoid blockage of the Eustachian tube.

5. Do not under any circumstances place pointed objects in your ear. As the saying goes, "Never put anything smaller than your elbow into your ear."

6. Blow your nose in the correct way. In essence, this means that you should not blow with too much force and gusto. A good way of implementing this caution is to blow one nostril at a time, and gently, with the handkerchief held loosely over the nostrils. Forceful blowing can drive mucous into the Eustachian tubes and up into the middle ear where infection occurs.

TECHNOLOGY, RESOURCES, AIDS, AND SERVICES

1. A *no-frills otoscope* can be ordered for $24.00 plus $2.00 postage from:
Medical Self-Care Catalog
P.O. Box 999
Pt. Reyes, CA 94956
A *professional-quality otoscope* that costs approximately $70.00 and comes with three speculate lenses can be purchased through a health care professional from:
Abbey Medical
13782 Crenshaw Blvd.
Gardena, CA 90249
(call [800] 421-5126 for ordering information, [800] 262-1294 in California)
(must be ordered through a health-care program)

2. A *portable audiometer* designed to test hearing ability can be purchased through Abbey Medical (see address above).

3. If you suffer from chronic ringing in the ears (tinnitus), the following organization provides consultation referrals to regional clinics as well as advice:
The American Tinnitus Association
P.O. Box 5
Portland, OR 97201
(503) 248-9985

4. A *self-help clinic for tinnitus sufferers,* sponsored by the Kresge Hearing Research Laboratory at the University of Oregon, is available through the American Tinnitus Association. Contact them directly (address above).

5. Those with hearing loss problems are advised to consult the following self-help organizations:
The National Association for Hearing and Speech Action
10801 Rockville Pike
Rockville, MD 20852

The National Hearing Aid Society
20361 Middlebelt
Livonia, MI 48152

6. A *self-help bimonthly newsletter* is published for people with chronic ear and hearing problems by a group called Self-Help for

the Hard of Hearing. They will also put you in touch with local self-help groups. Contact them directly at:

Self-Help for the Hard of Hearing
7800 Wisconsin Avenue
Bethesda, MD 20814

7. For individuals who are especially susceptible to ear problems during air travel, a pamphlet called *Ears, Altitude and Airplane Travel* is available from:

The American Council of Otolaryngology
Suite 602
1100 17th St., N.W.
Washington, DC 20036

8. The Alexander Graham Bell Association for the Deaf provides special *publications* and *audiovisual material* on deafness and hearing improvement. They also offer a large *catalog* of materials dealing with ear problems. Contact them directly at:

International Parents' Organization
c/o Alexander Graham Bell Association
1537 35th Street, N.W.
Washington, DC 20007

9. People who suffer from problems of the inner ear, especially dizziness, should obtain a pamphlet from the National Institute of Neurological and Communicative Disorders and Stroke called *Hope Through Research: Dizziness, Including Menière's Disease.* It can be obtained from:

National Institute of Neurological and Communicative Disorders and Stroke
Officer of Scientific and Health Reports
Building 31, Room 8A-08
National Institutes of Health
9000 Rockville Pike
Bethesda, MD 20014

CHAPTER 9

EYE PROBLEMS

Although glaucoma, trachoma, cataracts, direct injuries to the cornea, and any serious eye injuries should always be referred to a physician immediately, there are a number of minor problems that can often be treated at home. Certain eye disorders, for instance, stem purely from fatigue and strain. Others result from exposure to pollutants. In some cases, eye exercises can help restore blurred vision. In others, simple home remedies and good hygiene are all that is needed. In fact, vision in general can be both preserved and improved by proper eye hygiene and care.

Particles Lodged in the Eye

In city environments where the air is filled with innumerable waste particles, specks in the eye have become a major concern. If the object is small and smooth (most are particles from incinerators, cinders from waste plants, or eyelashes), and if it is visible on the pupil of the eye, it can usually be removed without trouble. Don't neglect these particles. There is some danger that they may seriously scratch the eye surface, become embedded in the cornea or white of the eye, and eventually cause corneal ulcers.

Self-Diagnosis of Particles Lodged in the Eye

Though usually self-evident, some specks are so small that their presence is not immediately felt. Common signs of objects in the eye include:

- A hot, burning sensation that is especially apparent when blinking.
- A sense that something is lodged or "stuck" in the eye.
- Excess moisture and watering of the eye.
- Redness or bloodshot eyes.
- A sudden over-sensitivity to light.

Self-Care for Particles in the Eye

What to Avoid When Removing a Particle from the Eye

1. Do not rub, push, or otherwise apply direct pressure to the sensitive areas. A lodged particle is best removed by movement of the eyeball and by irrigation, not by rubbing.

2. Never attempt to remove a speck from the eye with a match, toothpick, or any hard, pointed object. Permanent damage to the eye can result.

3. Never use dry cotton when removing objects from the eye. Cotton fibers tend to adhere to the moist surfaces of the eyeball and may become as much of a menace as the irritating particle.

Removal Tricks

1. Shut both eyes tightly for several minutes immediately after the speck has entered the eye. Squeeze the lids down firmly. Then open and blink rapidly. The slight moistening effect that these movements produce may wash the particle away.

2. Open your eyes, roll them vigorously, then shut them firmly for several seconds. Repeat this exercise several times.

3. If the particle remains, grasp the eyelashes of your upper lid firmly and pull it down over the lower lid, looking toward the floor as you do. Hold the lid down for several moments, then release. Repeat several times.

4. If you still have no luck, carefully splash lukewarm water directly onto the open eye.

5. For stubborn particles, an over-the-counter eye wash or irrigation preparation may be necessary. These products can be

purchased at any good pharmacy. Place one or two drops of the solution in the irritated eye, shut it firmly for at least a minute (this will prevent the liquid from dripping back into the nose), then open and move the eyes vigorously in circles for several more moments.

6. Some commercial eye irrigation preparations come packaged with an eye cup. This item can be a valuable tool. Make sure the cup is clean, then fill it halfway with the irrigating solution or with clean, cool water. Place the cup directly over your eye, tilt your head back, open and close your eye rapidly while it is immersed, rotating it in broad circles. In most instances, this maneuver will do the trick. If you want to clean your eye with special thoroughness, keep it shut tightly for a few minutes after irrigating.

7. If all else fails, take a piece of sterile gauze and, using a mirror to locate the speck, remove it with the tip of the gauze. Be sure not to poke or scrape the eyeball; a few gentle passes with the gauze should be all that is necessary. Aiming the beam of a flashlight directly at the eye will increase visibility and facilitate removal.

8. If the eye continues to water but close examination reveals no evidence of a lodged particle, it is possible that the offending speck is already out but that it has slightly scratched the surface of the eye. As a rule, these surface scratches heal quickly and are nothing to worry about. Keep the eye clean, bathe it once a day, and let it heal on its own.

9. If none of the above measures succeed, place a temporary dressing over the eye and seek professional help.

What You Should Know About Eye Irrigation Solutions

The FDA recommends that nonprescription eye wash solutions contain only sterilized water and inert chemicals such as preservatives, salt, and a weak solution of boric acid. Commercial brands that contain only these safe ingredients include A/K Rinse, Blinx, Collyrium Eye Lotion, Lavoptik Eye Wash, and M/Rinse.

WHEN TO CALL THE DOCTOR

- If the object lodged in the eye is large or has sharp surfaces.
- If there is any pain beyond mild irritation.
- If the particle entered the eye at rapid speed and/or is deeply embedded.

- If all attempts to remove the object have failed and the irritation has continued for more than several hours.

Black Eye

A black eye is nothing more than a bruise, a dramatic but usually harmless sign that the blood vessels in the delicate tissue surrounding the eye have been damaged. The blood released from the bruise collects in the soft pouchy areas of the eye and produces dark circles. A black eye can be treated more or less the same way as any other soft tissue contusion.

1. Apply an ice pack to the injured area immediately.
2. A compress or a beefsteak applied to the eye is an old favorite for reducing swelling, and still a worthy one.
3. After the first day, hourly applications of a towel soaked in hot water will help the healing process by speeding the absorption of blood under the skin.

WHEN TO CALL THE DOCTOR

Consult a physician if:
- There is indication of direct injury to the eyeball.
- There are any serious cuts or abrasions surrounding the eye.
- There is any sign of bleeding within the eye.
- Vision is impaired.

Note of Caution

Sometimes when the eye is struck directly by a foreign object, there may be no immediate signs of bruising. Later, after a week or more, the eye begins to blacken or redden, to swell, and generally to show signs of distress. If this condition occurs, see a doctor.

Eyestrain

The most common of all eye complaints, eyestrain, is produced by excessive or improper use of the eyes. It affects just about all of us at one time or another. As a rule, the problem is easily corrected—provided one can remember to practice the remedies.

Self-Diagnosis of Eyestrain

These are usually self-evident and are often accompanied by fatigue and stress. Symptoms include:
- A feeling of fatigue and tension in the eye muscles.
- Slight watering of the eyes.
- Redness of the eyes.
- A scratchy feeling in the eyelids.
- Twitching of the eyelids.
- Mild headache.

Prevention and Self-Care of Eyestrain

First, *prevention:*

1. Avoid straining your eyes when reading. Be especially aware of proper lighting. As a rule, the light source should come from *behind and from the side, preferably from the side that will cast no shadows.* Never face directly into the light while reading. The intensity of illumination should be sufficient but not so strong that it creates glare; glare is the enemy of the human eye. Be careful of hallogen lamps, which are often too strong for reading. Seventy-five to one hundred watts is an ideal intensity. When using your eyes for long periods, look up periodically and focus them on a distant point for a moment or so.

2. Practice regular eye exercises. There are, of course, many varieties of these exercises. One of the best and simplest is as follows. Practice it twice a day, morning and night, anywhere you wish—in an easy chair, waiting for a bus, on the job, etc. Start by focusing your eyes on a distant point. Keep your eyes fixed on this point for several seconds, then refocus on a point in mid-ground. Stay at this point for several seconds, then refocus again on an object no farther than a foot away from your eyes. Now return to the far point and repeat the cycle. Do five to ten cycles of this exercise, twice a day or more.

3. When watching television, keep at least one light on in the room. Don't sit too close to the TV (six to seven feet away is about right), and sit directly in front of the screen. Angle viewing is a strain. Always keep the picture in sharp focus.

4. When you are in a brightly lit environment for prolonged periods of time, wear sunglasses. Glare causes the eyes to tense up and quickly become fatigued.

5. Eyestrain is often a symptom of faulty vision. If your vision is at all blurred or distorted, you may want to visit an optometrist to be examined for a pair of glasses.

And now, *treatment:*

1. Rest your eyes for brief periods during the day, especially when they are being taxed. Close your eyes for a minute or two, covering them with your hands, and make a concerted effort to thoroughly relax the muscles in the upper and middle part of the face, the scalp, the eyebrows, eyelids, temples, and cheeks. After a minute, take a deep breath and picture a restful image—a beautiful landscape, the face of a loved one, a Christmas tree with candles, the sea—any image that is pleasing and relaxingly familiar. Take these brief rest stops at various intervals during the day, and the beneficial results will soon be apparent.

2. Practice the eye exercise described above in the prevention section.

3. When your vision feels strained, an over-the-counter eye-drop preparation will cool the eyes and rinse out irritating specks and airborne pollutants. Whether drops actually "soothe" the eyes, however, is open to argument in medical circles. It is generally believed that nonprescription eye drops will relieve minor eye irritations, reduce redness, and provide temporary relief for dry eyes. They will *not* necessarily relieve fatigue, make eyes look younger and more sparkling, or endow them with a "glamorous new luster." Nor will they help you relax.

There is no cut-and-dried answer to whether you should use eye drops. Personal experimentation is the only way to know for sure. Popular brands deemed safe and effective include Allerest Eye Drops, Clear Eyes, Tetrasine, Optigene II Eye Drops, Tear-Efrin Eye Drops, VasoClear, Clear & Brite, Murine Plus Eye Drops, Soothe Eye Drops, and Visine.

A final word of warning: Eye drops are *not* for daily use, contrary to the claims of some manufacturers, and excessive use over a prolonged period can be dangerous.

4. Eyestrain and physical fatigue are directly connected, and one can easily trigger the other. In the chapter on headache (page 39), a method for overall body relaxation is described. Try it.

5. When suffering from eyestrain, avoid all bright lights and glare. If you work indoors, stay away from work surfaces that reflect light. Sunglasses are, of course, a welcome benefit if you work outside, but don't waste your money on the brightly col-

ored ones or those with red or blue lenses; they are not designed to give adequate protection against ultraviolet rays. Amber, black, and brown are better.

WHEN TO CALL THE DOCTOR

Eyestrain is dangerous only when it is a symptom of a more serious ailment. Consult a physician if:
• Severe headaches consistently accompany eyestrain.
• Your vision has suddenly become blurred, double-imaged, or otherwise distorted.
• Eyestrain is accompanied by severe pain.
• One eye is consistently painful and the other feels normal.

When Should You Have Your Eyes Examined?

Generally speaking, have an eye examination if you have more than one of the following symptoms:
• Extreme sensitivity to light
• Chronic eye pains
• Blurred or otherwise distorted vision
• Constant watering of the eyes
• Light flashes
• Chronic bloodshot eyes

TECHNOLOGY, RESOURCES, AIDS, AND SERVICES

1. For people who work with computers and are worried about the effects of glare and radiation, Langley–St. Clair Instrumentation Systems (132 West 24th Street, New York, NY 10011) has developed a *special lead impregnated acrylic shield* that blocks X rays and ultraviolet light. The device fits easily onto the front of most computers. For information, call their toll free number: (800) 221-7070 (in New York call [212] 989-6876).

2. Eyestrain is often a result of ordinary tension and stress, and can be helped with *relaxation and antistress programs*. For a full list of such programs, consult the technology and resources section in the insomnia, headache, and stress chapters.

3. One of the best *pairs of sunglasses* on the market is a model known as "Wings," manufactured by Bausch & Lomb. These extraordinary glasses offer excellent glare protection and ex-

tremely low ultraviolet light transmission without the usual color distortion. They retail for $50 to $60 at most stores. Bausch & Lomb also offers a useful booklet on choosing sunglasses called *Sunglasses and Your Eyes: A Consumer Guide on Sunglass Selection and Uses.* Order it from:

Bausch & Lomb
One Lincoln Square
Rochester, NY 14601

4. There are a number of vision aids, lenses, and optical mechanisms on the market today to help people with eye disorders and damaged vision. The American Optometric Association (address listed in number 6 below) publishes a booklet called *Beautiful! Vision Information About Partial Sight,* which describes the most useful of these.

5. A catalog of large-type reading materials for the vision-impaired is offered by:

National Association for the Visually Handicapped
305 East 24th Street
17C
New York, NY 10010

6. Some useful booklets on the subject of eye care and eye disorders include:

I Care: Eye Care at Work, Home and Play
Physicians Art Service, Inc.
Marketing Department
343-B Serramonte Plaza Office Center
Daly City, CA 94015
(cost $1.25)

Answers to Your Questions About Vision Conditions
American Optometric Association
Communications Division
243 N. Lindbergh Blvd.
St. Louis, MO 63142
(enclose stamped, self-addressed envelope)

Answers to Your Questions About Seeing Spots and Floaters
American Optometric Association
(address above, enclose stamped envelope)

Your Vision—The Second Fifty Years
American Optometric Association
(address above)

Medical Eye Care
American Association of Ophthalmology
1100 17th Street
Washington, DC 20036

Seeing Well as You Grow Older
American Association of Ophthalmology
(address above)

First Aid for Eye Emergencies
National Society for the Prevention of Blindness
79 Madison Avenue
New York, NY 10016

7. Several lengthy catalogs featuring self-help products for the blind and for those with eye ailments are available from the American Foundation for the Blind, 15 West 16th Street, New York NY 10011. Ask for *Catalog of Consumer Products for the Blind and Visually Handicapped* and for *Products for People with Vision Problems.* Examples picked at random of items that can be ordered from these catalogs include *large-number clocks, large-print games and recreational materials, voice-activated thermometers, large-key calculators, talking money identifiers,* and many others.

8. A *free home eye chart* designed to test the sight of preschoolers and people who cannot read is also available from the National Society to Prevent Blindness (address above).

9. Eye Care Inc. is a nonprofit organization dedicated to providing consumers with the latest information on eye care. They publish a newsletter called *I Care Through Eye Care.* Contact them at: 523 8th Street, S.E., Washington, DC 20003 for details.

10. Two agencies will provide you with information on eye problems, eye care products, drugs, and referrals to specialists. Contact either The Eye Research Institute of Retina Foundation, 20 Stanford Street, Boston, MA 02114, or Fight for Sight, National Council to Combat Blindness, 139 East 57th Street, New York, NY 10022.

11. If you can't afford to buy a pair of glasses, either the Lions Club International, 300 22nd Street, Oakbrook, IL 60521, or New Eyes for the Needy, Short Hills, NJ 07078 will purchase them for you. Contact either organization for information.

CHAPTER 10

COLDS
AND FLU

As the saying goes, if you get plenty of rest, drink lots of liquids, take medicine, and sleep deeply, your cold will be gone in seven days. Otherwise, it will last a week.

Is there really nothing that can be done to help a cold? Must all cases of influenza be so prolonged and weakening? The answer is that certain remedies do seem to have beneficial effects for certain people at certain times. Nothing that works for everyone has been discovered yet, as we all know, but there are some little-known aids, tricks, and surprising shortcuts that can *sometimes* speed up the healing process.

SELF-DIAGNOSIS OF COLDS AND FLU

It is a common error to suppose that colds and influenza stem from only one or two varieties of virus. Not so. There are at least five major groups of cold-producing viruses, each with its own set of sub-strains, and one of these major groups, the rhinoviruses, contains more than ninety strains. Several types of flu virus also exist, the A variety being a good deal more debilitating than the B and C, and the worst of them having exotic names like "Hong Kong" or "Asian." Both flu and colds are highly contagious. They are spread by saliva or droplets of moisture that are coughed, sneezed, and breathed from one person to the next.

Incubation time for both is rarely longer than a few days, and both disorders can, if neglected, lead to more serious secondary infections such as bronchitis or pneumonia.

Interestingly, some of the more bothersome symptoms of colds and flu are actually part of the body's attempt to rid itself of the disease. Coughing is the lung's reflex for expelling excess mucous. Mucous itself serves to wash the invading organisms out of the system. Fever increases the body's amount of interferon, a natural influenza-destroying substance, and helps literally to burn up germs. There is also strong evidence that fever makes an infection less contagious and increases the power of antibiotics. Therefore, one must think twice before giving into the knee-jerk reflex of downing over-the-counter pills to suppress cold and flu symptoms.

	Colds	Flu
Incubation time	12 to 78 hours	12 to 78 hours
Contagious	Yes	Yes
Area of infection	Upper respiratory tract, nose, ears, throat, sinuses	Upper and lower respiratory tract
Fever	Mild, if present at all; sometimes sub-fever	Can range between 100° F to 104° F; occasionally goes higher, with chills
Headache	Mild, if present at all	Often severe
Nasal symptoms	Runny nose, sneezing	Usually absent
Cough	Mild, if present at all	Mild to severe; cough symptoms tend to worsen in last days of illness, and sometimes linger
Malaise, fatigue, and lassitude	Mild	Severe
Duration	Approximately a week	From several days to several weeks
Other symptoms	Watery eyes, sore throat, temporary loss of smell and taste, stuffed nose	Exhaustion, severe muscular ache, chills, runny nose, depression, vomiting, nausea, loss of appetite, diarrhea

Colds and Flu: How They Differ

The difference between the symptoms of colds and influenza is more one of degree than of kind.

Why Colds?

Why do some people catch colds and others don't? Though no one is quite certain, it seems a safe bet that fatigue, lack of sleep, poor eating habits, over-exposure to the elements, stress, depression, heavy drinking and smoking, and anything else that puts undue strain on the body lowers resistance. If you want to avoid colds and flu, the first and foremost rule is simple: *Take care of yourself.*

SELF-CARE FOR COLDS AND FLU

Conventional Wisdom for a Cold

1. Rest. Stay in bed if possible. The body needs all its energies to fight the invading virus. Don't strain if you can help it.

2. Drink plenty of liquids. There has recently been some scientific evidence showing that chicken soup has a therapeutic effect on colds and flu. Orange juice and lemon mixed with honey are good for sore throats; an acidic environment is unfriendly to viruses. Take lots of fresh water. The more you urinate, the better.

3. Place a vaporizer or humidifer in your room to make breathing easier.

4. Eat plain, bland foods. If your stomach is upset, go easy on the roughage, strong on soups and teas. No junk foods or solid foods of any type. Go very easy on the dairy, too; it's mucous-producing.

5. Two aspirin tablets every four hours will ease discomfort and take the edge off the malaise. Nasal decongestants will allow for easier breathing through the nose. If you have a sore throat, periodic gargling with warm saltwater may help.

6. Stay wrapped up in blankets or wear warm clothes. Avoid chills and drafts.

7. If fever is high, a sponge bath will be refreshing. Take your temperature frequently and remember that if you have recently eaten very hot or very cold food, this will affect the reading. Rec-

tal temperatures are at least one degree higher than oral. If the temperature goes above 102° F, a bath in a half-filed tub of tepid water or a brisk sponging down and drying should help bring it down. As a rule, a person's normal body temperature tends to be lowest in the morning, highest at night.

8. General body massage, if not too irritating to the patient, is a boon to circulation and can provide a sense of well-being.

9. Most especially, relax and allow your body's natural forces to cure you.

Unconventional Wisdom for a Cold

The following methods have all been used by innumerable cold sufferers through the years, sometimes with success, sometimes not. Why not try a few and judge for yourself?

1. Some people claim that one thousand milligrams of vitamin C taken twice a day when the cold or flu is in its early stages helps speed up the healing process. Since smoking depletes the body's store of vitamin C, this may be particularly valuable for smokers. Two tablets of calcium lactate and a high-potency vitamin B complex are also deemed useful by enthusiasts of the vitamin method. Many people take regular large doses of vitamin C during the cold/flu season as a preventive measure. This is safe because vitamin C is water soluble, and the body simply excretes what it cannot use. A kit to measure your body's level of vitamin C can be purchased for about $10.00 from Abroca, Inc., P.O. Box 5528, Maple Drive Annex, Beverly Hills, CA 90201.

2. Herbal teas are popular among afficionados of natural cures. Here are some popular mixtures (addresses for purchasing herbs will be given in the resource section):

• Mix the following: one ounce peppermint; one ounce rosemary; one ounce cayenne pepper; one ounce rose hips
  Boil a cup of water, allow the mixture to steep for fifteen minutes, add honey, and drink. Take twice a day.
• Mix the following: one-half ounce black elder flowers; one-half ounce peppermint leaves
  Boil water, steep for fifteen minutes, sweeten, and drink.
• Mix the following: two ounces peppermint leaves; one ounce ginger; one ounce goldenseal; one ounce boneset
  Boil water, steep for a half hour, sweeten, and drink three cups a day.
  Other herb teas that are reputed to help colds and flu include:

borage	dandelion greens	peppermint
camomile	ginger	rose hips
catnip	licorice	sage
clover	garlic	lemon
	goldenseal	

3. In the Slavic countries, garlic is known as "nature's anti-biotic" or "Russian penicillin." It is the custom there to chew three or four cloves a day while sick and constantly to inhale the vapors from crushed garlic. It is known that garlic does have some verifiable anti-germicidal effect, although how much has not been established. Another popular remedy is steamed milk cooked with crushed onions.

4. The old Yankee remedy, honey and apple cider vinegar, is another perennial favorite that really seems to work, especially for colds accompanied by sore throats. Mix three teaspoons of apple cider vinegar and three teaspoons of honey, and take the preparation six times a day. For a gargle, place three teaspoons of apple cider vinegar in a tumbler of water. Gargle the first mouthful and spit it out. Then swallow the next mouthful. Alternate until the glass is empty. Repeat every two hours.

5. Many people follow a liquid fast for several days when suffering from the flu or a severe cold. During this time they take only water, tea, fruit and vegetable juice, soup, and other easily digestible liquids. They abstain from solid foods entirely. At most, they will eat a puree of greens, carrots, and peppers. This allows the body to rest and to use its energies for healing.

6. The latest in wonder cures for colds is zinc tablets—not the regular zinc mineral supplements you buy at pharmacies, but a special, chewable variety. Believed to inhibit the growth of viruses, zinc's curative powers have received some support in recent laboratory tests. Many people swear by them. An address for procuring chewable zinc is included in the technology and resources section below.

The Lowdown on Cold Remedies

The first and most important thing to understand about over-the-counter cold remedies is that they suppress symptoms; they do not cure. The most popular cold remedies contain several basic ingredients—a decongestant, an antihistamine, a pain reliever, a cough suppressant. Almost always, however, you will find that these remedies contain the single ingredient that is of unquestionable value: aspirin, whose usefulness towers above the rest.

What of the others? As Joe Graedon points out in his book *The People's Pharmacy,* the antihistamine in so many nonprescription cold remedies has a very limited effect on colds. At best it helps dry the mucous membranes, and at worst it does nothing at all. Decongestant capsules can be effective, but the amounts found in combination cold remedies are often so small that they have a negligible effect. The same is true of cough suppressant syrups, although potential danger lies in the fact that by suppressing symptoms they can sometimes mask more serious ailments. Expectorants have little or no medicinal value. Mouth washes have no therapeutic value for sore throats.

Why then do people stand by their old remedies with dogged loyalty? For several reasons. First, because colds and flu respond to the placebo effect better than practically any ailment we know of: With colds, if you think it's going to work, it often does. Second, because of aspirin. Without question, aspirin relieves the headache and malaise that accompany colds, and, to a certain degree, even mitigates the heavy-duty aches of flu as well. Aspirin works, of this there is no question. And it is usually the aspirin in the cold pills that makes you feel better.

As for the other ingredients, well, maybe they're working, maybe they're not.

The upshot of it all, then, is that if you want to go the drug route for colds and flu, plain aspirin is usually your best bet. If you feel that something more is needed, treat the symptoms individually: aspirin for headaches, malaise, and fever; decongestants for nasal congestion; cough suppressants for respiratory congestion. Avoid any cold preparations that include more than three types of active ingredients or contain two types of active ingredients that are designed to relieve a single symptom, e.g., two types of decongestant in the same medication. Here's a list of how to fit the remedy to the symptom:

Symptom	Remedy
Cough	Cough suppressants Honey, candy
Headache, malaise, fever	Aspirin, acetaminophen (see section on headaches for information on aspirin substitutes)

Symptom	Remedy
Sore throat	Analgesics
	Decongestants
	Demulcents (elm bark, glycerin)
	Saltwater or apple cider vinegar
Nasal congestion	Decongestants
	Proper room humidification
Respiratory congestion	Cough suppressants

A word on nasal decongestant sprays and drops. Though sold without prescription, the power of these substances must be respected. It is necessary to follow the directions on the label. They should generally be used for no longer than three consecutive days. Overuse will not only decrease their effectiveness, but also may create a "rebound effect," whereby the decongestants *cause* congestion rather than relieve it.

For certain people, the active ingredients in cold pills can be a definite hazard.

• *Codeine,* included in some cold pills as a cough suppressant, can cause severe constipation and possible addiction, even in small doses.

• *Dextromethorphan,* a common antihistamine, may cause severe drowsiness and must be used with care by those who commute or who drive professionally.

• *Decongestants* in general, and *phenylephrine hydrochloride* and *phenylpropanolamine* in particular, are known to be potentially dangerous for people suffering from high blood pressure. If you are one of them, consult with a physician before using these medications.

• *Belladonna,* used as an anticholinergic (drying agent), can cause drowsiness, dizziness, and delirium when inhaled. *Atropine,* also a drying agent, can have a similarly dangerous effect.

• *Terpin hydrate,* an expectorant, causes nausea and vomiting in many people. So does another expectorant, *antimony potassium.*

• *Caramiphen edisylate,* a cough suppressant, has a drying effect on mucous membranes throughout the body and can irritate conditions of glaucoma and enlarged prostate glands.

• *Caffeine,* used to offset drowsiness, can contribute to insomnia and make it difficult to relax.

Read the labels. If you have a chronic ailment of any kind, if you are using birth control pills, or if you are pregnant, consult your physician before using even the most common cold remedies.

A Brief Warning on Mouthwash

Studies have shown that the high rates of cancer of the mouth and throat among alcoholics can be traced to the carcinogenic qualities of alcohol. Since many commercial mouthwashes also contain large amounts of alcohol, the same risk may apply to daily mouthwash use. It is best to gargle with these products sparingly. They have, as mentioned, no therapeutic value, and if used regularly to disguise halitosis, they may in fact be hiding symptoms of gum disease or digestive problems that would be better referred to a doctor. A safer and cheaper alternative is to make your own nonalcoholic mouthwash blend. Add two tablespoons of baking soda and a teaspoon of salt to a glass of warm water. If you wish, steep a mint tea bag in the mixture for flavor and gargle as you would with any commercial mouthwash.

A Word on Symmetrel

Symmetrel is a little-known drug that has been used with apparent success against type-A flu for some years. It can still be purchased with a doctor's prescription and is said to be one of the very few antiviral medications that really work, both as a preventive drug and as a cure. If your doctor doesn't know about it, have him or her look into it.

WHEN TO CALL THE DOCTOR

A cold will never kill you. A flu can and occasionally does; the great influenza epidemic of 1918 accounted for between six to ten million deaths throughout the world, including half a million in the United States. Vaccines have, of course, been developed against certain strains of flu, but their value is conjectural, and some people maintain that these innoculations harm more people than they protect. The symptoms of colds and flu are sometimes not due to colds or flu at all, moreover, but to entirely different ailments like measles or strep throat, or to more serious conditions like mononucleosis or pneumonia. Therefore, it pays to keep a close eye on the intensity of symptoms and to watch for unusual or disquieting developments. In general, you should consult a doctor if:

- The symptoms continue intensely for more than two weeks or seem to worsen after a week.
- The fever rises above 102° F.
- The patient is in unusually great discomfort.
- There are skin rashes or breakouts.
- The glands swell and remain swollen for a prolonged period of time.
- There is blood in the sputum.
- The cough becomes particularly insistent and severe.
- There is any indication of a secondary infection such as an earache or strep throat.

TECHNOLOGY, RESOURCES, AIDS, AND SERVICES

1. Ace Brand manufactures both *a single-use and permanent cold compress* that is an excellent aid for cooling fevers. The compresses can be purchased at most good pharmacies. Though the single-use compress is cheaper, it represents a greater saving in the long run to buy the permanent kind. It's good to have such a health aid around the house not only for colds, but also for insect stings, joint injuries, headaches, and so forth.

2. *Automatic digital thermometers* with LCD digital displays are faster and more accurate than the old mercury thermometer, and there is no chance of broken glass or mercury spillage. They cost from $15 to $25, depending on brand and elaborateness. Many pharmacies now carry them. You can order one for $17.50 plus $2.00 postage from *The Medical Self-Care Catalog*, P.O. Box 999, Pt. Reyes, CA 94956.

3. Since the symptoms of colds, flu, and mononucleosis are similar, you may wish to buy a home test that determines whether antibodies for the virus are present in your bloodstream. The name of the test is the *Monosticon-Dri-Dot*. It costs about $20 and provides enough materials for fifteen re-tests. The kit includes full instructions; be aware that it requires you to take a blood sample (see number 4 below). For details, contact Organon Diagnostics, West Orange, NJ 07052.

4. *Lancet mechanisms* are designed to allow you to take your own blood sample quickly and (almost) painlessly. They can be

purchased from the manufacturers. A device called the Autolet costs about $20.00 from Ulster Scientific, P.O. Box 902, Highland, NY 12528, (914) 795-2522. A smaller device, the Penlet, costs about $12 from LifeScan, P.O. Box 1118, Mountain View, CA 94042, (415) 969-5720.

5. *Heating pads* are an old standby for chest cold and flu sufferers. *The Medical Self-Care Catalog* (address listed in number 1) offers a particularly nice model called the Therm-O-Lax, which applies a steady, moist heat, useful not only for chest congestion, but also for muscular and joint pains. It costs about $59 plus $2 for postage.

6. *Zinc pills* for colds can be ordered from Quantum Research, P.O. Box 2791, Eugene, OR 97402, (503) 345-5556.

7. Information on obtaining *a kit for setting up a do-it-yourself cold self-care clinic* complete with plans, signs, instructions, brochures, teaching materials, etc., can be ordered from John Betinis, M.D., University Health Services, University of Wisconsin at Stevens Point, Stevens Point, WI 54481, (715) 346-4646.

8. Perhaps the best book on self-care for colds is *Cold Comfort: Everybody's Guide to Self-Treatment of Colds and Flu* by Hal Z. Bennett (New York: Yolla Bolly Press/Clarkson Potter, Inc., 1979).

9. A few interesting free pamphlets on the subject of self-help for colds and flu include: ˜

Common Cold
Consumer Information Center
Pueblo, CO 81009
(Write the word "FREE" on the envelope)

The Facts About Your Lungs: Common Cold
American Lung Association
1740 Broadway
New York, NY 10019

Infectious Diseases Research: The Common Cold
National Institute of Allergy and Infectious Diseases
Information Office
Room 7A-32, Bldg. 31
9000 Rockville Pike
Bethesda, MD 20014

CHAPTER 11

HAY FEVER (RHINITIS)

Hay fever, known medically as either *allergic, seasonal,* or *perennial rhinitis,* is an inflammation of the nasal mucous membranes caused by allergic response. It is a sensitivity to allergy-causing substances, especially plant pollens, molds, dust, animal dander (often thought to be the hair or fur of a pet, but actually dry skin scales that flake off), grasses, and several other airborne particles. Collectively, these allergy-producing particles are known as *allergens.*

Hay fever is a misnomer because it rarely causes a fever and is almost never triggered by hay (because hay is harvested in spring when the sneezing season is at its height, people once assumed there was a link between the two). Hay fever sufferers with symptoms that come and go with the seasons are said to have the seasonal variety of rhinitis. Those with symptoms that last all year round have the perennial variety. Perennial rhinitis sufferers, moreover, are usually sensitive not only to seasonal plants, but also to household inhalants such as dust, animal dander, and molds.

SELF-DIAGNOSIS OF HAY FEVER

In order to become allergic to any substance, a process that allergists term "sensitization" must occur. This means you must first come into contact with a specific allergen, such as a mold or pollen. Then your immune system must produce a set of antibodies against that substance. These antibodies are known as *IgE Immunoglobulins.*

Most nonallergic people have very low levels of IgE antibodies in their bloodstream. However, those sensitized to a specific pollen or mold produce inordinately large amounts of IgE's whenever they come into contact with these allergens, and the IgE's and allergens then interact in such a way that *mediators* are released directly into the bloodstream. The best known of these mediators is *histamine* (note the name of the allergy drug: antihistamine). It is these mediators—especially histamine—that trigger hay fever.

What are these symptoms?
- Constant and sometimes uncontrollable sneezing.
- Watery discharge from the eyes and nose.
- Nasal congestion and possible sore throat.
- Inflammation and burning of the eyes and nose.
- Elimination or reduction of smell.
- Dark circles under the eyes (called allergic "shiners").
- Tickling and itching in the nose, throat, and mouth.
- Possible photosensitivity (sensitivity to light).

Hay fever sufferers often find themselves sneezing repeatedly in the morning, especially during the first hour after waking. The severity of the symptoms may ease up during the day, then return with a vengeance at night. Extremely high or low temperatures, strong winds, high humidity, or bright light may aggravate the symptoms of those who are particularly sensitive.

While hay fever symptoms are quite evident, there may be some confusion in telling them apart from the symptoms of a cold (infectious rhinitis). This is especially true in the winter months. There are some basic differences, however, and this is how the two conditions can be distinguished:

HOW TO TELL HAY FEVER FROM THE COMMON COLD

Symptoms	Hay fever	Colds
Fever	None	Low grade
Color of nasal membranes	Pale or dark purple	Red and dark

Symptoms	Hay fever	Colds
Itching	Severe itching of nose, eyes, throat, and roof of mouth	Little or none
Sneezing	Common	Occasional
Nasal discharge	White, loose, watery, and not irritating to the nose and lips	Yellow, brown, greenish in color; causes irritation to nose and lips
Malaise and fatigue	Rare	Common
Duration	Weeks to months	7 to 10 days

Testing at Home for Hay Fever Allergies

Patch testing, a common diagnostic test used by both allergists and dermatologists, involves such a simple and direct procedure that it can be applied at home. Needless to say, the home version will be neither as efficient nor as accurate as the test administered by doctors. While no guarantees are offered, and while this procedure is mainly used to test for skin disorders, it can under certain circumstances be useful in identifying hay fever–causing allergens as well.

As its name implies, this test involves placing an allergen on a patch—in this case, the patch can be made from a simple gauze bandage—fastening the bandage onto the skin for a forty-eight-hour period, and then examining the spot beneath the bandage for redness, inflammation, or swelling, all of which indicate a positive response to the tested substance. Here's how to perform the test, step by step:

1. Procure the suspected allergen. If hay fever is the problem, you will want to gather and test local weed pollens: ragweed, goldenrod, etc., as well as the various molds and danders common to your environment.

2. Take a tiny amount of the suspected allergen, say the size of a broken pencil lead, and mix it with several drops of mineral oil. Carefully wash a smooth, hairless section of your forearm or back, place three or four drops of the solution onto a bandage, and fasten the bandage onto the chosen spot. As a control, to be certain that you are not allergic to the gauze, place a second untreated bandage somewhere near the first. Allow the "patches" to remain in place for at least forty-eight hours, then remove.

3. Examine the area beneath the treated bandage. Is it red? Swollen? Blistered? Itchy? Irritated in any way? If so, then you are most likely allergic to the tested substance. Be sure to look underneath the untreated bandage as well to determine whether the skin beneath it is normal. If it is also irritated, you may suspect the gauze in the bandage as well as—or instead of—the tested allergen. Even if no irritation is apparent, continue to observe the test site for several days after removing the bandage. Delayed reactions are not uncommon. If, on the other hand, the test site becomes irritated quickly after applying the patch, remove it immediately and consider the response to be decidedly positive.

HAY FEVER PREVENTION

1. *Pollen and dust proof your home*
Dust is the accumulated breakdown of organic materials found throughout the house. It also includes a little-known intruder from the insect world known as the dust mite. This ubiquitous creature resides mainly in household bedding—in pillows, sheets, and blankets. *It is probably the chief allergic ingredient in household dust and must be subdued if the home is to be allergy free.* Happily, dust-mite control is not a difficult chore. It requires that the mattress be vacuumed once a week, that the sheets, mattress cover, and blankets be thoroughly washed, and that pillows receive regular airings.

Further dust control can be achieved by in-depth household cleaning. Carpets, curtains, and upholstered furniture are especially rife with household allergens. These should be thoroughly vacuumed several times a week. Bedrooms demand frequent once-overs, including attention to woodwork, windows, lampshades, shelves, and anything stuffed or padded.

Beds with metal springs or platforms beneath them are best for allergic persons, along with foam rubber mattresses and pillows filled with synthetic fibers. Avoid down comforters and chenile bedspreads. Hardwood or linoleum floors are preferable to thick carpeting. If you do have wall-to-wall carpeting, be sure that the under rugs are made of foam and not the highly allergenic hair pads.

Books gather dust like magnets and cry out for a regular feather dusting. (In homes where the inhabitants are particularly allergic, books should be covered in plastic for extra protection.) Forced air heating will channel strong currents of hot air into your rooms and cause dust to blow about. Remedy this situation by covering the vents with filters or with cheesecloth. Check all venetian blinds and window shades; also, any inside doormats. Go over all corners, hidden crannies, closets, and crawl spaces. Is your cellar damp? Hay fever-causing molds may be living there. Has your attic been cleaned lately? Dust may be filtering downstairs.

2. *Pets can be a menace*

Many people are highly allergic to dander, especially if it comes from dogs or cats. The saliva of the animal may also cause reactions. If you are a hay-fever sufferer, chances are you may be allergic to your pet, and this means you must make the difficult choice of whether or not to remove it from the house. If you live in a rural environment, a good compromise is to keep the animal out-of-doors. Another approach is to "quarantine" it in one area of the house and to clean this area with extra care. You might also try giving the animal away for a three-week trial period, then cleaning your house from top to bottom to eliminate whatever dander it left behind. If your hay fever does not improve during this time, you know the pet is not at fault and you can take it back with impunity. When and if it is determined that an animal is at fault, and if it must be given away, be sure to give your house a thorough cleaning following its removal. Lingering dander and residues will otherwise continue to cause trouble many months after the pet has gone.

3. *Control your indoor atmosphere*

There are several ways of accomplishing this task. Plain air conditioning will help to some extent, although most air conditioners do not filter out the finer pollens and molds. For this you will require an electronic filtering device. HEPA filters (High Efficiency Particulate Air) are probably the best machines for this purpose, having been originally developed to purify the air in spacecrafts. They are capable of removing around 95 percent of all offending particles. Unlike certain less expensive air cleaners, HEPA units do not emit ozone, a potentially allergenic gas. Large-model HEPA filters fit into the main heating unit, and smaller models can be used as freestanding room units. All varieties are expensive.

Less costly are regular electrostatic air cleaning units that contain a built-in high voltage plate that exerts an electromagnetic charge on the room air, removing all dust particles in the same way a magnet draws metal fillings. There are some drawbacks to these machines, however, including the facts that they produce the potentially toxic ozone and that their filtering efficiency varies greatly, especially as the machine ages. Nonetheless, some people report great success with them. Sources for air cleaning devices will be provided in the section on technology and resources.

Negative Ion Generators

A new machine appeared several years ago that generates large numbers of negatively charged molecules (ions) into the local environment. Manufacturers claimed that negative ions helped to restore and maintain health and to combat depression. No one has proved very much one way or the other, although the general attitude of users is not particularly enthusiastic. All the same, there is some evidence that negative ionizers can help hay fever sufferers by capturing pollens and removing them from the air. If you are interested, consult the addresses in the resource section below.

4. *Stay away from the source of your problem*

If you discover you are allergic to ragweed, avoid walking in fields and grassy areas during the ragweed season. If you know you are sensitive to molds, do not spend time in dark basements or damp areas where stagnant waters collect. If you start sneezing when you walk into strong sunlight, wear a hat and sunglasses. And so forth. While there is no way of avoiding contact with allergens entirely, especially since they are airborne inhalants, you can work at minimizing this contact, and the effort will usually help.

SELF-CARE FOR HAY FEVER

Hay fever is a difficult ailment to control. For many sufferers, partial symptomatic relief with drugs is the best that can be expected. Although for an unfortunate minority, strong drugs such as prescription antihistamines or even steroids may be necessary, most people are helped by simple over-the-counter medications, specifically antihistamines and decongestants.

Antihistamines

Antihistamines are just what their name connotes—substances that counteract symptoms caused by the chemical mediator histamine. In medical use for more than forty years, there is little question that the mild drying effect these drugs exert on the tissues of the mucous membranes are, except in certain specific instances we will mention below, both safe and effective in controlling hay fever reactions. Antihistamines are one of the best and safest of all over-the-counter medications.

Out of the six principal antihistamine families, some are quite strong and require a prescription; others are mild and can be purchased without a prescription. Among the most popular over-the-counter antihistamines are:

1. *Chlorpheniramine maleate*

Brands: Chlor-Trimeton, Teldrin, Chlo-Amine, Chlor-Niramine, Histrey

Benefits and Drawbacks: Will effectively stop sneezing and general allergic symptoms. Low incidence of side effects. Does not always effectively clear up nasal congestion, but a formula is available that also contains a decongestant.

2. *Pyrilamine maleate*

Brands: Pyrilamine maleate (generic name)

Benefits and Drawbacks: General relief of most hay fever symptoms. Has a relatively high incidence of side-effects such as nausea, depression, and drowsiness, most of which are mild.

3. *Brompheniramine maleate*

Brands: Bromphen (generic name), Dimetane

Benefits and Drawbacks: Especially helpful for runny nose. Low incidence of side effects.

4. *Doxylamine succinate*

Brands: Decapryn

Benefits and Drawbacks: Gives general symptomatic relief for hay fever symptoms. Has the highest incidence of drowsiness (50 percent of all users) of all popular nonprescription antihistamines.

5. *Diphenhydramine hydrochloride*

Brands: Benylin

Benefits and Drawbacks: Primarily for use with coughs. Produces drowsiness in around 50 percent of users.

Warning

The foremost negative side effect of antihistamines is drowsiness. If you drive professionally, if you are involved in a dangerous profession, or if you commute to and from work, consult with your doctor before using this drug regularly. Note also that over-the-counter antihistamines are often mixed with caffeine. Anyone not able to tolerate this substance should read labels carefully.

Decongestants

The second line of defense—and for some the first—against mucous drip and sneezing is the drugstore decongestant. Whereas antihistamines dry the mucous membranes of the nose and sinus areas, decongestants shrink the swollen blood vessels that block the nose. Decongestants come in two forms:

1. *Topical* (local) preparations such as sprays, inhalers, jellies, and drops.

2. *Oral* preparations (tablet and liquids).

Generally speaking, topical preparations cause fewer side effects than oral ones because a good deal less of the topical medicine reaches the bloodstream. However, topical medications can cause decongestant *rebound effect* in which the medicine increases symptoms rather than suppresses them. More on such potential hazards below.

Topical Decongestants

Be especially careful to read the labels when using topical decongestants. Match up what you know about the listed ingredients with any disorders you have (e.g., you will see that a warning appears on most decongestant labels for people suffering from high blood pressure and heart disease).

As a rule, however, decongestants are harmless. The following substances used in topical decongestant medications have been judged safe and effective by the FDA:

1. *Ephedrine*

Brands: ephedrine sulfate (generic name), Vatronol

Benefits and Drawbacks: Generally considered safe and effective if used for no longer than three days. Use two to three drops or spray in each nostril approximately once every four or five hours.

2. *Oxymetazoline hydrochloride*

Brands: Afrin, Duration

Benefits and Drawbacks: A long-acting medication that lasts five to seven hours between applications, and is usually taken once in the morning and once at night. It can occasionally produce a severe rebound effect (see below).

3. *Naphazoline hydrochloride*

Brands: Privine

Benefits and Drawbacks: This decongestant works quickly and lasts from five to six hours. For some people it can become habit-forming, and overuse will exacerbate symptoms rather than relieve them.

4. *Xylometazoline*

Brands: Neo-Synephrine II, 4-Way Long-Acting, Dristan Long-Lasting, Otrivin, Sinutab, Sinex Long-Acting, Sine-Off, Chlorohist-LA

Benefits and Drawbacks: This decongestant is long-acting and, if used properly, its risk of causing rebound effect is low. Minor side effects have been reported in some cases.

What Is the Rebound Effect? Have you ever known a person who seems never to be without an inhaler? You know the type, the runny-nosed fellow who is constantly blowing his nose, the nasal-voiced woman forever popping mentholated sprayers out of her purse. Such people are practically married to their decongestants yet, despite the ever-present medication, they continually nurse a running nose that never improves. What's happening?

The fact is that after a certain amount of clinical use, three or four days at most, the beneficial effects of decongestants wear off and then, by "rebound," start to *cause* the very symptoms they are designed to control. What's more, some decongestants contain substances that are actually physically addictive. Therefore, the user becomes dependent on the very substance that is making him or her sick. Doctors have a term for such a condition—*rhinitis medicamentosa.* It was coined specifically to describe nasal symptoms that result from the misuse of decongestants.

How to deal with this problem? Easy. *Never* use a topical decongestant for more than three or four days in a row. If you see any signs of rebound effect even in the first or second day, quickly discontinue the decongestant and seek professional medical advice.

Oral Decongestants

Oral decongestants can be taken in tablet, capsule, or liquid form. Because the ingredients in these drugs pass directly into the bloodstream, when side effects do occur, they may occasionally be severe. Be sure to check the label of any oral decongestant for warnings. Here is a list of the most popular, effective, and safe oral decongestants on the market:

1. *Phenylephrine hydrochloride*

Brands: Neo-Synephrine, Super Anahist, Allerest Nasal, Rhinall, Alconefrin

Benefits and Drawbacks: Quite effective for symptomatic relief, especially for clearing a stuffy nose. Persons with high blood pressure and heart disease, however, should take this drug only with a doctor's recommendation.

2. *Phenylpropanolamine*

Brands: Propadrine (capsules and elixir)

Benefits and Drawbacks: Generally quite effective for symptomatic relief, it causes few side effects and is one of the safest oral decongestants. Still, persons suffering from diabetes, high blood pressure, or heart disease should be monitored closely if given this drug.

3. *Pseudoephedrine hydrochloride and sulfate*

Brands: Afrinol Repetabs, First Sign, Sudafed, Novafed, Symptom-2, Cenafed Syrup

Benefits and Drawbacks: An extremely effective nasal decongestant that has a very decent safety record. People suffering from heart disease and hypertension should consult a physician before using. Some drowsiness may be experienced.

A Few Other (Possible) Remedies for Hay Fever

Here follows a list of natural remedies that *may* help relieve the symptoms of hay fever:

• Bee Pollen—One hypothesis holds that you can protect yourself against hay fever by chewing pieces of comb honey taken from a local apiary. The theory is that since the honey and wax come from the weeds and flowers in your area, eating a small amount of local pollens every day allows the body slowly to build an immunity to them.

• Vitamin C—Certain tests have shown conclusively that vitamin C helps fight hay fever by acting as a natural histamine-inhibitor. Certain other tests have shown conclusively that vitamin C is of no value whatsoever in relieving allergies, and that taking too much of it will worsen the condition. You have nothing to lose by taking a hefty dose of vitamin C daily, say one thousand milligrams, starting about a month before hay fever season and continuing until the season has passed. Some hay fever sufferers believe that a one-thousand-milligram pill of pantothenic acid each day helps, too.

• Eucalyptus Vapors—A natural decongestant can be made by boiling eucalyptus leaves in water for ten to fifteen minutes, then (carefully) inhaling the steam during an attack.

• Herb Teas—Again, why not try? The following mixtures are used and endorsed by naturopaths and herbologists. Addresses listing sources for purchasing herbs are given in the resource section. Here are some useful formulas:

Mix: one ounce vervain; two ounces boneset; four ounces valerian; two and one-half ounces yarrow; one ounce hyssop.

Drop the ingredients into boiling water and allow to boil for twenty minutes. Strain, add honey to taste, and drink twice a day.

Mix: one-half ounce fenugreek; one-half ounce anise; one-fourth ounce cubeb berries.

Add boiling water to the ingredients and let simmer a half hour. Strain, mix with honey, and drink three times a day.

Take several fresh leaves from the comfrey plant, grind them up into a mush, add several teaspoons of honey plus a teaspoon of grated orange peel. Take the mixture once a day, starting several weeks before allergy season begins.

• Acupressure—Applying finger pressure across the upper lip to stop sneezing works for many people.

Interestingly, this area is an acupoint that has been used in Oriental medicine for many centuries to control hay fever. Another point that controls sneezing is located on the inner crease of the elbow. Next time you're sneezing from hay fever, press the point situated approximately one inch to the outside of the hollow (i.e., on the side away from the body) formed at the inner joint of the elbow. Stimulate this point on both arms for twenty seconds, stop, and repeat until the sneezing stops. This trick really works.

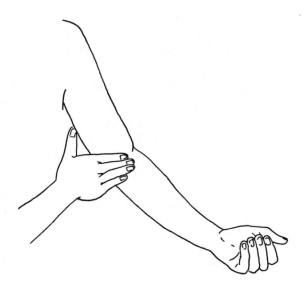

WHEN TO CALL THE DOCTOR

Hay fever is not a dangerous ailment, but it should not be neglected. If allowed to go untreated for several years, especially in children, the constant sniffling and nasal pressures can lead to changes in the dental arch (resulting in a high-arched palate), as well as permanent damage to the tender membranes of the nasal areas. The worst scenario, rare as it may be, includes serious lower respiratory tract symptoms such as wheezing and shortness of breath. Asthma and hay fever, in fact, often go hand in hand, and if any signs of wheezing or breathing difficulties accompany hay fever attacks, the sufferer should be referred to a physician.

TECHNOLOGY, RESOURCES, AIDS, AND SERVICES

1. *HEPA air purifiers* can be purchased at pharmacies that specialize in respiratory equipment or they can be bought directly by mail. Contact Bio-Tech Systems, P.O. Box 25380, Chicago, IL 60625, or Vitaire Corp., 81-13 Broadway, Elmhurst, NY 11373 for further information. *Small, room-sized HEPA filters* can be ordered from Allergen-Proof Encasings, Inc., 1450 E. 363 St., Eastlake, OH 44094, or Air Techniques, Inc., 1717 Whitehead Rd., Baltimore, MD 21207. Regular air purifiers can be bought from almost any good pharmacy or surgical supply house.

2. *Nonallergenic housewares* can be purchased via mail order from The Cotton Place, P.O. Box 59721, Dallas, TX 75229. The price of their catalog changes frequently. Write them for information. Nonallergenic housewares (kitchen equipment, napkins, linens, towels, etc., and furniture) are also available from Futon Designs, P.O. Box 4217, St. Paul, MN 55104, and Garnet Hill, P.O. Box 262, Franconia, NH 03580. A good source for nonallergenic household products such as soaps, bedding, air cleaners, infant care items, etc., is The Allergy Store, 7345 Healdsburg Avenue, #511, Sebastopol, CA 95472.

3. *Nonallergenic bedding* is available through the mail from Shinera, P.O. Box 528, Boston, MA 02102, from Scope Natural Fibers, 3578 Stacy Circle, Lumberton, NC 28358, and from Dona Shrier, 825 Northlake Dr., Richardson, TX 75080.

4. *Special cleaning supplies and equipment for allergic persons* (products such as mold killers, nonirritating detergents, and anti-pollen soaps) can be ordered by mail from Bio-Tech Systems, P.O. Box 25380, Chicago, IL 60625. Also from Allergen-Proof Encasings (address in number 1); write for information.

5. Special *air filters for forced air heating and kitchen exhaust fans* can be purchased with the help of health-care professionals from Research Products Corp., 1015 E. Washington Ave., P.O. Box 1467, Madison, WI 53701.

6. Rexair, Inc. makes a *"water reservoir" vacuum cleaner* especially designed to remove dust from the environment. Write to them at 900 Tower Drive, Suite 700, P.O. Box 3610, Troy, MI 48098, for information about where you can purchase one in your area.

7. Special *allergen-proof masks* to filter pollen and irritating particles can be purchased from Allergen-Proof Encasings (address in number 1). Also from Bio-Tech Systems (address in number 1).

8. *Medicinal herbs* can be ordered by mail from Aphrodisia Products, 282 Bleecker Street, New York, NY 10012. Write for their catalog.

9. *Allergy identification necklaces and bracelets, along with medical alert cards* for the wallet and a *medical alert information kit* for the home can be ordered from Health Alert Foundation International, P.O. Box 1009, Turlock, CA 95380.

10. Some free or inexpensive booklets on hay fever:

Moving or Traveling? Consider Your Hay Fever
American Allergy Association
P.O. Box 7273
Menlo Park, CA 94025

Hay Fever: How to Escape the Ragweed Season
Abbot Laboratories
Public Relations Dept.
Abbott Park
North Chicago, IL 60064

Pollen Allergy
National Institute of Allergy and Infectious Diseases
Information Office
Room 7A-32, Bldg. 31
9000 Rockville Pike
Bethesda, MD 20014
11. If you are looking for referrals to a physician for hay fe-
ver, the following organizations will help:
American Academy of Allergy
Insect Committee
611 East Wells St.
Milwaukee, WI 53202

CHAPTER 12

SKIN PROBLEMS

Skin is the body's first line of resistance, serving both as protective covering and as the "screen" on which signs of internal problems—rashes, discolorations, lumps, and various surface irritations—first appear. In this sense, the skin both covers the workings of the body and reveals them.

Accessible as the skin may be, many dermatological problems are extremely difficult to cure. Palliation of symptoms is often the best that can be achieved. The positive side of the situation is that self-care is an easy and appropriate means of gaining relief from many simple skin ailments.

Athlete's Foot (Ringworm of the Feet)

Not limited to athletes or even to the locker room, athlete's foot is a form of *ringworm* known to doctors as *tinea pedis,* and to soldiers and explorers as "jungle rot." While the feet and especially the webs in between the smaller toes are a prime location for tinea, it is by no means exclusive to these areas, and can grow on the dead skin cells of practically any part of the body, particularly the armpits and groin. Athlete's foot is fairly contagious, quite common, and rarely dangerous. But whatever you do, don't let it go untreated. It spreads quickly and can become a chronic source of irritation.

SELF-DIAGNOSIS OF ATHLETE'S FOOT

Whether or not you get athlete's foot depends largely on your body's powers of resistance to the fungus responsible for it. While this fungus can live practically everywhere, it thrives in the warm, damp, enclosed areas of the body like the armpits, crotch, anus, under the toenails, and between the smaller toes. It is found in great concentrations in steam rooms, gymnasiums, indoor swimming pools, public showers, health clubs, and dormitories—in any dark, warm place where people go barefoot. Symptoms of athlete's foot include the following:

• The first signs are usually small blisters on the soles of the feet or on the toes.

• The involved area is red and/or dull white. If the blisters pop, the skin becomes fissured, soft, and scaly.

• If untended, the fissures deepen and are accompanied by itching, burning, and general discomfort. Walking may become painful.

• Friction, rubbing, and wetness tend to worsen the disorder.

SELF-CARE FOR ATHLETE'S FOOT

The following steps will help mild cases of athlete's foot:

1. Treat the irritation while the lesions are still small and dry and while the condition is uncomplicated by bacterial infection. You will know that a secondary infection has occurred if the lesions become moist, whitish, highly irritated, deeply fissured, and start to emit an unpleasant smell.

2. The athlete's foot fungus thrives on dampness. Keep the feet *dry* at all times. Take special care to dry the area between the toes after every shower and bath.

3. Wash the infected area thoroughly with soap and water, then dab a mild alcoholic solution onto the sores. Repeat this procedure several times a day. You can also shake unperfumed talcum or tolnaftate powder (such as Aftate or Tinactin) into your socks and over the irritated area. Make sure that no irritating fabrics or fibers are touching the sores while they heal. Wear open-toed shoes, ventilated sneakers, or sandals.

4. Be careful of sweat buildup in shoes or sneakers, and avoid tight-fitting panty hose. Wear absorbent socks, but make sure they

are not so thick that they induce extra sweating, not so rough that they irritate the lesions. Change your socks once a day. Make certain that all socks are laundered in between wearings. If possible, abstain from strenuous activities and sports that cause your feet to perspire. Avoid using anyone else's towels or bath mats. While the lesions are healing, avoid places where the fungus tends to breed.

5. Expose the irritated areas to sunlight as often as you can. Elevate the feet frequently. In many instances, mild cases of athlete's foot will disappear in a few weeks without medication.

6. As a preventive measure, always wear rubber zorries or sandals in public showers, gyms, or any place where the athlete's foot fungus abounds.

Treating Stubborn Cases

The following measures should be taken for persistent and severe athlete's foot:

1. Follow all directions as above.

2. To fight secondary bacterial infections, treat the lesions with a 30 percent solution of aluminum chloride that can be prepared for you at most good pharmacies. Apply twice a day with cotton.

3. Any of the following over-the-counter fungicides should help. (Creams should be used twice or three times a day, especially at bedtime. Powders work well in the morning. Powders are also effective as preventives when used after a shower. Although aerosols are effective, as well, the chemicals in them may sometimes act as irritants.)

- *Tolnaftate*—Found commercially in spray, powder, gel, and cream. Generally considered the most effective of all athlete's foot preparations. Commercial brands include Aftate and Tinactin.

- *Iodochlorhydroxyquin*—Found commercially in ointment form. Brands include the generic form (called iodochlorhydroxyquin), Torofor, and Vioform.

- *Undecylenic acid and salts*—Found commercially in cream, spray, ointment, powder, liquid, foam, and soap. Commercial brands include undecylenic compound (generic), Cruex, Desenex, Deso-Creme, Fungex, Fung-O-Spray, Medaped, NP-27, Podiaspray, Quinsana Plus, Sal-Dex, Ting.

- *Miconazole nitrate*—Recently okayed by the FDA as a non-prescription drug, it is highly effective. Look for it commercially in Micatin.

When to Call the Doctor

Untreated and unprotected athlete's foot lesions often spread to other parts of the body. (If they do not spread but linger stubbornly for many weeks, the problem may not be athlete's foot at all but an allergic skin condition with similar symptoms.) Also be warned that athlete's foot can become chronic, recurring regularly and resisting all attempts to eliminate it. Untreated athlete's foot offers an open invitation to secondary bacterial infections that can be far worse than the original problem. Consult a physician for any of the following symptoms:

- The lesions recur on a regular basis and do not respond to nonprescription medications.
- The condition impairs your ability to walk.
- There is indication that a secondary bacterial infection has set in.
- The lesions are excessively red, fissured, oozing, and painful.
- The infection spreads under the toenails.
- You have a history of skin allergies.
- The condition does not clear up within a month.

Ray's Ointment

A natural remedy marketed by the followers of the psychic healer, Edgar Cayce, is composed of a combination of witch hazel, sassafras oil, kerosene, and other ingredients. It is known to have helped many chronic cases of athlete's foot. For information, write directly to Membership Services, ARE, P.O. Box 595, Virginia Beach, VA.

Jock Itch

The evocative name of this ailment (or the even more picturesque term "crotch rot"), has gained a unanimous if somewhat embarrassed acceptability in medical circles. The term migrated from the locker room to the doctor's office mainly because it so accurately states the case: Jock itch, known as *tinea cruris,* is a fungus infection of the pubic regions. Contracted mostly by athletes through unwashed athlete equipment, locker-room benches, dirty towels, and sweaty undergarments, jock itch develops almost exclusively in the groin area and spreads to the penis, scrotum, or vagina only on the rarest occasions. As a rule, it is quite self-treatable. Happily, women are usually immune to its discomforts.

SELF-DIAGNOSIS OF JOCK ITCH

Unlike athlete's foot, jock itch rarely if ever spreads to other parts of the body. It is found exclusively in the groin and thighs, and can be recognized there by:
• Light red sores with dark red edges.
• Itching.
• Possible oozing and scaling of sores.

SELF-CARE FOR JOCK ITCH

Like athlete's foot, jock itch goes away in several weeks with proper care:
1. Keep the infected area clean.
2. Make sure all undergarments are clean, not too tight or binding, and made of smooth, nonirritating material.
3. Avoid wearing an athletic supporter until the condition clears up.
4. Avoid wearing tight clothing.
5. Keep the infected area dry and well powdered during the day. Tinactin powder is especially effective for jock itch.
6. If medication is required, use the same nonprescription preparations listed above for athlete's foot.

WHEN TO CALL THE DOCTOR

Jock itch is rarely serious. However, if any of the following conditions develop, it is wise to get medical advice:
• The condition becomes chronic.
• The sores become excessively red, oozing, and painful.
• There is evidence of a secondary bacterial infection.
• The condition does not clear up after a month.

Ringworm

Like its close relatives, athlete's foot and jock itch, ringworm is a fungus infection of the skin. It develops on the trunk, arms, legs, or—more problematically—on the scalp and under the nails. Often it is passed to human beings from a pet dog or cat. It is not produced by worms; the name comes from the wormlike roundness of its characteristic lesions.

SELF-DIAGNOSIS OF RINGWORM

You will recognize ringworm from the following symptoms:
• The development of a small, red sore, usually somewhere on the trunk, abdomen, chest, legs, or back; around it a red ring or circle forms. As the sore heals and disappears, the ring continues to spread in red, concentric circles.
• The infected area is red, round, itchy, and scaly.
Ringworm of the scalp is present if:
• Mangelike patches form on the back of the head. These irritated areas may cause hair loss and even spotty baldness.
• Small boils or pustules form on the sores.
• The condition spreads rapidly.

SELF-CARE OF RINGWORM

Take the following steps:
1. Wash the irritated areas regularly and keep them clean and dry.
2. Expose the sores to light as frequently as possible.
3. Any of the medications listed above in the athlete's foot section will be effective against ringworm.

Note: Ringworm of the *scalp* can become a chronic condition that is not easy to heal, even with prescription medications. Because its ugly patches quickly become a psychological burden, and because the infection spreads easily, it is best to refer it to a physician's care.

Boils

A boil or *furuncle* is a potentially serious skin eruption that should be self-medicated only when it is small, not intensely inflamed, and in its earliest stages. If improvement is not soon apparent, antibiotics may be necessary to kill the infection (usually a staph bacteria such as *Staphylococcus aureus*) and to reduce the risk of secondary infections.

Basically, bacterial infections of the hair follicles, boils grow on practically any part of the body, although they tend to appear primarily on the back, buttocks, armpits, neck, and face. Potentially contagious, they usually do not spread unless there is prolonged contact. A related condition, the carbuncle, is a cluster of boils linked under the skin by tubelike connections. Carbuncles can be an extremely severe disorder and should *always* be looked at by a doctor.

SELF-DIAGNOSIS OF BOILS

- Boils tend to form in hair roots such as those located on the neck, face, armpits, buttocks, and back.
- Mechanics, machinists, and laborers who work with oily chemicals are especially prone to boils. Viscous substances like oil trap the staph bacteria under the skin and expose the hair follicles to easy infection.
- Ordinarily, a boil starts as a small, hard, hot, red pimple that grows larger and more nasty looking as the inflammation progresses, eventually forming a yellow head at its center. In the beginning, the sore is only slightly tender. As the boil swells and "ripens," the tenderness turns into a burning pain and throbbing begins. Sometimes simply touching the irritated spot can send a person into spasms of agony. Eventually, the eruption may burst, releasing copious amounts of pus, blood, and other secretions, and instantly relieving the pain. Boils can be as small as a pimple or as large as a half-dollar.

SELF-CARE FOR BOILS

If the boil is small, not too painful, not located on the face, and other symptoms such as fever are absent, you may proceed with self-medication. Start by observing the following DON'TS:

1. Don't ever squeeze the boil. Squeezing will invariably drive the infection deeper into the bloodstream. This warning is especially appropriate if you have facial boils, which can be connected by tiny vessels directly to the brain.

2. Don't scrub, towel, or rub the boil too vigorously.

3. Don't ever attempt to lance a boil on your own.

4. Don't let the boil come in contact with dirty, rough, or irritating surfaces.

5. Don't allow the secretions from a boil to come in contact with other persons. Wash all garments, towels, utensils, and especially hands that have touched the sores.

And some DO'S:

1. Wash the boil carefully several times a day. Keep it immaculate. Use antiseptic soap and hot saltwater.

2. Wash your whole body carefully at least once and preferably twice a day while the wound is festering. This prevents the staph bacteria from spreading.

3. Cover the boil with hot compresses for fifteen to twenty minutes several times a day, being careful not to make them so hot that they burn the skin. The compresses will draw blood to the surface and will hasten bursting or the reabsorption of the infection before it ruptures. Some people find that epsom salts added to the water (a spoonful per cup) is helpful.

4. When not applying compresses, keep the boils covered with gauze bandages and adhesive tape.

5. Eat simple, nutritious foods, and get plenty of sleep and rest while the boils are present. The body requires all the help it can get to fight this infection.

6. After the boil has ruptured, encourage draining. Wash the infected site immediately with soap and hot water, then cleanse it with cotton soaked in hydrogen peroxide. Continue regular cleanings and keep the wound lightly covered with a gauze bandage until the healing is complete. Antiseptic creams like Bacitracin may help healing and decrease the chances of secondary infections. With small boils, there will usually be no scars left on the skin. Larger eruptions sometimes leave traces.

Be Especially Careful of Contracting Boils When:

• It is summertime and you sweat a great deal. If you are boil-prone, take plenty of soapy showers, wear loose-fitting clothing, and be immaculate about your personal hygiene.

• Hygienic conditions are poor in your environment. Clean bed linens and undergarments are particularly important in this respect.

• Your resistance is low. Low resistance means that the body is less capable of fighting off the staph bacteria or any other infectious agent.

• You are in contact with other persons suffering from boils.

• You are in contact with dirt, oil, or grease. Keep your skin as clean as possible.

WHEN TO CALL THE DOCTOR

As mentioned, a boil can be serious. If any of the following symptoms occur, get a physician's help immediately:

- More than one boil appears at a time.
- The eruptions appear simultaneously on different parts of the body.
- The boils come in crops.
- There is high fever, chills, sweats, severe malaise, and overall fatigue.
- The pain becomes extremely intense.
- The boils appear on the face.
- There is suspicion that the patient has diabetes or anemia.
- The boil does not go away on its own after a week or more.
- Recurrence of the boils becomes chronic.
- The boil feels hard and full, is red and painful, yet will not rupture and drain on its own.
- There is a red streak emanating from the boil, a possible sign of blood poisoning or lymphangitis. Get help *immediately*.

Heat Rash

Heat rash, or prickly heat, is a skin condition that occurs in the closed areas of the body—the armpits, groin, and lower parts of the neck—where sweating is profuse. It is caused by temporary blockage of the sweat ducts. Mainly an affliction of young children, heat rash is almost never serious and is ordinarily manageable at home.

SELF-DIAGNOSIS OF HEAT RASH

A heat rash can be identified by the following symptoms:
- Clusters of small, red, raised spots in areas of the body that tend to sweat frequently.
- A sensation of itching, burning, or "prickling" in the irritated areas.
- A rash that comes and goes with relative abruptness.

SELF-CARE FOR HEAT RASH

Heat rash tends to go away on its own when:
1. The irritated areas are exposed to air and light.
2. Sweating stops.
3. Sweat is removed with soap and water.

A cold shower followed by a brisk toweling and a sprinkling of talcum powder will usually do the trick. Calamine lotion or cornstarch can be applied to sooth the itching, although this treatment is often unnecessary and sometimes ineffective. During the summer months, avoid activities that produce excessive sweating. Loose-fitting clothes and air-conditioned rooms will help, too.

WHEN TO CALL THE DOCTOR

A trip to the doctor is warranted only if the heat rash does not go away when treated as above or when a secondary infection sets in. With children, *any* type of chronic skin irritation that does not heal quickly should be referred to a pediatrician or a dermatologist.

Impetigo

Another skin irritation that appears primarily on children, impetigo is a rapidly spreading, highly contagious bacterial infection, usually of a staph or strep variety. It requires quick attention and usually an antibiotic. Home care is advisable only when there is no fever, few lesions, and a localization of the sores, preferably on the arms and legs.

SELF-DIAGNOSIS OF IMPETIGO

The symptoms of impetigo include:
• Small red spots located on the face, hands, legs, or scalp that turn into thick, brown, crusty blisters.
• Sores that weep a yellowish pus when opened or picked at. Blisters that break and crack, causing constant discharge.
• Sores that are self-spreading and proliferate with disconcerting speed. Squeezing or scratching makes them spread faster.
• Impetigo sores tend to form on the sites of previous skin injuries such as insect bites, scratches, or rashes.
Note: If the impetigo crusts are hard, brownish or blackish, painful, and bleed easily, a skin irritation similar to impetigo called *ecthyma* may be the culprit. A deeper and potentially disfiguring infection, ecthyma should be referred to a physician.

SELF-CARE FOR IMPETIGO

1. Clean the blisters with antiseptic soap and water. Though some doctors recommend an antibiotic ointment, the effectiveness of these preparations is questionable; besides, mild impetigo often clears up on its own after several days if kept scrupulously clean.

2. Place gauze dressings over the blisters to contain spreading. Do everything in your power to discourage the patient from rubbing, itching, picking at, or otherwise handling the blisters.

3. Make sure that all utensils, towels, linens, and handkerchiefs touched by the person are laundered carefully before allowing other members of the household to handle them.

WHEN TO CALL THE DOCTOR

Impetigo should be referred to a physician if:
- The sores do not heal quickly or they become profuse and severe.
- Signs of secondary infection become apparent.
- The sores become severely painful.
- The person cannot stop itching and scratching the sores.
- A fever, chills, sweat or general malaise accompanies the condition.
- The sores are located near the eyes.

Warts

Warts are caused by a virus and usually clear up on their own within a year. Occasionally, however, they form in embarrassingly conspicuous places (like the end of the nose) or linger on the fingers or feet where they are continually rubbed and irritated. Finally comes the wish to have it removed. But how? Cut a wart and it soon grows back. Pick at it and it often becomes infected. Drugstore wart-removal preparations work only sometimes. All you can do to treat yourself in this instance is approach the process of wart-removal with the knowledge that it is an unpredictable and at times unsuccessful undertaking.

SELF-DIAGNOSIS OF WARTS

Warts are small skin eruptions that vary in size from one sixteenth to one fourth of an inch, and tend to grow primarily on the hands, feet, neck, and face. They can be hard and horny or soft and spongy with a scaled, cauliflowerlike texture. The color ranges from brown to gray to translucent beige. They frequently grow in clusters, and occasionally they hurt. Contrary to popular misconceptions, warts are *not* tiny skin cancers. In most cases they are entirely harmless.

Plantar warts, a somewhat more serious disorder, are so named because they grow on the soles or "plantar" areas of the feet.

These unpleasant growths are flat, have a "mosaic" appearance, can be exceedingly painful, and are difficult to remove. They create a rubbing sensation on the foot, as if a stone were caught in the shoe. The irritation slowly turns into a steadily worsening pain, which eventually becomes agonizing. Particularly serious cases can impede a person's ability to walk. As a rule, plantar warts should be taken care of by a foot specialist immediately.

SELF-CARE FOR WARTS

There are three approaches to the treatment of ordinary warts:
• Try to remove them with drugstore remedies.
• Try to remove them with home remedies.
• Let them be.

1. *Treating Warts with Drugstore Remedies*

These wart-removers require repeated, regular applications, and hence time and patience. They do not always work; after months of painstaking application, and after the outer shell of the wart has finally peeled off, a new wart may quickly spring up in its place. *Never* use wart-removers on moles or other growths other than normal warts.

Salicylic acid is the basic keratolytic (skin peeling) agent found in over-the-counter wart medications, and it is generally considered safe and effective. Usually the wart-removers must be painted onto the growths several times a day, without fail; forgetting even one or two applications can interfere with the removal process. Be prepared to bring patience and consistency to this boring task, and don't expect instant results. Brands that are known to be effective include Calicylic Creme, Wartgon, Off-Ezy and Wart-Off.

When applying wart-removal preparations that contain salicylic acid, be sure to avoid the skin surrounding the growth. These areas can become easily irritated and even burned. Sometimes the removal substances wash off with water, sometimes not—check the label on the package for specific instructions. Certain brands combine salicylic acid with other substances such as calcium pantothenate or lactic acid, although the value of these chemicals has not been fully substantiated.

2. *Treating Warts with Home Remedies*

As you probably know, home remedies abound in this department. Some of the more popular methods include the following:
• Soften the wart by covering it for a day (or a night) with a

plaster containing 30 percent salicylic acid solution. Remove the dressing, soak it for a half hour in hot water filled with epsom salts, then file the wart carefully with an emery board or pumice stone. At each filing session, a bit more of the wart will peel off, though you may have to repeat the routine for some weeks before it entirely disappears.

• Puncture a gelatin capsule of vitamin E and one of vitamin A and squeeze their liquids onto the wart. Do this twice a day, morning and night. Regular application of castor or olive oil work in some cases, too. The oil may eventually dissolve the wart.

• An even older and more primitive method is to slice an onion or a potato in half and hold the fresh-cut part on the wart for twenty minutes, twice a day.

• A favorite wart remedy of the healer Edgar Cayce calls for making a paste of baking soda mixed with castor oil. Apply the paste to the wart frequently during the day.

3. *Let the Warts Be*

As mentioned, many warts disappear on their own after six months to a year. Unless they are a cosmetic embarrassment or are growing on tender places, it may be best to leave them alone and let nature take its course.

A Surprising Fact About Warts

You may or may not know it, but warts are contagious—at least within the area of one's own body—and scratching, picking, or rubbing can cause the wart virus to spread from, say, the hands to the face, or from the knees to the toes. It is, therefore, wise to keep all warts clean, dry, and well protected (some people cover them with a permanent bandage, although this seems unnecessary), and to not scrape them, cut them, or otherwise irritate the wart's volatile inner tissue.

WHEN TO CALL THE DOCTOR

A physician should examine a wart if:
• It is a plantar wart on the foot that is steadily growing in size and sensitivity.
• It becomes larger after being traumatized by a blow or cut.

- It undergoes sudden enlargement or any curious change, or becomes severely painful.
- It is located on a spot that is subjected to constant rubbing, friction, or trauma.

Diaper Rash

Diaper rash is an early childhood skin irritation—occasionally appearing on incontinent older persons—that is confined to the lower abdomen, buttocks, and genital regions. Scarcely any child has not suffered from some form of it. Closely related to prickly heat, it is caused by friction between the diaper and the skin, by ammonia in the urine trapped inside diapers, or funguslike yeast infections. It can usually be cleared up at home with appropriate care and medication.

Self-Diagnosis of Diaper Rash

Simple diaper rash, caused by friction between the diaper and the skin, shows the following symptoms:
- A bright red rash with highly delineated borders.
- The skin over the irritated area is rough, inflamed, and slightly scaly.
- The pattern of the rash conforms to the areas in contact with the diaper or rubber pants.

An *ammonia diaper rash,* caused by the ammonia in a child's urine, can be identified by:
- Reddened, scaly, inflamed skin, as described above, in combination with a pronounced smell of ammonia emanating from the child's genital areas.

Self-Care for Diaper Rash

1. Keep the child's genital and buttocks area as dry as possible.
2. Frequently wash and powder the problem areas.
3. Change the child's diapers frequently. Make certain the child does not walk about with wet diapers, as friction will aggravate the condition.
4. Avoid diapers that are too tight or too loose. If possible, do away with the tight plastic coverings that fit over diapers.
5. Make sure the rash is not due to the soap you are using to wash the child's bottom. If you use linen diapers, check the in-

gredients used in their laundering. You might consider changing soap or detergent.

6. As an experiment—perhaps a last-ditch one—try using linen diapers from a diaper service. Linen diapers allow air to reach the skin more easily than disposable ones.

7. If it is appropriate, let the child go naked. Air and light will help the healing process immensely. Instead of diapering before nap time, try placing a plastic sheet over the mattress. It is messy, but it will help the rash heal faster.

Medications

Two types of medications are available: *skin protectants* and *skin healers.*

Protectants are best used when the rash is mild. Some parents even use them as a preventive when the skin is clear. Protectants such as cocoa butter, cornstarch, petroleum jelly, Calamine lotion, zinc oxide, and glycerin (for children over six months) are all acceptable.

Commercial skin healers, useful if the rash is more serious, include commercial preparations such as Desitin, A and D Ointment, Bacitracin, and RASHanual.

WHEN TO CALL THE DOCTOR

A doctor's attention will be necessary for diaper rash only if:
- The rash becomes chronic and does not respond to any of the above home treatments.
- The rash becomes progressively worse despite treatment.
- The rash is accompanied by fever, malaise, and general signs of sickness.
- The child is taking other medications.
- The rash shows signs of secondary infection.

CHAPTER 13

FOOT PROBLEMS

Considering the distances we walk every day during our lifetime, our feet are sturdy, uncomplaining stalwarts that require relatively little care. Even so, they do develop problems from time to time. Here are a few of the most prominent ones.

Corns

The most prevalent of all foot complaints, corns are thickenings of the outer layers of skin caused by rubbing and friction, specifically between foot and shoe. After a prolonged period, small sections of the feet become thickened, irritated, and eventually—due to pressure from the enlarged skin masses on the nerves—painful. This unpleasant condition may have been many years in the making and it may put up a stubborn battle.

Corns come in two varieties, hard and soft. The hard corn is usually located on the outside of the toe (especially the little toe), the soft corn *between* the toes. They are essentially similar except that soft corns are bathed by perspiration between the toes. Corns are thick and slightly yellowish (soft corns are sometimes white) and taper into the skin like upside-down cones. Unlike calluses, corns have a central core or point, which can make them painful.

Self-Care for Corns

If the corn is relatively small and painless, you might want to try to remove it without medication.

1. Soak your toes in hot water for fifteen or twenty minutes until the corn becomes soft and pliable.

2. Gently file the corn's horny outer layers with a pumice stone or emery board. Stop filing if any pain or redness occurs. Soak and file every day.

3. After each day's filing, anoint the corn with mineral oil, olive oil, baby oil, or castor oil. Cover the irritated spot with a bandage. This method should get rid of the corn in a few weeks.

Note: During treatment, wear only sandals or open-toed shoes that do not abrade the healing skin surface. Keep the corn covered during this time and be on the lookout for infection.

Though several chemicals are used in commercial corn-removers, there is really only one keratolytic (skin peeling) agent that does the trick safely and efficiently: salicylic acid. You can purchase this substance from any pharmacy in a 10 percent solution. Take the mixture home, cover a plain cornpad with several drops, and apply the dressing to the corn. Leave it in place for four or five days, then remove. The corn should be dissolved so thoroughly that it will lift out easily. Commercial preparations that contain salicylic acid and seem to work well include Mediplast plaster, "2" Drop Corn/Callus Remover, and Wart-Off.

Corn-Prevention Techniques

1. Loose and tight-fitting shoes alike can cause corns. Avoid the problem entirely by wearing shoes that really fit.

2. If soft corns are a problem, wear lamb's wool pads between your toes. These will absorb perspiration and prevent rubbing.

3. Wear cotton socks to absorb sweat. Go barefooted as much as possible. Many studies indicate that in countries where shoes are not worn, corns are practically unknown.

4. Do *not* attempt to cut away the corn. When corns become severe and surgery is required, it should be performed by a podiatrist or general surgeon.

5. If you have diabetes, do *not* attempt to remove your own corns. Self-treatment in this case can easily lead to infections.

WHEN TO CALL THE DOCTOR

Corns should receive professional attention if:
- They are bleeding or turn red or blue.
- They do not respond to home treatment.
- They become excessively large or painful.
- You suffer from poor circulation or diabetes.

Bunions

A bunion is an advanced corn that tends to form on the outside part of the foot just below the base of the big toe. Like a corn, it is caused by ill-fitting shoes, especially the pointed kind. A bunion exerts excessive pressure on the big toe, squeezing it and exposing the metatarsal joint to friction. The skin in this area gradually becomes thickened and the underlying bursa swells. A bunion is lumpy, hard, and sometimes aches dully. Once developed, it is difficult to miss. Poor posture may contribute to the problem by placing stress on the wrong parts of the feet.

SELF-CARE FOR BUNIONS

When a bunion is small and in the beginning stages, self-treatment may help. Here's what you can do:

1. *Most important,* wear shoes that do not rub problem spots and that fit perfectly.

2. To help separate the big toe from the second toe, keep a cotton pad or a swatch of lamb's wool between the toes during the day.

3. A number of orthopedic devices can be used to correct balance, relieve pressure on the bunion, and help healing. Toe jackets or toe sleeves are designed to redistribute the balance of the foot. Latex shields and gauze pads can be worn to protect the bunion from friction. Pharmacies that specialize in orthopedic and podiatric equipment will be able to suggest other aids as well.

4. Twice a day, morning and night, soak the bunion in a hot water bath in which some epsom salts have been dissolved. Stick to this routine faithfully for several weeks. It has helped many bunion sufferers.

See a physician or podiatrist about your bunions if:
- They do not respond to home care.
- They become especially large and painful.
- They interfere with proper walking.

Ingrown Toenails

An ingrown toenail, usually (but not invariably) located on the big toe, does not actually grow into the surrounding flesh. Rather, the flesh from the surrounding nail bed grows over it and results in infection. The condition is caused by poorly fitting shoes and faulty nail-clipping technique.

You'll recognize this problem by the burning pain it causes and by the appearance of the toenail itself—close inspection will reveal that the skin of the nail bed has grown over the nail and slightly overlaps it. The skin on these flaps may be red, swollen, and inflamed. Pus may drip from the infection, especially if it has gone untreated for some time.

SELF-CARE FOR INGROWN TOENAILS

There are three approaches, one of them therapeutic, two of them preventive.

1. *Therapy for an Ingrown Nail*
- First, wash the toenail and keep it clean. Already infected, it is now a prime target for serious secondary infections.
- Soak your foot twice a day in lukewarm water containing a tablespoon of epsom salts. This bath will help shrink the inflamed tissue and relieve pain. Continue until the irritation and redness subside.
- Soak a bit of cotton in castor oil and insert it under the ingrown edge of the nail. Cover the nail with a gauze pad and fasten it on with adhesive tape. Allow the irritation to heal on its own. Change the dressing daily.
- Cutting a one-fourth-inch notch in the center of the infected toenail to help the nail grow straight is an old trick and a controversial one. Although most foot specialists feel it has little or no value, the technique has seemed to help many people through the years. If done carefully and if the cut is not made

too deeply, this trick is harmless and may prove of some value.
* Wear sandals or open-toed shoes while the irritation is healing. Keep your feet exposed to air and light (especially sunshine) as much as possible.
* Over-the-counter substances such as Dr. Scholl's Oxinol or Nail-A-Cain are designed to harden the skin surrounding the toenail, soften the nail, fight infection, and shrink inflamed tissues. As with many such products, the reviews are mixed. Some people swear by them, and it wouldn't hurt to try one and see.

2. *Prevent Ingrown Nails with Proper Footwear*

Poorly fitting shoes cause the flesh on either side of the toes to be squeezed inward and eventually to grow inward. Avoid shoes that bind, cramp, or rub, especially in the toes. Tight socks and panty hose can irritate, if not cause, ingrown toenails, and both should be avoided.

3. *Prevent Ingrown Nails with Proper Nail Clipping*

This is especially important.

Observe the following DON'TS:
1. Cut the nail lower than *one fourth of an inch* below the tip of the toe.
2. Cut the toenail in a half-moon shape with rounded edges.

And some DO'S:
1. Cut straight across the top of the toenail.
2. Square the corners.

When to Call the Doctor

* If the infection does not heal after following the above instructions or is causing a great deal of pain.
* If there is sign of serious infection with oozing of blood and pus, or a boil at the site.
* If you are having difficulty walking.

Blisters

Another extremely familiar foot problem, blisters are pockets of lymph that form under the skin in response to rubbing and friction, usually from ill-fitting shoes or from jagged objects trapped inside the shoes.

The irritated spots are small, sensitive, raised mounds of red or translucent skin located anywhere on the foot's surface, especially on the sides and soles. When popped, they leak copious

fluid and reveal a loose, wet, red flap of skin. While not dangerous, they should be attended to quickly to prevent infection.

SELF-CARE FOR BLISTERS

It's your choice whether or not to pop the blister or let it be.
Some doctors recommend popping, others caution against it. If
you decide to lance the blister yourself, be careful to:

1. Swab the inflamed area with alcohol. Never neglect this step.

2. Sterilize a needle in a flame and carefully prick the blister
at its outermost edge. A surprisingly large amount of fluid will
pour out. The blister will then deflate.

3. Wash the blister carefully and cover it with an adhesive
bandage. Try not to walk on the wound or otherwise irritate it
for a day or so. Expose it to air as frequently as possible while it
is healing.

WHEN TO CALL THE DOCTOR

- If there is any sign of infection.
- If the blister is particularly large and painful.

Sore, Aching Feet

Although it is not a disease, sore, aching feet keep a lot of
people awake at night and cause plenty of discomfort during the
day. Sometimes the problem comes from easily remedied habits
such as wearing tight shoes. At other times, it is simply the result
of the daily pavement pounding that is part of modern life. Here
are a few suggestions:

1. *Treat your feet well*
- Wear properly fitting shoes, not only to keep feet from getting
  sore, but also to prevent podiatric problems such as bunions,
  corns, and blisters (see entries above). Don't be tempted by cheap
  shoes. Carefully crafted, properly fitting shoes are a luxury you
  can't afford to deny yourself.
- Avoid tightly binding socks, garters, and panty hose. They reduce circulation to the feet.
- If foot odor is a problem, alternate shoes daily to allow the
  perspiration in each pair to dry thoroughly. Wear leather shoes;
  leather has a greater "breathing" capacity than synthetics. Wear
  socks made of a light, absorbent material such as cotton, and

change them frequently. A daily airing, washing, and dusting of the feet with talcum powder will usually eliminate odors entirely.

2. Keep the toenails properly clipped

See the section on ingrown toenails for instructions.

3. Go easy on your feet when you're standing up

The best position for standing is with the feet pointing straight ahead, parallel to each other, with a predominance of weight resting on the heels. The so-called military position, in which the feet slant smartly outward in a "V," will tire you quickly and stress the instep. If your job requires you to stand for long hours, arrange your schedule so that you can take many short breaks throughout the day rather than (or as well as) one or two long ones. When you get home at night, elevate your feet for ten or fifteen minutes before eating dinner. This will increase circulation in your legs as well as in your feet. Those who are desk-bound should try making small circular movements with the feet frequently throughout the day, wiggling the toes whenever possible, and taking the shoes off when no one is peeking to pamper the feet with a quick massage (see number 6 below).

4. Foot cramps

If foot cramps are a problem, proper nutrition may be the answer. According to laboratory tests, leg cramps may be due to a lack of calcium and/or vitamin B_6. Massage will also help (see number 6 below).

5. Soak your feet

One of the best antidotes ever designed for tired feet is a twenty-minute soak in a hot water bath. Try adding a little epsom salts to the bath for a bonus. Mechanical appliances that swish the water around are often helpful as well.

6. Massage your feet whenever possible

Massage increases circulation, invigorates the feet, and relieves the soreness and tension that build up in the ankles and toes. Get into the habit of massaging your feet whenever you can. Aside from the benefits mentioned above, foot massage creates a strange sense of overall well-being. Here are some simple techniques:

• Grip your foot in one hand, make a fist with the other, and run the knuckles firmly up and down the middle of the sole. Push especially hard in the central areas. Repeat several times.

• Knead the flesh on the sole of the foot, the ball of the foot, the ankle, and the webs between the toes.

• Pull the toes on both feet, ten seconds per toe. Grip the big toe firmly and rotate it for several seconds. Wiggle the toes freely, crunch them up, extend them forcefully, and wiggle them again.

TECHNOLOGY, RESOURCES, AIDS, AND SERVICES

1. *"Rest and Roll" wooden foot massager* is a useful appliance for relieving foot and back strain and for increasing circulation in the feet. Designed with desk jobs in mind, the massager is a tilting wooden platform that contains rows of wooden balls on one side for foot massage and a plain surface (or optional rotating base for range of motion exercises) on the other. There are two models, which retail from $100 to $125. For information write R and R Concepts, 241 Conejo Road, Santa Barbara, CA 93103.

2. *"The Foot Fixer," a portable foot soak and massage appliance,* provides either a plain hot bath for the feet or a whirlpool bath. It costs from $50 to $60. Contact the manufacturer, Clairol Inc., at 90 Commerce Rd., Stamford, CT 06902, for information on finding one in your area, or call them toll-free at 800-447-4700. Most pharmacies now carry one or more brands of foot baths/massagers.

3. *A portable whirlpool foot bath* with a six-gallon capacity and a ten-gallon pumping action can be purchased for around $120 from Cleo, Inc., 3957 Mayfield Rd., Cleveland, OH 44121, (800) 321-0595 (in Ohio call [800] 222-CLEO).

4. The *Cushi-Heel Pillow,* a special appliance for sore heels designed to fit directly into the shoe, costs from $7.00 to $10.00. For information contact Calderon Products, P.O. Box 5117, Akron, OH 44313.

5. A good *adhesive covering developed especially for preventing blisters and calluses* is made by Spenco. It's called the Adhesive Kit and can be purchased directly from the Spenco Medical Corporation, P.O. Box 2501, Waco, TX 76702-2501, (800) 433-3334. Spenco also makes a *Blister Kit,* two absorbent and deodorant foot preparations called *Dry Feet* and *Fresh Feet,* and *insoles for sneakers, heel cushions, arch supports, and corn and blister padding.*

6. Available for runners and frequent walkers are *custom-fitted orthotic foot supports for sneakers or walking shoes.* Used primarily to reduce foot fatigue and ease heel spurs, bursitis, shin splints, and other foot and leg problems, these fitted plastic supports must be custom fitted. Carolina Biological Supply Company, 2700 York Rd., Burlington, NC 27215, offers a do-it-your-

self kit for this purpose. First, you order a "Foot Impression Kit" for around $20. You take your foot measurement with the kit and mail the imprint back to Carolina with another $59.95. The company then sends you the custom-made supports for a sixty-day home trial. Call them toll-free for further information at (800) 334-5551 (in North Carolina call [800] 632-1231).

7. One of the best ways to massage your feet is with a hand-held *vibrating massager*, the kind barbers used to use on a customer's scalp after a haircut in the good old days. A particularly good Swedish hand massager can be purchased from Carolina Biological Supply Company (address and toll-free number in number 6) for around $60.00. Call them for details.

8. Various orthopedic equipment for foot injuries such as *foam rubber heel protectors, prefabricated foot splints, elastic bandages, ankle-joint shoe inserts, moleskin,* etc., can be ordered from Fred Sammons, Inc., P.O. Box 32, Brookfield, IL 60513-0032, (800) 323-5547 (in Illinois, call [800] 942-2129).

9. *Corn and blister padding—polymer pads to absorb friction and pressure* along with *corn, callus, and blister treatment kits* can be ordered from HSA, P.O. Box 288, Farmville, NC 27828, (800) 334-1187 (in North Carolina call [800] 672-4214).

10. A wide assortment of *foot health literature, including pamphlets, reprints, charts, and educational materials,* are described in an *annotated catalog* from the American Podiatry Association. Their address is 20 Chevy Chase Circle, N.W., Washington, DC 20015.

11. Good books and pamphlets on foot care include:
Foot Owner's Manual
Krames Communications
312 90 St.
Daly City, CA 94015-1898
$1.25 plus $1.50 postage

Keep Your Feet Working Around the Clock
American Podiatry Association
20 Chevy Chase Circle, N.W.
Washington, DC 20015
Free

Advice from Your Podiatrist: Step Up to Foot Health
American Podiatry Association
(address above)
Free

Memo to: Parents
Re: Your Child's Foot Health
American Podiatry Association
(address above)
Free

Light on Your Feet
Public Affairs Committee, Inc.
381 Park Ave.
New York, NY 10016
$.50

CHAPTER 14

MOUTH, TEETH, AND GUM PROBLEMS

Although most of us assume that problems of the teeth or gums should be immediately and automatically referred to a dentist, self-care movements throughout the country are stressing the fact that many minor oral/dental problems can be self-medicated, and that costly trips to the dentist are not always necessary. Of course, you shouldn't pull your own teeth, but specific oral/dental problems such as pyorrhea or gingivitis can, up to a point, be dealt with at home. More serious difficulties like toothaches and dental abscesses can be kept under control until help is available.

Your At-Home Dental Kit: The Best Prevention

The first line of defense against dental problems is to be well equipped. The following items are helpful:

Dental floss—The best of all cavity preventives, it comes in two styles, waxed and unwaxed. The waxed is easier and more pleasant to use; the unwaxed feels a bit like chalk on a blackboard between the teeth but does the job better than the waxed.

Toothbrush—Contrary to popular opinion, the best brush is not the stiffest. The bristles on a good toothbrush should be firm yet have plenty of give. A rounded head on the end of the brush can prevent the tissue injury sometimes caused by toothbrushes with square ends—these can literally rip open the delicate gum tissue if misused. If the bristles are worn down, bent, or broken off, replace your brush immediately: It has become all but useless for getting the teeth really clean.

Dental mirror—You've seen the dentist use one. It's great for performing an oral self-exam, for finding cavities, and for studying gum and tongue irritations. Pharmacies, many hardware stores, and dental supply houses stock them.

Dental toothpick—You've seen dentists use this, too—the long, hooked metal instrument used to scrape teeth and to pick at plaque. You can purchase one at a dental supply store or at some pharmacies. Hardware stores and hobby shops sometimes stock them as well.

Aspirin or acetominophen—Still the best over-the-counter medications for controlling toothache pain.

Oral irrigating device—Although there is some controversy over the value of these appliances, many dentists feel that the gentle streams of water they generate are better than either floss or toothbrushes for cleaning between the teeth and for stimulating the gums. Some people use both, the oral irrigating device first, then the toothbrush and floss. Oral irrigating devices can be purchased at almost any pharmacy or appliance store.

Disclosing agent—This is a harmless, temporary dye rinse that—when rubbed over the teeth—turns plaque a bright color so that it can be pinpointed and removed. It is particularly effective when used with a dental mirror. You can purchase a disclosing agent at most pharmacies.

Home dental first aid kit—The Medical Self-Care Catalog (see page 160 for address) offers an emergency first aid dental kit that contains, in their words, "all the tools you need to eliminate pain from common dental emergencies until professional help can be obtained."

Performing a Self-Examination on Your Mouth, Teeth, and Gums

Like any medical self-examination, this checkup is not meant to replace a dentist's visit but to supplement it, to alert you to the fact that a trip to the dentist is or is not necessary. There are many obvious and subtle things that you can identify while performing this exam, and the information gathered will help your dentist do his or her job better and faster. Proceed as follows:

1. Start by opening and closing your mouth several times. Is

there pain in the jaw or muscles of the mouth? If so, where is it located?

2. Examine your gums in a mirror. Healthy gums are a pleasant pink color, unhealthy ones have a drab, dark, or even greenish tinge. The gum tissue should be firm, should encase each tooth tightly, and should not bleed when brushed or flossed (except, perhaps, if you haven't flossed for a while and are just beginning again). If your gums do bleed, which sections of your mouth bleed the most? Do you see signs of spotting, redness, puffiness, swelling, or unusual coloration on the gums? Is there indication that your gums have receded to any great extent? Make special note of this last fact if the answer is yes.

3. Check your teeth in the mirror. Adults should have thirty-two teeth, sixteen in the upper jaw, sixteen in the lower, minus, of course, those lost to extractions, accidents, etc. The sharp teeth located in the four corners of the mouth are called *incisors*. Directly behind come the *cuspids,* followed by the first and second *bicuspids,* then the first, second, and third molars. The enameled top of a tooth is known as the *crown,* the section below the gum is the *root.* The root is sheathed in the *periodontal membrane,* which keeps the tooth tightly fixed to the jaw socket and absorbs the pressure and friction of chewing. Inside the tooth is the *pulp chamber* containing all the many nerves and blood vessels which keep the tooth alive.

Although the front teeth can be examined directly in a wall mirror, the labyrinthine spaces behind and between the molars are best studied with a dental hand mirror. Use a strong spotlight or flashlight. Look for decay, breakage, abscess, or strange discolorations. If you have any chronically sore or irritated spots, examine them carefully. Are your wisdom teeth still in place? If so, be aware that the gums surrounding them tend to encroach on the tooth surface and to form pockets ripe for trapping bacteria. These can become easily inflamed, especially around the lower wisdom teeth. If you have repeated soreness or irritation in these areas, call it to your dentist's attention; it may be wise to extract the wisdom teeth instead of keeping them around as a perpetual source of infection.

4. The mouth lining: The tissue here should be a healthy and somewhat subdued pink color. Potential trouble spots are pock marks, fissures, dark patches, skin flaps, mucous deposits, lumps, sores, swellings, growths, white coating, or white and red spots.

5. Now check for breath odor. Halitosis can stem from several sources. Stomach problems or poor oral hygiene are the most common culprits. If the latter is to blame, it is usually due to sulfurous gases released from failure to brush properly, gum disease, or bacterial infections in the teeth. More on dealing with halitosis below.

6. Last, the tongue. Check for impaired movement by sticking the tongue out and moving it in circles. Any pain or difficulty of movement should be noted. A healthy tongue is pink (but not too bright a pink), smooth, soft, moist, and not too heavily coated with mucous. Raised whitish patches on the tongue can indicate a fungus infection. A dry, furred (coated) tongue with white, brown, or black coloration can herald fever or a more serious underlying ailment. A bright red tongue may warn of a nutritional deficiency such as chronic lack of vitamin B. Check the fold of membrane beneath the tongue that connects it to the floor of the mouth (it is called the *frenum*). If it grows too far out toward the front part of the tongue it can cause the condition known as "tongue tie."

Gum Disease

It is popularly believed that most tooth loss in adulthood is due to tooth decay, but the major reason so many of us walk around wearing dentures or dental plates is that we were once delinquent in caring for our gums. In fact, it has been estimated that 90 percent of all tooth loss after the age of forty-five is due directly to lack of preventive care for the gums, and that more than three quarters of the dental extractions that take place each year might be avoided with proper oral hygiene.

Gum disease, known as *pyorrhea* or *periodontal disease,* usually develops in two stages. The first stage, *gingivitis,* is mild and self-treatable; the second, *periodontitis,* is usually too severe to be treated at home. The purpose behind self-applied gum therapy is to prevent the first condition from turning into the second.

Gingivitis

Gingivitis is the medical term for irritated or bleeding gums. Bleeding in this case does not mean that the gums are continually bloody (although in some cases they are), but that they bleed when exposed to slight pressures such as eating, using a tooth-pick, or brushing the teeth.

SELF-DIAGNOSIS OF GINGIVITIS

• Gums that bleed easily, sometimes on their own and some-times at inappropriate times such as when biting into a piece of hard fruit, rinsing the mouth, using an irrigating device, etc.

• Gums that are sore, red, swollen, and inflamed, usually at the point where the teeth and the gums meet. These areas are highly tender and sensitive to pressure.

• Occasional secretions of pus from the irritated spaces be-tween the teeth, giving the breath a foul odor.

Note: Be careful to make the distinction between gums that bleed from external irritants such as poorly fitting dentures, trau-mas to the mouth, cuts, sores, and burns, and gums that are un-naturally tender, chronically inflamed, and bleed on their own without external stimulation.

PREVENTING GINGIVITIS

1. *Good oral/dental care*

The keystone is keeping your gums, and hence your teeth, free from bacterial buildups of plaque. It consists of regular rinsing, proper brushing, and correct flossing.

• A simple and often neglected aid to oral health, rinsing dis-lodges decay-causing food particles, washes out sugars, and gen-erally cleanses the mouth. (Think of how many food particles come out from between your teeth whenever you rinse after meals.) After each meal, fill a glass with warm water. Take a sip, rinse, and gargle for about fifteen seconds. Repeat until you have fin-ished the glass. A little salt added to the water will add a pleasant astringent quality to the rinse.

• Tooth decay begins when bacteria forms in the mouth as a by-product of digestion, producing an acidic film known as plaque. This ubiquitous substance works its way down into the lower gums where it eats away tooth enamel. Brushing is still the best method to remove plaque.

Start with a good, soft-bristle brush. Toothpaste is by no means necessary for getting your teeth clean or for preventing cavities (the fluoride in toothpaste is generally considered to be a cavity preventive only for children), and you can use it or not, accord-ing to your preference. Set the brush at a forty-five-degree angle to the teeth. Brush in short, gentle circles with an emphasis on horizontal movement, then switch to a rapid up-and-down movement (there are two schools of tooth brushing, the horizontal and the vertical method; we combine them). Make sure to clean the teeth near the gums as well as along the crown. If possible, let the bristles slide gently under the edge of the gums. Also brush the back of the teeth, the corners of the mouth, and the tongue itself (brushing the tongue will help prevent halitosis). A disclosing agent (see section on home dental kits above) used in conjunction with brushing will help you locate plaque.

• If done correctly, flossing will remove the food particles missed by rinsing and brushing. Dental floss (or the slightly wider dental tape) comes waxed and unwaxed. The waxed kind slides through the teeth easily, but for this reason it fails to capture as much debris as the more abrasive, unwaxed kind. Pull off a piece of floss approximately twenty inches long. Tautly stretch about five inches of it between your thumbs or index fingers, slide it between two teeth, then work the string vigorously back and forth, side to side, up and down, making sure to floss the edges of both teeth and to slide it up under the gum line. Continue in this manner through the upper and lower jaw. If you want to be particularly thorough you can brush again after flossing.

2. *Proper eating habits*

The two enemies of the gums are sugar and smoking. Sugar literally feeds the bacteria that form plaque, and eating large amounts of it will speed up the process of plaque formation under the gums at an amazing rate. If you are a heavy sugar eater, rinse immediately after each candy bar, soft drink, or ice cream cone. Better still, try taking your sugar quotient in natural carbohydrates such as apples, carrots, pears, grapes, or other fruit.

Besides staining the teeth, the smoke from cigarettes, pipes, and cigars irritates the gums, causing them to bleed easily and frequently. Cutting down on your smoking, or better, stopping entirely, will produce gratifying and unexpected results.

3. *Bleeding gums*

Bleeding gums may derive from factors other than poor oral hygiene. For instance, bleeding gums may be a sign of general physical debility. They may indicate that you are poorly nourished or overtired, that you are stressed or otherwise ailing. They may also be caused by poorly fitting dental plates or dentures, by pregnancy, by the side effects of medications, or by certain blood diseases. If you have any questions about this, confer with your physician.

SELF-CARE FOR GINGIVITIS

1. As a rule, it is best to see a dentist relatively quickly for chronic bleeding gums, even if the condition is mild. Though the ailment may seem to be a trifle at this point, a good deal is going on under the surface where plaque may be inexorably ruining your gums and destroying your teeth.

2. Until you see a dentist, however, constant rinsing and gargling with lukewarm water will help keep the bleeding under control.

3. Some people stimulate their gums by massaging them with their fingers, although there is no conclusive evidence that this helps very much.

4. Increased intake of vitamin C, vitamin E, and calcium seems in some instances to stem chronic gum bleeding.

5. An herbal remedy devised by Edgar Cayce called Ipsab, consisting of salt, prickly ash bark, peppermint, and various other chemicals and herbs, also seems to help in certain cases.

Gum Medications

Over-the-counter gum medications palliate symptoms but do not cure them. You can use these preparations to relieve the distress of chronic gum bleeding, but you should not rely on them. Instead, allow a dentist to examine you and prescribe the proper long-term course of action.

Nonprescription gum medications fall into several categories:

1. *Antimicrobial agents:* Designed to kill infectious bacteria. There are many mouthwashes and over-the-counter oral hygiene drugs (such as boric acid, benzoic acid, and menthol) that claim to rid the mouth and gums of gum-infecting bacteria. These claims have been largely discredited by the FDA, and to date few if any drugstore antimicrobials are believed to work. If you're going to use them at all, the best of the lot is probably hydrogen peroxide.

2. *Analgesics:* Designed to relieve specific pain of gum disease. Effective pain-killing solutions for gum infection include Benzodent ointment, Rid-A-Pain gel, and Orajel gel.

3. *Gum protectants:* Designed to coat raw, open areas on the gum, protect them from further infection, and help healing. Approved gum protectants include tincture of benzoin and benzoin compound tincture. Both can be purchased from any pharmacy.

4. *Gum wound cleaners:* Designed to keep mouth and gum irritations clean and antiseptic. The best of these is probably hydrogen peroxide. Other effective preparations include Peroxyl Mouthrinse, Gly-Oxide drops, and Periolav drops. Both Amosan powder and Proxigel are considered unsafe and ineffective.

Periodontitis

Periodontitis is gingivitis in its advanced stages. It should be referred to a dentist as soon as possible. It should *not* be home-medicated. Delay could cost you your teeth and a good deal in dentist's bills.

SELF-DIAGNOSIS OF PERIODONTITIS

You will know that your gum disease is reaching the advanced stages from the following symptoms:
• The gums bleed easily, often, and at the slightest provocation. Sometimes bleeding continues for many minutes.
• There is a noticeable buildup of hardened plaque, called calculus, along the gum line of one or more teeth.
• One or more teeth are loose in their sockets and can be easily wiggled about.
• The gums appear to be rapidly shrinking and receding, with large areas of the lower tooth exposed.
• The breath is consistently bad.
If any of the above symptoms appear, get dental help immediately.

Toothache

Toothaches are usually the result of cavities or of infections beneath the gums. There is not much you can do about them at home except ease the symptoms and pray that the dentist will soon be in his or her office. As a rule, toothaches are brought about by long-term neglect, sometimes *decades* of neglect. The best way to prevent them is to review the regimen of oral hygiene suggested above and stick to it faithfully.

SELF-DIAGNOSIS OF TOOTHACHE

Symptoms include:
• Pain. Toothache discomfort starts as a dull intermittent ache, then works its way into a constant throbbing, searing pain.

• When infected, a swelling and reddening of the gum around the irritated tooth. Look for such signs especially in impacted wisdom teeth. (If the toothache is caused by a cavity the gums may show no sign of inflammation or swelling.)

• Sensitivity of the tooth and jaw.

SELF-CARE FOR TOOTHACHES

Never assume that a toothache will get better on its own. It probably won't, especially if the problem is a cavity or infection. Get help right away. While you're waiting, any of the following measures should help keep the pain under control:

1. Gargle with warm salt water every hour.

2. Apply an ice pack directly to the jaw. Do *not* apply heat, especially if the tooth is throbbing. It will increase the pain.

3. Take aspirin or an aspirin substitute to deaden the pain.

4. Keep away from all sweets. These irritate cavities and increase pain. Also, avoid hot and spicy foods and any type of soft drink. Keep foreign objects like gum and toothpicks out of your mouth. In fact, it is probably best not to eat at all until help is found.

5. Over-the-counter toothache medications are ineffective and in some cases irritating to teeth and gums. Avoid them.

6. If the problem is an aching cavity, you can pack it with a bit of sterile cotton soaked in oil of cloves. Oil of cloves is available at any pharmacy. Be careful handling it, however, and don't get it on your lips or tongue—it burns. Some people simply suck on a fresh clove, although the taste is strong and the juice has a numbing effect on the entire mouth.

WHEN TO SEE THE DENTIST

As mentioned, you should *always* see a dentist for a toothache. Don't put it off, even if the problem is small and the pain is mild. It will probably return again if it goes untreated, next time with more vengeance than before. If you develop a fever along with a toothache, it is likely that the tooth is abscessed. Get professional help immediately.

Canker Sores

Canker sores are small ulcers located in the mouth or on the lips. They come and go on their own schedule without causing more than minor irritation, although they occasionally indicate a more serious underlying infection. No one is quite sure what causes them, but it is supposed that heavy smoking, stress, menstruation, and perhaps an unidentified virus may bring them on. The sores are not contagious.

SELF-DIAGNOSIS OF CANKER SORES

Canker sores can be recognized by:
• Long, sunken, sensitive sores located on the inner lip, below the gums, and on the insides of the cheeks.
• Upon examination, the sores appear red and swollen.
• Although they occasionally arrive in crops, they tend to come one at a time.

SELF-CARE FOR CANKER SORES

1. There is not a great deal you can do about these irritating sores other than keep them clean. Meanwhile, don't eat acidic fruits (oranges, lemons, limes, tomatoes) and vegetables; they irritate the sores.
2. Some people use warm saltwater gargles, although the salt tends to irritate the sores.
3. Glyoxide drops occasionally prove helpful, as does a weak solution of hydrogen peroxide.

WHEN TO CALL THE DOCTOR

While canker sores are not serious, they can be a symptom of a more serious disorder, especially if they become chronic. Consult a physician if a canker sore has not disappeared after two or three weeks.

Halitosis

The archetypal social no-no, chronic bad breath, is a common annoyance that is more often than not the result of sloppy oral hygiene and diseased gums. Other causes include indigestion, onions and garlic, cigarettes and cigars, nasal and sinus infections, fasting, and, in some rare cases, lung or liver disease. Mixing many types of foods at a single meal (e.g., meat, dairy products, sweets, vegetables, and fruits) causes much fermentation during digestion, and this can also produce halitosis.

SELF-DIAGNOSIS OF HALITOSIS

An unfortunate characteristic of halitosis is that it is almost impossible to detect its traces on your own breath, while those around you may be too polite or too timid to give you the terrible news. Mouthwash manufacturers have, of course, made millions out of this uncertainty, and sold millions of gallons of the stuff to people who probably never needed it. So before you become too concerned about what your best friends won't tell you, take a simple home test: Find a confidant or family member whose judgment you trust, and breathe in his or her face. Then ask how your breath smells. If you pick the right person, an honest answer will be forthcoming.

SELF-CARE FOR HALITOSIS

Here are the most effective ways to go about controlling this problem:

1. Practice regular and conscientious oral hygiene. This includes rinsing after each meal, regular brushing, flossing, and plaque removal, and trips to the dentist to have your teeth cleaned. While this method is not guaranteed to make halitosis vanish forever, it will certainly go a long way toward removing the bacteria that cause the problem.

2. Gargle regularly. A controversial subject. While regular gargling with a commercial mouthwash or even a natural substance like baking soda does clear up halitosis, the bad odor tends to recur relatively soon, within the hour certainly, making mouthwash a temporary remedy at best. Moreover, mouthwash simply hides mouth odor with sweet-smelling chemicals; it does not eliminate it. In some instances, the disguise can camouflage symptoms of stomach or gum problems that are better left revealed. What's more, there is evidence that alcohol, a primary ingredient in most commercial mouthwashes, may be carcinogenic, contributing directly to the incidence of mouth and throat cancer. We know for sure that alcohol dries up the mucous membranes, thus making the mouth and throat particularly vulnerable to infections.*

---

* Mouthwashes containing the largest amounts of alcohol include Astring-O-Sol, Dalidyne, and Odora. Those with the least include Proxigel, Lavoris, Alkalol, Greenmint, and Betadine.

If you are going to use commercial mouthwashes at all, use them sparingly. Both salt and baking soda make good natural dentifrices and rinses and create the alkaline state that helps neutralize decay-causing acids. You might also consider chewing anise seeds, cardomon seeds, and Sen-Sen, gargling with fenugreek or mint tea, or eating vegetables such as parsley and watercress that contain large amounts of chlorophyll. A fresh apple kept by the bedside and eaten upon arising is still one of the best breath-improvers there is.

When to Call the Doctor

It may seem silly to visit a doctor purely because you have halitosis, and you shouldn't—unless the halitosis becomes chronic and persists despite all preventive measures you may take. In this case, it may signal a serious underlying illness and should be called to the attention of a physician whenever you have the chance.

Serious Mouth and Gum Diseases

The following ailments require a doctor's care and supervision. They should *not* be self-medicated. You can, however, act as your own physician by recognizing these conditions and arriving at a tentative diagnosis.

Trenchmouth

Known formally as Vincent's Disease, the infection forms in the gum webs between the teeth. These areas become soft and red, emit a gray secretion, and develop small ulcers that quickly spread throughout the mouth. The breath smells foul as a result of infection. Hydrogen peroxide gargles are sometimes recommended for this problem, although they bring little relief for most people.

Thrush

A fungus infection found primarily in infants, it begins with patchy white spots over the palate, tongue, and lips. Nausea and fever sometimes accompany the spots. In adults, thrush can be caused by antibiotics, diabetes, and certain types of cancer.

Primary Herpetic Stomatitis

Symptoms include inflammation of the mouth tissue, blisterlike sores throughout the mouth (especially on the tongue and the floor of the mouth), increased saliva production, pain, and swollen, bright pink gums. The condition is caused by a viral infection of the herpes family, but improperly fitting dentures, poor diet, decaying teeth, and frequent oral exposure to heavy metals such as mercury can all make a person vulnerable to it.

Secondary Herpetic Infections

Causing sores to form on the roof of the mouth and the lips, this is a less serious version of the same virus that produces primary herpetic stomatitis.

Aphthous Stomatitis

Known as Bechet's Syndrome, it is characterized by an inflammation of the oral mucosa and the presence of small, painful white ulcers throughout the mouth. The sores tend to recur, and the ailment can quickly become chronic.

Herpangina

This is a viral ailment that tends to strike younger children, especially in late summer and early fall. It is typified by small, grayish-white papules (small, somewhat pointed bumps) located on the palate, tonsils, tongue, and uvula. These rupture easily and cause a good deal of pain when they do. A fever may be present as well.

Resources, Technology, Aids, and Services

1. A *dental first aid* kit can be bought from *The Medical Self-Care Catalog*, P.O. Box 999, Pt. Reyes, CA 94956. It costs around $20.00 plus postage. Contact them for ordering information. Another *home dental kit* can be purchased from Murtex, P.O. Box 55621, Houston, TX 77055. Write for information. A special *dental emergency kit* for broken teeth, dislocated braces, bleeding, painful decayed teeth, etc., can be purchased for around $20.00 plus postage from Dental Aides Products, P.O. Box 1164, Rahway, NJ 07065. Write directly for information.

2. A special high-tech toothbrush called the *ROTA-DENT* is meant to imitate the motion of the dentist's drill, with mechanically revolving brushes that reach into hidden spaces behind and between the teeth. It costs around $64.00 plus postage from *The*

Medical Self-Care Catalog (address in number 1).

3. The *ORAPIK* is a professional-quality metal dental pick that can be used to scrape off plaque and clean out hard-to-get-at places in the teeth. It costs around $12.50 plus postage from The Medical Self-Care Catalog (address in number 1).

4. Information on *Ipsab*, an herbal gum medication, can be obtained by writing to The Heritage Store, P.O. Box 444, Virginia Beach, VA 23458.

5. A *free list of dental newsletters*, some of them concerned with dental self-care, can be ordered from Jerome S. Mittleman, D.D.S., 30 East 60th St., New York, NY 10022.

6. The *Nutrition and Dental Health Activities Program* is a large and costly teaching package designed to guide a classroom full of young people toward proper oral/dental habits. The kit contains a teacher's guide, activity folios and folders, charts, and enough toothbrushes, trays, dental reflectors, disclosing tablets, mouth molds, molding supplies, etc., to go around. It costs $440 plus postage from Delta Education, P.O. Box M, Nashua, NH 03061-6012. Call their toll-free number for further information: (800) 258-1302.

7. A number of *self-help recordings on dental problems* such as plaque, tooth decay, choosing the right toothpaste, reducing dental costs, canker sores, teething, warning signs of gum disease, replacing teeth, dealing with toothache, dental insurance, saving abscessed teeth, selecting a dentist, proper flossing techniques and diet, and lots more can be dialed directly via the Tel-Med Library. See page 319 for information on how the library works and the Tel-Med number nearest you.

8. The book *Dental Self Help*, published by ADI, a nonprofit organization, explains how to re-mineralize teeth, heal inflammed gums, and beat plaque on your own. The emphasis is on natural methods of dentistry. It costs around $10.00 from American Dental Institute, 2509 N. Campbell, #9F, Tucson, AZ 85719.

9. Free and inexpensive booklets providing answers to some of your questions about oral/dental care include:

Your Teeth and What They Do
American Dental Association
Bureau of Dental Health Education
211 East Chicago Ave.
Chicago, IL 60611
Free

How to Become a Wise Dental Consumer
American Dental Association
(address above)
Free

Dental Care: Questions and Answers
Metropolitan Life
Health and Welfare Division
One Madison Ave.
New York, NY 10010
Free

Periodontal Disease
National Institute of Dental Research
Office of Scientific and Health Reports
Bldg. 31, Room 2C-34
4000 Rockville Pike
Bethesda, MD 20014
Free (booklet #NIH 76-1142)

Research Explores Pyorrhea and Other Gum Diseases
National Institute of Dental Research
(address above)
Free (booklet #NIH 72-271)

How to Keep Your Teeth After 30
Public Affairs Committee
381 Park Ave. South
New York, NY 10016
$.50 (booklet #433)

Publications (a list of booklets on dental health and care)
American Academy of Periodontology
211 East Chicago Ave.
Room 924
Chicago, IL 60611
Free

CHAPTER 15

CONSTIPATION

Constipation—infrequent or difficult bowel movements—is generally more a symptom than a disease. Depending on the situation it can be due to:

- Stress
- Depression
- Poor eating patterns
- Insufficient exercise
- Inattentive toilet habits
- Lack of fiber in the diet
- Reaction to drugs
- Low fluid intake

A variety of other possible conditions can also be involved, a few of which are serious, most of which are not. This means that what cures one person will not necessarily cure the next. It also means that in many cases chronic constipation takes years to develop; as a result, it resists treatment with the tenacity of an ingrained habit. A wide variety of treatments have arisen through the years to treat this bothersome and stubborn disorder. In most cases simple constipation can be treated quite successfully at home. Patience and a willingness to experiment may both be necessary, however, before success is achieved.

SELF-DIAGNOSIS OF CONSTIPATION

It's not difficult to tell when you're constipated. You will know the problem when you have:

• Infrequent bowel movements and/or difficulty moving your bowels.

• A bloated, full feeling in the stomach much of the time.

• Small, compact, hard and/or leathery stools.

• Occasional pain during bowel movements due to rubbing of the hard outer exterior of the stool along the anus.

• A possible case of hemorrhoids (these are often associated with chronic constipation).

A FEW QUESTIONS ABOUT CONSTIPATION

How many bowel movements are enough bowel movements? This question depends to an extent on each person's physiology. Certain men and women simply have less active peristalsis than others, and in general it is believed that you do *not* have to eliminate every day to be healthy. Every other day is acceptable, though even once or twice a week is considered to be within the normal range.

When is the best time for a bowel movement? In the morning, about a half hour after breakfast. Residual food has worked its way down to the lower colon during the night, ready to be removed, and peristaltic activity is at its strongest.

What internal processes actually cause constipation? After food has been broken down in the digestive tract, the residues pass into the colon where some of their water is absorbed. When too much water is removed, the fecal matter hardens and stalls in the colon.

Is constipation mental? It *can* be, depending on the situation. Depressed persons often find that their alimentary functions mirror the sluggish, stagnant state of their feelings. The parallel can be more than coincidental, as an improvement in the depression often coincides with a lessening of the constipation. Some chronically constipated persons trace their problem back to early parental influence whereby they were made to feel that bowel movements were dirty or disgusting.

How does one's response to the urge to eliminate affect regu-

larity? Habitual refusal to move the bowels when the need arises can, over time, have an inhibiting effect on regularity. It is imperative that you do not postpone going when nature calls. Choose a time of day, preferably shortly after breakfast, for toilet activities. Go at this time every day, even if the urge is not present. With a little patience, the bowels can be trained to perform at specific hours.

SELF-CARE FOR CONSTIPATION

First, a sensible, easy-to-follow, five-step method for alleviating constipation based on both conventional and nonconventional wisdom. This program is holistic, in the sense that it addresses both the constipation itself and the life-style that may be causing it. You can put this program into operation whenever you wish with a minimum of dramatic change in your daily habits. Here's how it works:

1. *Modify your diet*

Perhaps the best way to beat constipation is by selective nutrition. This means both addition and subtraction: addition of unprocessed, high-fiber foods; subtraction of highly processed, low-fiber foods.

Fiber is the nonmetabolized residue of plant tissue, the parts that pass through the body undigested and exit largely intact. You won't find this substance in meats, fish, or dairy products. It comes exclusively from the plant kingdom, specifically in vegetables, fruit, grains, and nuts.

Fiber's ability to improve constipation is well known, and with good reason. Fiber exerts a strong absorbent action in the gut, drawing local stores of water into the feces and swelling their size and weight. These stores add both bulk and softness to the stool and make it pass more swiftly and easily through the digestive system. Tests show that those who eat a high-fiber diet eliminate more frequently than those who do not. Furthermore, their feces are larger and fuller, and more wastes are excreted at each bowel movement.

The following foods, in their fresh, unrefined/unprocessed states, are all high in fiber and should be placed on your menu if constipation is a problem. Sometimes their addition alone will cause immediate improvement. The starred items are especially rich in fiber:

Apples*	Green beans*	Prunes
Avocados*	Grits*	Pineapples
Bananas	Kidney beans	Peaches
Beets*	Lentils*	Potatoes in their skins*
Bran*	Lettuce	Raspberries*
Broccoli	Mangoes*	Rice (brown)
Cabbage	Okra	Rolled oats*
Carrots	Oranges	Raisins
Cauliflower	Parsnips*	Strawberries*
Celery	Pears	Tomatoes
Corn*	Peas	Whole wheat bread

Refined carbohydrates—polished rice, white sugar, white bread—have the majority of their fiber removed and tend to be soft and pulpy, without coarseness or body. Inside the digestive tract this mealy, denatured residue moves ponderously along. Because it contains no fiber it does not stimulate the linings of the gut in the way that fiber-bearing foods do, and is digested especially slowly. Soon it stagnates and grows hard, resulting in constipation. To remedy this situation, incorporate the following measures into your eating habits:

• Substitute unrefined, unprocessed grains and nuts (in breads, cakes, rice, peanut butter, etc.) for the refined varieties. Eat only whole wheat breads and cereals.

• Eliminate foods that can cause constipation: tea, chocolate, fatty meat, drugs, hot and spicy foods, and especially alcoholic drinks. The latter are notorious for causing bloat and impacted bowels.

• Eat more fresh vegetables. See the list above.

• Eat more fresh fruits. See the list above.

• Eat foods that ferment quickly in the gut such as sauerkraut, sauerkraut juice, cabbage juice, sourdough bread, miso, and pickles. For some people the addition of sauerkraut alone restores regularity. Sample a drink made up of half sauerkraut juice, half tomato juice, and a squeeze of lemon. If it helps you, use it every other day.

• Don't cook with cheap oils. Visit a natural foods store and splurge on cold-pressed, unrefined safflower, olive, sesame, corn, or wheat germ oil. The difference will be apparent in everything you eat.

• Add natural laxative foods to your diet such as yogurt, garlic, rhubarb, bran products, kefir, pumpkin seeds, papaya juice, prunes, apricots, sauerkraut, prune juice, and ground flaxseeds. They can all be purchased at any natural foods store.

2. *Drink more liquids*

This easy step is often neglected. But it will really help. When you get up in the morning, drink a glass of tepid water. During the day drink eight to ten glasses of water, at least two of these between each meal. Stick to this regimen faithfully as long as constipation is a problem.

3. *Exercise regularly*

Inactivity leads directly to sluggish bowels. If you hold a desk job, if you are housebound, if you are sedentary for any other reason, then exercise is a must. Yoga is a particularly good choice for alleviating constipation. Its stretches and lifts are designed to gently tone the gut and to increase circulation in the areas responsible for digestion and elimination. Regular calisthenics and aerobics are also helpful, as are running, swimming, brisk walking, sports like tennis, racquetball, basketball, the martial arts—any invigorating activity that provides physical stimulation. Whatever exercise you enjoy, however, be regular about it. That's the key. Three times a week is the minimum, once a day is ideal. When you get up in the morning, run through a few stretching exercises to get your blood flowing and the gastrointestinal system working quickly, just in time for your morning elimination.

4. *Apply stomach and bowel massage*

Direct pressure and external stimulation of the stomach and bowel areas have been recognized for centuries as effective ways to promote regularity. Use the following massage techniques on a daily basis. They can be practiced alone or by another person. Combined with steps one through three above, massage can be quite effective:

• Place your palms over the navel, one on top of the other. Keeping the hands stationary, move them in a clockwise motion (the direction in which the food passes through the digestive tract), applying deep, regular pressure. Continue for several minutes.

• Locate a spot approximately three inches below and in line with the navel. Keeping the fingers of one hand straight, press directly into this spot for thirty seconds. Release, then repeat twice more. The hand remains stationary, applying deep, steady pressure.

• Apply long, deep vertical strokes to the lower abdomen with both palms. All movements should be made in a firm, steady downward direction, toward the groin.

• Place both hands over the abdomen. Shake and vibrate this area lightly and steadily for thirty seconds. Stop for a moment, then repeat.

• Starting at a point approximately three inches below the navel, draw an imaginary line from hip to hip across the lower abdomen. Keeping the fingertips stiff and together, push carefully but firmly along this line, moving from left hip to right hip and then right hip to left. Repeat for several minutes. If the stomach is too painful in this area, do not continue.

• Stand up. Bend over. Put your hands on your knees. Exhale forcefully and at the same time suck in your stomach. Continue to exhale as long as you can. When all the air is forced out of the stomach, use your abdominal muscles to push the stomach in and out alternately, in waves. Suck in each side, the right, then the left, push out, pull in, move the muscles in a circle, up and down, side to side—in other words, use the abdominal muscles to massage the internal organs of the gut. Catch your breath, and repeat. Practice this exercise for five minutes twice a day, once in the morning and once at night. It is used in both Chinese and Indian yoga, and is very powerful.

The Laxative Question

Many members of the medical community regard over-the-counter laxatives with a dubious eye: They easily become habit-forming, many brands irritate the lining of the colon, and prolonged overuse can cause constipation rather than cure it. Laxatives sap the vigor of the digestive system, and excessive use can literally atrophy key digestive organs. In the end, the eliminative system loses its ability to function without the stimulation of a laxative chemical. Then: addiction.

Nevertheless, the use of laxatives may occasionally be a necessary evil, particularly if travel, strange foods, or sickness cause the bowels to become seriously slowed, and if less dramatic methods of therapy prove ineffective. In such cases, one should begin with the most gentle variety, the so-called *bulk-forming laxatives*. These include:

Wheat bran

Oat bran (also good for lowering cholesterol, recent tests have indicated)

Psyllium derivatives (Metamucil, Siblin, Konsyl, Mucilose)
Malt soup extract (Maltsupex)
Polycarbophil (Mitrolan tablets)
Take these preparations with plenty of water, and be careful not to mix them with aspirin or prescription drugs. If you have any questions along these lines, consult your doctor.

A word on bran: The chaff of the wheat or oat kernel removed during the refining process, bran contains small amounts of vitamin B and trace minerals in addition to its laxative properties. If sprinkled over cereal or taken by the teaspoonsful with a glass of water, it will indeed promote regularity. Bran works by absorbing water and expanding the size of the feces, thus irritating the lining of the colon and increasing peristalsis. When used now and then to relieve constipation, it is an excellent medicine. However, if you come to depend too heavily on bran's laxative powers and if you eat too much of it every day, it may compact into large watery lumps within the gut, eventually obstructing the intestines and *creating* constipation. In particularly severe cases of bran overdose, surgery may be necessary to remove these lumps. So—like any laxative—use bran sparingly.

Other Laxatives

If bulk-forming laxatives do not do the job, *stool softeners* such as Bu-Lax, D-S-S, Colace, and Laxinate will help, but take them only for one day, or two at most. *Lubricant laxatives* such as mineral oil are sometimes useful, too, although overuse will interfere with proper nutrient absorption (taking mineral oil at bedtime can cause some older people to aspirate the oil from the stomach into the lungs). Suppositories work for some people. *Saline laxatives* such as milk of magnesia and tartar salts can cause loss of important body salts and are not frequently recommended.

The most powerful laxatives of all are *stimulant laxatives*. These act directly on the intestines, artificially reducing the transit time of food through the bowels. This category includes:
Castor oil
Dehydrocholic acid (Cholan-DH, Decholin)
Bile salts (Ox Bile Extract)
Bisacodyl (Cenalax, Fleet Bisacodyl, Dulcolax, Bisco-Lax)
Phenolphthalein (Ex-Lax, Feen-a-Mint, Phenolax, Evac-U-Gen)
Cascara sagrada

Senna (Senexon, Senokot)

In general, it is suggested that you take stimulant laxatives only on the rarest occasions, and then only when they are absolutely needed. Never use them for more than three or four days. They work too well, and the bowels will quickly become dependent on them.

WHEN TO CALL THE DOCTOR

Nine times out of ten, constipation is a minor problem. If any of the following conditions exists, however, a consultation with a doctor is advisable:

- Extreme abdominal pain.
- Bloody stools.
- Thin, "squeezed" stools (these may be a sign of an obstruction in the bowels).
- Constipation that appears suddenly, stays longer than usual, and does not respond to any of the above treatments.
- Vomiting of feculent material.
- Signs of pus or mucous in the stools.
- Any sudden change in bowel habits.

TECHNOLOGY, RESOURCES, AIDS, AND SERVICES

1. One of the best forms of exercise for stomach problems and especially for constipation is bicycling. If for any reason you can't bicycle, you can duplicate the experience on a *home bicycle exerciser*. These come in all varieties and can be purchased in most department and sporting goods stores for $50 to $500. A relatively well-made, inexpensive model can be purchased for $69.95 plus postage from Carolina Biological Supply Company, 2700 York Road, Burlington, NC 27215. Call them toll-free at (800) 334-5551 (in North Carolina call [800] 632-1231) for details. They carry a complete line of therapeutic exercise equipment.

2. Another excellent exercise for constipation is jogging. Again, if conditions don't permit, you can derive similar benefits at home from a *rebound exerciser* (read: small trampoline). They cost from $35 to $100 at sporting goods or health foods stores. Carolina Biological Supply Company (see address and phone number above) has one for around $100.

3. *A telephone hotline for people with digestive and stomach ailments* is available for the price of the call. A gastroenterologist will answer all your questions about symptoms, medications, side

effects, etc. Call GUTLINE (301) 652-9293. The hours are 7:30 PM to 9 PM Tuesday.

4. *The Digestive Disease Information Center,* located at 6410 Rockledge Drive, Suite 208, Bethesda, MD 20034, will answer your questions about the care, prevention, and treatment of digestive disorders. They also publish a free newsletter.

5. *The videocassette "I Am Joe's Stomach"* details the intricate workings of the digestive system with vivid three-dimensional animation and live sequences. This film and others on similar subjects are available from the Medcom Film Library, P.O. Box 116, Garden Grove, CA 92642, (800) 854-2485 (in California call [800] 472-2479).

6. Useful books and booklets on constipation include:
BOOKLETS
Constipation
American Medical Association
535 North Dearborn Street
Chicago, IL 60610
$.35 (there is a $1.00 minimum on all orders)

Hints on How to Avoid Constipation
Hoechst-Roussel Pharmaceuticals
Publications Officer
Route 202-206 North
Somerville, NJ 08876
Free

Constipation and What You Can Do About It
Searle Educational Systems
P.O. Box 5110
Chicago, IL 60680
Free (pamphlet #7602)

BOOK
Save Your Stomach by Lawrence Galton (New York: Crown Publishers, 1982).

CHAPTER 16

DIARRHEA

Like constipation, diarrhea can be a symptom of a number of ailments ranging from stress to food poisoning. It is the body's way of getting rid of toxins quickly. Minor cases usually come and go quickly and respond well to home therapies. Although diarrhea may begin as a minor reaction, prolonged bouts can lead to severe mineral depletion, electrolyte imbalance, and dehydration. For children it may even turn into a life-threatening situation. Here are tricks to treating it yourself:

1. Do not let the condition continue for too long without attention.

2. Find out what is causing the diarrhea and determine whether or not this cause is potentially hazardous.

3. Seek medical help quickly if the condition continues despite treatment or if it is caused by dangerous factors. Diarrhea is especially dangerous for infants—they can become dehydrated from runny bowels within a matter of a few hours.

Self-Diagnosis of Diarrhea

While the symptoms of diarrhea and its accompanying side effects may vary, the most common include:

• Loose, watery, abnormally frequent bowel movements.

- Much gas.
- General abdominal discomfort with sharp cramping.
- Possible accompanying nausea, headache, and vomiting.

Self-diagnosis of diarrhea is often easy, primarily because loose bowels are frequently traceable to something you have recently eaten or drunk. Hot, spicy foods, new or unusual foods, ethnic foods, large amounts of alcohol, apple juice, coffee, indiscriminate mixing of foods (e.g., ice cream and chili) or foods that are contaminated with bacteria or viruses are possible culprits.

Think back over the past forty-eight hours:

- Have you eaten in places where conditions were less than sanitary?
- What unusual sweets, fruits, drinks, meats, vegetables, etc., have you ingested?
- Have you recently changed your diet in any way? Are you on a diet?
- Are you taking new medications?
- Did you recently gorge on sweets or on rich foods? Did you eat a lot of junk foods? Greasy foods? Fatty foods?
- Do you suffer from any food allergies?
- Have you recently drunk large amounts of alcohol?
- Do you take massive doses of vitamin C?
- Have you eaten large amounts of raw fruits like prunes, plums, rhubarb, or green apples?
- Have you eaten uncooked foods of any kind?
- Have you recently dined out at a restaurant? Do you remember eating anything that seemed suspicious at the time?
- Often the diarrhea will be accompanied by an unpleasant aftertaste in the mouth and throat. Pay attention to this taste; it may provide a clue to the trouble-causing food.

If the cause of the diarrhea cannot be traced to particular foods, consider your activities over the past several days:

- Have you traveled recently? Are you feeling sick?
- Do you have a cold or flu?
- Have your received upsetting, sad, or frightening news? Are you anticipating a particularly stressful experience?
- Have you been rushed and harried?
- Have you had a particularly stressful encounter with another person?
- Are you depressed? Worried? Overtired?

All these factors can affect the sensitive eliminative system.

SELF-CARE FOR DIARRHEA

Self-care *for adults* is as follows:

1. Rest your stomach by not eating solid foods for at least a day. Weak, thin soups are fine, but go easy on the juices, especially orange juice, and any liquids that contain milk.

2. During the fast, drink plenty of pure water to maintain electrolyte balance. If you are vomiting, suck on ice to keep the fluids coming in. For some people, ginger ale or cola syrup settles the stomach. The Federal Center for Disease Control in Atlanta suggests the following method be used to treat diarrhea*:

Take two glasses. In the first, mix:

- eight ounces of orange, apple, or any other fruit juice rich in potassium (large amounts of potassium and magnesium are lost during periods of diarrhea)
- one-half teaspoon honey or corn syrup to promote absorption of essential salts
- a pinch of table salt

In the second glass, mix:

- eight ounces of water
- one-half teaspoon baking soda

Alternate sips from each glass throughout the day.

3. After the first day, return to mild, semisolid foods like Jell-O, applesauce, baked potatoes, soft-boiled eggs, brown rice, crushed bananas. Avoid foods high in roughage like lettuce, peanut butter, and raw fruits. Remain on this diet for at least a day or two, being careful to avoid coffee and alcoholic drinks.

4. A popular naturopathic aid for diarrhea is to place ice packs on the lower and middle parts of the spine. Keep the packs in place for about ten minutes at a time and repeat once every half hour. The theory is that cold applications along the spine stimulate the nerves responsible for controlling the excretory functions. Pepsin tablets, magnesium (500 milligrams a day), and a strong B-complex vitamin will also help in some situations. Warm-water enemas given morning and night will replace body fluids, clean the intestinal tract of harmful bacteria, and allow the body to absorb the liquids lost during the episode of diarrhea.

* As mentioned in David R. Zimmerman, *The Essential Guide to Nonprescription Drugs* (New York: Harper & Row, 1983), pp. 238–239.

5. If fasting does not control the diarrhea, a kaolin/pectin compound (commercial brands include Kaopectate or Donnagel) may help. For some people activated charcoal and tablets (Charcocaps) or acidophilus tablets (Bacid) are helpful. Paregoric, an opium-derivative available without a prescription, has a more dramatic effect on slowing the propulsive movement of the digestive tract and should be used only if the milder medications fail.

Home treatment for diarrhea *in children* is as follows:

1. If the child is an infant, dilute his or her regular formula to half-strength, or use skim milk diluted to half-strength. Feed it to the baby in frequent small amounts. For an older child, replace solid foods with liquids. Clear broth, bouillon, tea, gelatin, and water from boiled down rice can all be given. Remember that the child needs salt; add a pinch or two to anything he or she eats. If the diarrhea is particularly severe, or if it occurs more than once an hour, get your doctor's advice immediately.

2. Do not give paregoric or any antidiarrheal until you have consulted a physician. These medicines may be too strong for a child and may do more harm than good.

3. Follow the fluid regimen outlined in number 3 above in the adult treatment program. Children are more susceptible to dehydration than adults and it is vital that they receive adequate liquids during bouts of diarrhea. If liquid loss is a particular problem, an oral hydration solution known as Infalyte is available over-the-counter at most drugstores and can be given to counteract salt imbalance and fluid loss.

4. After the first day, return to mild, semi-solid foods such as applesauce, brown rice, whole wheat toast, and bananas.

5. For some children the so-called BRAT diet works well (Bananas, Rice, Applesauce, and Toast). Give small portions of these foods together every four hours. The combination will stimulate digestive enzymes that help control diarrhea.

WHEN TO CALL THE DOCTOR

A doctor should be contacted if:
- There is blood, pus, or mucus in the feces.
- The diarrhea continues intensely for more than two or three days despite home treatment (twenty-four hours in children).
- There is severe abdominal cramping and continuous stomach pains.

- The diarrhea is accompanied by bloody vomit.
- The person is diabetic or suffers from a chronic disease.
- There are signs of dehydration.
- The person urinates frequently.
- The person is pregnant.

CHAPTER 17

BACKACHE AND STIFF NECK

A wide variety of neck and back problems plagues people, especially those over thirty (a majority of back injuries occur between the ages of thirty-one and forty). Luckily, there are therapeutic techniques that can correct, or at least palliate, these disorders no matter what area of the back or neck they affect. We will acquaint you with a few of these therapeutic methods, along with the latest self-help appliances and technology that have been developed specifically for neck and back pain.

A special word of warning is necessary before we begin, however. The spine is one of the most resilient yet sensitive organs of the body, and it can become vulnerable to a number of unpredictable muscular and neurological disorders. While minor neck and back ailments usually respond well to home treatment, see a doctor immediately if a problem appears to be chronic, if it returns with predictable regularity, or if it really hurts. Once you have been diagnosed, self-treatment can be tailored to your specific needs.

SELF-CARE FOR STIFF OR STRAINED NECK

The following methods for the relief of a stiff or strained neck are by no means mutually exclusive.

1. *Consider your sleeping habits.* Many, perhaps most, stiff necks are caused by improper sleep positions. Particularly harmful is sleeping on the stomach with the face buried in the pillow. It is also dangerous to sleep sitting up, especially on an airplane or a train. The best sleep postures are on the back, with the legs slightly bent or elevated or on the side, tucked up in a semifetal position.

You might try sleeping without a pillow or finding a better back and neck support (pillows designed especially to reduce sore necks are described on page 197). Perhaps you have a tendency to remain in one position too long while sleeping; to break this habit, try giving yourself verbal suggestions before going to sleep. Tell yourself as you doze off that you will shift positions regularly throughout the night. Sometimes several weeks or more must pass before self-suggestion takes effect, so don't get discouraged.

Finally, what about your mattress? Is it firm? Is it too firm? Has it started to sag? Do the springs rub your underside? If you have any doubts about the quality of your mattress, you should replace it.

2. *Apply heat.* A heating pad is excellent for reducing pain and for speeding up the healing process. (Don't fall asleep with the pad underneath you, though; it can burn you if the temperature goes too high.) Take a hot shower, pointing the nozzle directly at the back of your neck for ten to fifteen minutes. Whirlpool baths and hot compresses are other options.

3. *Pad and protect your neck while you sleep.* Fold a thick towel lengthwise four times and pack it snugly around your neck, fastening the ends with a safety pin. Try sleeping with this home-made neck brace every night. The pad will keep your neck warm and immobile enough to prevent it from twisting into awkward positions.

4. *Use massage.* Both self-massage and applied massage are helpful. Here are some good techniques:

• Place your hands on the back of the neck just below the ears. Rub and knead for several minutes in the morning and at night.

• Place your thumbs in the hollows beneath the ears. Rub in small circles for approximately thirty seconds.

• With both hands stiff (as if giving a "karate chop"), apply a gentle chopping movement up and down the back of the neck.

• Apply deep, penetrating kneading and pinching massage along the shoulders and lower parts of the neck.

• Massage the vertebrae of the upper and lower neck.

You can, if you like, use a warming oil while you apply self-massage. Regular rubbing of the neck area will increase circulation of blood and lymph, tone the muscles, and generally speed up the healing process. An electric vibrator or a hand-held infrared heat device (see technology and resources section below) may also be useful.

5. *Exercise.* Unless you strengthen the muscles in the neck area with exercise, you can expect to see neck problems returning with predictable regularity. Here are some useful exercises:

• Take your head in your hands. Gently pull it up and away from your shoulders, giving your neck a vigorous stretch.

• Slowly turn your head from one side to the other, looking as far over each shoulder as you can. Don't strain.

• Rotate your head clockwise for several turns, then reverse and rotate it counterclockwise. Let your head hang limp and totally relaxed during this exercise. Let it fall by its own weight as it goes slowly round. This exercise is extremely relaxing and can be used to fight tension.

• Place your palm over your ear. Push your ear firmly against it, increasing the resistance for thirty seconds. Do this twice on each side.

• Lace your fingers together and grip your forehead. Press your head forward, resisting with your hands. Continue for thirty seconds, stop for a moment, then repeat twice again.

• Nod your head slowly downward, dropping your chin as far toward your chest as it will go. Hold for thirty seconds. Now reverse, dropping your head as far back as it will reach comfortably. Hold this position for thirty seconds, pointing your chin toward the ceiling. Return to normal position and repeat.

• Stand up, spread your feet to shoulder width, bend forward and let your head hang down. Swing both arms simultaneously in wide circles, ten rotations forward, ten back. Let your head hang as loosely and freely as possible while performing the rotations, and sense the pleasant stretch on the neck this exercise produces. You can increase the number of rotations as this exercise becomes increasingly comfortable.

6. *Don't be too inactive, even if your neck is in spasm.* Prolonged bed rest is not necessarily good for an acute sore neck and occasionally can make it worse. More than a day in bed is probably too much. Be careful, but move about. Alternate rest periods with gentle activity.

7. Practice common-sense preventive techniques.

• Avoid holding your neck at strange angles for prolonged periods. Sit directly in front of the TV. Make sure to hold your book or magazine at a comfortable angle. Do not sit too low in the seat when driving. If you frequently talk on the telephone, a shoulder rest will spare the neck muscles. Remember, if your neck is misused during the day, it is more likely to stiffen at night.

• Avoid drafts on the neck and face. Be especially careful of nighttime drafts from fans and air conditioners.

• If your vision is poor and you do not wear glasses, consider a trip to the optometrist. Blurred or distorted vision may cause you to crane and stretch your neck. If one eye is stronger than another, you may unconsciously tilt your head to get a better look at things.

• If you are prone to stiff necks, keep away from sports and other activities that cause neck strain. Wrestling, boxing, karate, and contact sports of any kind are obviously not for you if your neck is sensitive.

• Learn to sit in positions that are comfortable and ease strain on your neck.

• Make a habit of intentionally relaxing the muscles in your neck throughout the day and at night before bed. Tighten the neck muscles for thirty seconds, then relax them. Repeat. This exercise may help you to sleep better, too.

SELF-CARE FOR BACKACHE

Volumes have been written about treating back problems. We can only scratch the surface here, describing: 1) a few of the most effective and accessible methods for reducing both upper and lower back stress, 2) self-care methods for treating back pains when they occur, and 3) methods for preventing back troubles with exercise and posture control. Before you begin, however, take Dr. David Imrie's simple National Back Fitness Test to determine just how strong or weak your back really is.*

The National Back Fitness Test

This series of four self-tests is designed to assess the back's flexibility and muscle strength. If you have a bad back, the test

---

*Presented in Dr. David Imrie and Colleen Dimsen, *Goodbye Backache* (New York: Arco Publishing Company, 1983), pp. 65–76.

results will show how bad it really is. If your back seems sound, the results will indicate what the chances are of developing problems in the future. The tests are standardized—a chart at the end compares your scores with those of others who have taken the test. Finally, a word of warning: If you are currently suffering from back pains or recuperating from a back injury, do *not* take these tests. They are designed for men and women whose backs are in normal condition.

EXERCISE ONE: SIT-UP

1. Lie on the floor. Flex your knees approximately forty-five degrees and clasp your hands behind your head. Do a sit-up.

2. If you can't sit up all the way, try folding your arms across your chest and doing a sit-up.

3. If you still can't sit up all the way, try extending your arms in front of you and doing a sit-up.

4. If you can't sit up all the way, try keeping your arms at your sides and doing a sit-up.

   Scoring:
- If you did number 1, score it as excellent.
- If you did number 2, score it as good.
- If you did number 3, score it as fair.
- If you could *not* do 4, score it as poor.

EXERCISE TWO: LEG RAISE

Lie on your back and place your hands behind you in the hollow of the back. Push your lower back tight to the floor. Raise both feet ten inches off the floor and hold them suspended for a count of ten. Don't curve your lower back or raise it from the floor.

   Scoring:
- If you completed the above directions as indicated without difficulty, score it as excellent.
- If you raised your legs for a few seconds but could not keep your back tightly to the floor, score it as good.
- If you could raise your legs, but your back curved immediately, score it as fair.
- If you could not raise your legs at all, score it as "Poor."

EXERCISE THREE: TRUNK LIFT

Lie on your right side, legs straight. Have another person hold your legs tight to the floor; or hook your legs under a nearby overhang (the edge of a bed, the bottom of a desk, etc.) to prevent them from raising while you perform this exercise. Fold your arms across your chest. Remaining on your side, slowly raise your shoulders and upper part of your body off the floor. Remain raised for ten seconds, then slowly return to the floor. Reverse sides and repeat the same movement.

Scoring:
- If you performed the exercise as described on both sides without difficulty, score this as excellent.
- If you raised your body but could not keep it up for the full ten counts, score this as good.
- If you raised your body a few inches off the floor but could not hold it there, score this as fair.
- If you were unable to raise your body at all, score this as poor.

EXERCISE FOUR: HIP FLEXOR

Lie on your back, legs extended. Hug your right knee to your chest. Note the position of your left leg as your raise the right one. Is it still firmly to the floor? Is it slightly raised? Is it considerably raised? Repeat the same maneuver with the other leg.

Scoring:
- If you hugged your knee to your chest without raising the other leg at all, score this as excellent.
- If you hugged your knee and the other leg raised a little, score this as good.
- If you hugged your knee and the other leg raised entirely off the floor, score this as fair.
- If you hugged your knee and the other leg raised high off the floor, score this as poor.

YOUR FINAL ASSESSMENT BASED ON A NATIONAL AVERAGE
(Circle the score you received for each exercise)

	Excellent	Good	Fair	Poor
Test 1	1	2	3	4
Test 2	1	2	3	4
Test 3	½ (right leg)	1	1½	2
	½ (left leg)	1	1½	2
Test 4	½ (right leg)	1	1½	2
	½ (left leg)	1	1½	2

Scoring yourself:
- 4 to 5 means your back is in excellent shape.
- 6 to 9 means your back is in average shape.
- 10 to 13 means your back is in fair shape.
- 14 to 16 means your back is in poor shape.

Men and women over forty-five can subtract two from their final score.

Preventing Back Problems

There are many things you can do to strengthen your back and help it resist stress. The following techniques are based on sound preventive procedure, and if practiced diligently are almost sure to work.

1. *Improve your sleeping conditions.* Sleep position and mattress quality are as important for the back as for the neck (see page 178). If your mattress is too soft, consider placing a 4-foot x 8-foot plywood board beneath it for better support. Special therapeutic mattresses for bad backs are available at most bedding and orthopedic supply stores. See the technology and resources section below.

2. *Exercise.* Exercise is one of the best ways to prevent back problems. The more you strengthen the muscles of the back with daily exercise, the more flexible and resilient they become.

The following exercises have proven especially effective through the years. Start them slowly, a few minutes a day, and build from there. If you feel any pain or discomfort, discontinue the exercise immediately.

Warning

Never continue an exercise that hurts, *especially* if it involves your neck or back.

Exercises for the Lower Back

1. Lie on your back. Press your pelvis and the small of your back firmly to the floor for five seconds, tightening your buttocks and abdominal muscles as you do. Relax and release. Repeat ten times. When practicing this exercise, your stomach should be

sucked in. The more downward pressure you apply the better. This is especially good for reducing lower back spasms.

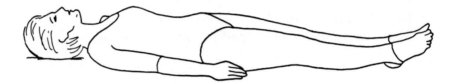

2. Lie on your back. Take your right knee, pull it smartly to your chest and hug it, keeping your left leg on the floor, slightly flexed. Lift your head as close to the hugged knee as you can. Hold it there for ten seconds and return it to the floor. Repeat with the other leg. Repeat five times.

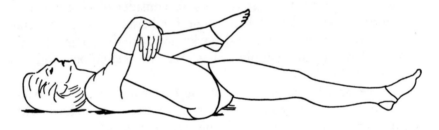

3. Lie on your back with the small of your back pressed tightly to the floor. Take both knees, hug them simultaneously to your chest, and release. Do not raise your head. Repeat ten times.

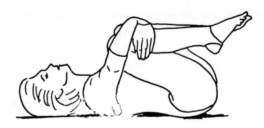

EXERCISES FOR THE LOWER AND MIDDLE BACK

1. The humble sit-up is excellent not only for toning and tightening the stomach muscles, but also for relieving pressure and stress from the spine. Lie on your back, bend your knees at a

forty-five-degree angle, extend your arms in front of you (experts can clasp their hands behind their heads), and lift from the waist. Do ten to twenty sit-ups every morning and night.

2. Stand in a doorway with your feet about five inches from the door frame. Tighten your stomach and press your back and neck against the frame, bending your knees slightly. Keep your chin tucked in to your chest. Press the small of the back to the frame for five seconds, then relax. Repeat several times.

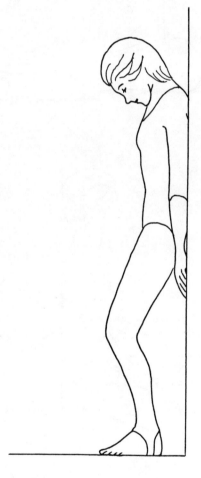

3. Sit on the floor with your legs extended in front of you. Clasp your hands behind your back. Keeping your arms straight, squeeze your shoulder blades together, trying to make your elbows touch. Hold this position for five seconds and release. Repeat several times.

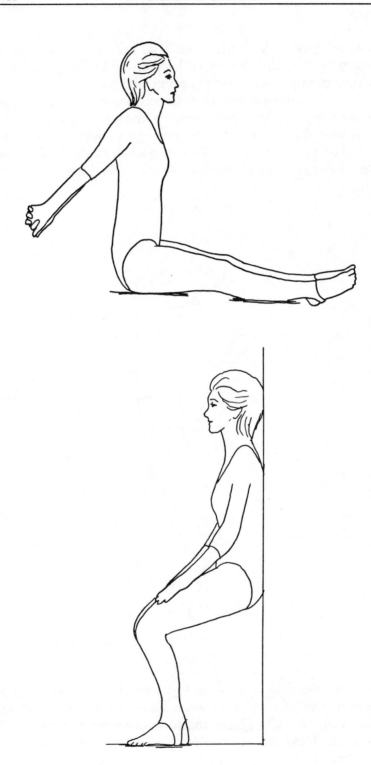

4. Stand with your back against a wall. Bending your knees and keeping your spine against the wall, slowly slide to a sitting position—back straight, legs bent as if seated in a chair. Hold this position for five seconds, then slide back up. With a bit of practice, you should be able to remain in this posture for twenty or thirty seconds at a time. It is an excellent exercise for increasing back strength and flexibility.

5. Lie on your stomach with your hands clasped under your chin. Slowly raise your left leg, keeping your pelvis and right leg flat on the floor. Hold the leg suspended for five seconds, then bring it down slowly. Repeat the same movement with right leg. Do several sets in a row.

While exercising, be alert to the DO'S and DON'TS of back exercise:

• *Do* practice your exercises every day. Regular exercise is the key to an improved back.

• *Don't* exercise strenuously one day, skip three or four days, then exercise twice as hard on the fifth to make up for the omission. Lost exercise cannot be compensated for by periodic exercise binges. Remain faithful to a regular schedule and avoid inconsistency.

• If you work standing up, *don't* stand for prolonged periods of time on a hard surface. A soft rubber mat, a rug, or a pair of well-padded shoes will help absorb some of the stress on the spine.

• *Don't* perform vigorous exercises or potentially back-straining movements the moment you wake up. Warm up first.

• *Don't* hold your breath for long periods of time while exercising. Certain yoga exercises, it is true, require holding one's breath. But breathing should generally be deep and regular—breathing in on the exertion, out during the pause.

• *Don't* exercise immediately after eating. Wait at least an hour.

• *Don't* exercise for at least three hours after drinking alcohol.

• If you suffer from insomnia or sleep problems, *don't* exercise at bedtime. Exercise raises the body temperature and may interfere with the sleep process.

• *Do* drink plenty of water before and after exercise sessions. Liquids help muscles to work more efficiently. *Don't,* however, drink ice water after working out.

• *Don't* sit for long periods of time with a wallet in your back pocket. It has recently been discovered that a wallet can exert pressure on the sciatic nerve and may ultimately contribute to the development of sciatica.

• If you work at a desk, *do* get up and walk around during the day and shift your sitting position as frequently as possible.

• If you carry a briefcase or purse, *don't* overload it, and take care to shift it frequently from one arm to the other.

• *Do* try to produce a warm stretching sensation in your muscles when you exercise, but avoid straining your muscles.

• *Don't* lift weights or do pull-ups, push-ups, or stiff-legged toe touching. *Don't* participate in violent contact sports such as karate, football, wrestling, etc.

• *Do* supplement your regular exercise with nonstrenuous activities, especially swimming and brisk walking.

• If you are currently suffering from acute back pains, *don't* exercise unless given special instructions by an informed health care professional.

• *Do* warm up for a few minutes before doing your back exercises. Practice simple stretches, arm lifts, jogging in place, jumping jacks, etc.

3. *Reduce stress and depression.* Stress, overwork, worry, depression—all of these can take a toll on your back. See section on stress for suggestions.

4. *Work on improving your posture.* A good standing posture means that the shoulders are level with one another, held slightly back, and the buttocks are tucked in. The pelvis is thrust slightly forward, avoiding any swayback or exaggerated "S" curve posture. The chin is drawn slightly in and the chest is comfortably high and open, allowing room for the lungs to contract and expand comfortably.

5. *Learn to lift things properly.* More backs are thrown out by lifting things the wrong way than by any other activity. When you reach down to lift an object—whether heavy or light—bend from your knees. Do *not* keep your legs straight.

6. *And a few other hints:*

• Make sure your shoes fit. High heels are notoriously hard on the spine and should be avoided by anyone with a vulnerable back. If you are a runner, be certain to wear well-padded, impact-absorbing shoes.

• Support your back firmly while sitting. Especially if you have a desk job, the type of back support you choose is of vital importance. Avoid over-soft seats and chair backs that give too easily. Try placing a pillow or rolled up towel between the back and the chair. Consult the technology and resources section for information on locating special chairs and backrests.

• Watch your weight. Be especially careful about developing a large belly. Too much poundage, especially when located in the abdomen, places severe stress on the back.

• Be careful when you sneeze, cough, or make any violent forward motion. Sneeze with your head up. Hold your stomach in when you cough. Never cough or sneeze when your back or neck is twisted. When looking over your shoulder, turn your whole body, not just your neck.

• Damp, cold, and wet weather can aggravate back conditions. The Japanese wrap a special cummerbund around the stomach and lower back during the winter months. You might try the same trick, using any warm, snug material.

• Make sure that your bathroom and kitchen sinks, cabinets, shelves, work benches, and desks are placed at a convenient height.

ACUTE BACK PAINS: SELF-CARE WHEN ACTIVE BACK TROUBLES BEGIN

Once trouble starts and your back goes into acute muscular spasms, treatment must be swift and sure. Many of the preventive measures outlined above become irrelevant in this instance and even potentially damaging. For example, stretching exercises, an excellent preventive, will worsen acute back conditions.

The following measures are all effective for temporary relief of acute back spasms. Needless to say, if you have any suspicion that the pain originates from a serious underlying problem such as a ruptured disc, osteoarthritis, spondylolisthesis, etc., see a health-care professional quickly for advice. As a rule, however, simple acute back pain can be treated effectively at home. Here are some of the best techniques:

1. *Rest.* Backaches need rest, sometimes bed rest, for at least a day and sometimes two or three. Rest immobilizes the injured area, minimizes irritation, and helps control inflammation. While in bed stay on your back as much as possible. Make sure your mattress is firm (placing a 4-foot x 8-foot piece of plywood under the mattress will provide the extra support your back needs while healing). You can also try sitting up in bed with a pillow under your knees. Don't stay flat on your back longer than is necessary, as too much bed rest can have a reverse effect, weakening rather

than strengthening your back. If you're resting your back in bed for a day or so, don't reinjure it by getting up or lying down too hastily. The best method for safely getting out of bed is to lie on your side at the edge of the bed and, keeping your back straight, push your body up into a sitting position with your arm, simultaneously pivoting your feet onto the floor. Get back into bed by reversing this maneuver: Sit on the side of the bed and bring your legs up onto the mattress while you ease your body down with your arm.

2. *Apply heat.* Heat applied to the painful area will increase circulation of healing blood, relax the muscles, and ease overall discomfort. Although there are several schools of thought on the subject, moist heat is generally considered better than dry. Moist heat can be applied with hot water compresses, a whirlpool bath, hot towels, a hot tub, or a hot water bottle. Try standing in a hot shower for ten to fifteen minutes with the spray aimed directly at the sore spot. Dry heat can be applied with a heating pad or heat lamp. (Occasionally, it should also be added, heat applied to an injured back will cause both the spasm and the pain to increase in severity. If you have any questions along these lines, consult with a health care professional.)

3. *Apply ice.* For some members of the bad back club, ice is a more efficient agent than heat. You will have to experiment in this regard. Try applying ice packs to the inflamed area or use wet towels that have been chilled in the freezer. Repeat this procedure at least three times a day and more if it helps.

4. *Use an "ice massage."* A therapeutic technique recommended by the Department of Rehabilitation Medicine at New York Hospital–Cornell Medical Center* consists of placing several paper cups filled with water in a freezer overnight. Next day, remove and tear off the bottom of one of the cups, exposing an inch or so of ice. Grip the cup, and using circular and up-and-down strokes, massage the injured areas with the frozen ends. When a burning feeling develops along the massaged areas, stop the treatment until the sensation ceases, then begin again. Continue applying ice until the massaged area becomes numb, using as many frozen cups as are necessary. Once numbness sets in, this means the beneficial effects have taken place: end the mas-

---

* Shirley Linde, *How to Beat a Bad Back* (New York: Rawson, Wade, 1980), p. 22.

sage. In general, do not continue ice massage longer than seven minutes.

5. *Apply massage.* Gentle Swedish massage of the injured area can provide temporary pain relief in some cases. Sometimes the massage will relax the person and increase his or her sense of well-being but nothing more. Massage techniques include:

• Long, deep strokes up and down the entire back.

• Light slapping and pounding over the sore areas.

• Short circular pushing motions applied to the sore spots with the heel of the hand.

• Deep thumb and finger kneading over the problem areas.

Information on massage therapy is included on page 178.

6. *Apply acupressure (Shiatsu).* Pressure point therapy is often helpful in relieving back pain. Specific pressure points along the back and elsewhere are stimulated by applying concentrated pressure with the balls of the thumbs. Each point is pushed for ten to fifteen seconds, two or three times in a row. The thumb pressure should be reasonably firm. One practitioner describes the pushing process as producing sensations half-way between pleasure and pain.

The theory behind acupressure (and acupuncture) is that the health of the body is determined by the circulation of subtle energies that move along twelve defined lines or *meridians* throughout the body. There is, for instance, the lung meridian, the liver meridian, the stomach meridian, and so forth. When these energies are moving freely, the body is healthy. When they are blocked, illness results. Located along these meridians are certain points or centers—the acupressure/acupuncture points. Properly stimulated, these points disperse, concentrate, stimulate, or subdue energy along their corresponding meridians, sending energy to aid the healing process and restore balance to the system.

• Position yourself as if to give a massage. Palpate the person's spine to locate the spaces between the vertebrae. With the thumbs, simultaneously stimulate the points approximately two inches to the left and two inches to the right of these spaces, as shown in the illustration. Start at the top of the spine and work your way down to the lower lumbar region. Repeat. Work slowly, applying pressure for ten to fifteen seconds at each point. You are stimulating the energies of the so-called bladder meridian, which has been known to make the back feel better in an amazingly short period of time.

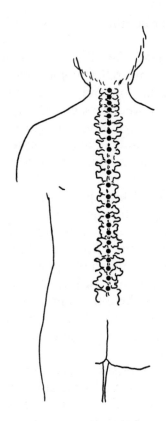

• Stimulate the points on both shoulder blades halfway between the base of the neck and the bottom tip of the shoulder bone.

• With the person on his or her stomach, arms to the side, draw an imaginary line across the back from elbow to elbow. Apply simultaneous thumb pressure along this line on the points located a hand's width distance to either side of the spine.

• Massage the lower back over the lumbar vertebrae and the buttocks area. Then apply deep thumb pressure to the points indicated in the illustration.

• Have the person be on his back. Measure the width of one hand down from the bottom of the kneecap on the shin. From here measure the width of two thumbs toward the outside of the leg. The point is situated between the shinbone and a large adjacent muscle, and will probably be sensitive when touched. Deeply probe this point several times in a row on both legs.

Note: Consult with a health-care specialist or a professional acupressurist before applying acupressure for back pains if:

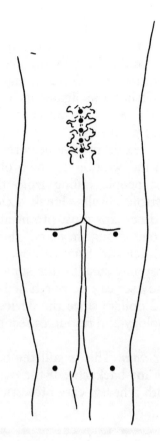

• The person is pregnant.
• The person is taking a prescription medication.
• The injury is related to a chronic degenerative disease such as arthritis, diabetes, etc.
• The designated acupressure point is located on a large mole, wart, open sore, etc.

7. *Lie on a slantboard.* This helpful piece of apparatus can be made from any sturdy piece of wood or formica capable of supporting a person's weight (such as a piece of 1-inch thick plywood). Position it with one end on the ground, the other end raised a foot or more, and lie on it with feet up, head toward the floor. Remaining in this posture for a few minutes is said to aid circulation, reduce swelling, relax the muscles, and flatten the back. The board should be slanted so that it elevates the feet at least fifteen inches above the head. Lie on the slant board for ten or fifteen minutes a day.

8. *Use a gravity inversion device.* Similar to vertical traction,

versions of which have been used for centuries by doctors around the world, inversion consists of hanging upside down for extended periods of time on a specially designed piece of exercise equipment. Suspension from this device elongates the spine, stimulates circulation, stretches the ligaments and muscle sheaths (fascia), and takes pressure off the vertebrae. It is said to be especially helpful for disc problems.

While few adverse side effects have been reported from gravity inversion, getting into the position can be problematic, and there have been reports of people falling from these contraptions, sometimes with disastrous results. Freak accidents aside, inversion is the newest and perhaps most promising self-care method of back therapy to come along in years. The cost of the apparatus, which can be purchased from orthopedic supply stores or by mail, has been dropping steadily for some time, and though still not cheap, a sturdy set can be purchased for $150 to $300, down several hundred dollars since the device first came on the market. See the technology and resources section below for information.

9. *Take aspirin for pain.* This is still the best of all over-the-counter pain relievers for backache. If the pain becomes too in tense, get in touch with a health-care professional immediately.

When You See a Specialist: Who Can Help?

There are a number of options. Basically, the back specialists best known for achieving positive results include:
- Chiropractors
- Sports medicine specialists
- Acupuncturists
- Kinesiologists
- Shiatsu (acupressure) specialists
- Osteopaths
- Orthopedic surgeons
- Massage therapists
- Rolfers
- Mensendieck System therapists
- Feldenkrais System therapists
- Alexander Technique therapists

WHEN TO SEE A DOCTOR

See a doctor for back problems if:
- Your backache does not improve after applying the above self-care remedies.
- Your backache recurs with increasing frequency.
- Your backache is severe.
- You are immobilized.
- You have a fever and/or headache along with back pains.
- You are experiencing a sensation of numbness or tingling in the injured areas.
- Your range of motion in the back, neck, or shoulders is seriously (and uncharacteristically) limited.

Exercise Systems That Work for Backs

Methods that are most popular and seem to work best include:
- Yoga
- Tai chi
- Modern dance
- Standard orthopedic exercises
- Isometric abdominal and back exercises
- Mensendieck exercises
- Feldenkrais exercises
- Alexander exercises

TECHNOLOGY, RESOURCES, AIDS, AND SERVICES

An entire book could be filled with the commercial back aids and home therapeutic devices currently flooding the market. There are stores that sell nothing but back-care equipment and specialize in every imaginable type of back-oriented merchandise. The following list, although far from exhaustive, provides a good sampling of the array of high-tech, low-tech, and old-fashioned orthopedic self-care equipment available to home consumers. If you are interested in learning more, write directly to the companies listed below for catalogs and/or specific items.

1. Special chairs engineered for back sufferers include the *Balans Vital Swivel Chair* designed to tilt the hips and maintain pos-

ture, and the *Multisit* office chair that adjusts automatically to the shape and curve of the sitter's back. Information on both can be obtained from The Backworks, 2051 Walnut Street, Philadelphia, PA, (215) 864-0877. A third option is the *Inversion Chair* from Carolina Health and Fitness, 2700 York Road, Burlington, NC 27215, (800) 334-5551 (in North Carolina call [800] 632-1231). It was designed by medical experts to follow the line of the back, seat a person in the natural position of rest, and elevate the feet higher than the head. The *Bear Chair,* also obtainable from Carolina Health and Fitness, was designed for children by a team of doctors to fit the natural contours of a child's bone structure and to provide support. Finally, there is the *massage lounger,* an expensive (around $1,200) but luxurious cushioned lounge chair that vibrates electronically to stimulate the acupressure points located along the neck and back. The chair is made by Panasonic.

2. *Inverse gravity traction equipment* can be purchased from several sources. The *Pal-Relax-Bar* is a sturdy traction unit available from Pal-Relax-Bar Company, Inc., 233 Oak Knoll Rd., Ukiah, CA 95482, (707) 462-1444. *The Medical Self-Care Catalog,* P.O. Box 999, Pt. Reyes, CA 94956, offers a small A-frame model especially designed for individual adjustment and extra safety. It retails for around $260 plus postage. Abbey Medical Supply Company, 13782 Crenshaw Blvd., Gardena, CA 90249, (800) 421-5126 (in California call [800] 262-1294), sells inversion boots and an inversion bar separately for under $100; you can use them together to set up your own home system. Abbey also offers a large wall traction unit that includes a plated steel frame, an oscillation bed, two parallel side bars, a chin-up bar and a lower assist mechanism unit for around $1,300, as well as a regular lightweight inverse gravity unit for $450. (Any materials from Abbey must be ordered through a health-care professional.) Still another gravity inversion mechanism is sold by Carolina Biological Supply Company, 2700 York Rd., Burlington, NC 27215, (800) 334-5551 (in North Carolina call [800] 632-1231), for around $280. Plans for *building your own traction device* can be purchased for $10 to $15 from T&G Enterprises, P.O. Box 725, Black Mountain, NC 28711.

3. A special *air belt* designed to fit around the waist and provide weightless support to the lower back is available for around $115 plus postage from Delaware Valley Safeguards Company,

Inc., Leisz Rd., R.D. 1, Lessport, PA 19533, (215) 926-5232. The belt is inflated with a special detachable hand pump, and it can be worn under pants, a suit, or a dress. A noninflatable model called the *lumbar support* fits around the waist and fastens with Velcro. Order it from Edmunds Scientific, 101 East Gloucester Pike, Barrington, NJ 08007, (609) 547-3488.

4. *Special pillows* for the neck and back can be purchased from a number of stores and companies. Walter Drake, Drake Building, Colorado Springs, CO 80940, (303) 596-3140, sells an *inflatable bath pillow* that cushions both head and neck while you bathe. Also available from Drake is the *knee pillow*, designed to elevate the knees while you're lying on your back. The *Wal-Pil-O Cervical Pillow* from Carolina Biological Supply Company (address in number 2) allows you to customize your neck support four ways by placing your head on the "soft," "medium," "firm narrow," or "firm wide" section of the pillow. The Wal-Pil-O comes in a regular size (around $36.00) or a travel model (around $24). Carolina also features a variety of *posture back support pillows* designed to support the spine in the car, office, home, etc. Other special *back pillows for automobiles*, such as the *contour cushion* and the *adjustable back-aid seat*, both of which conform to the back's contours, are available through a health-care professional from Fred Sammons, Inc., P.O. Box 32, Brookfield, IL 60513-0032, (800) 323-5547 (in Illinois call [800] 942-2129). A pillow called the *lumbar wedge* is especially useful for lower back problems. It tucks into the curve of the lower back while you lie flat and provides support to the entire lumbar area. It is available from the Spenco Medical Corporation, P.O. Box 2501, Waco, TX 76702-2501, (800) 433-3334. For raising the back or legs while you are sleeping, the wedge-shaped *inflatable Incline Pillow* can be useful. Order it from Cleo, Inc., 3957 Mayfield Rd., Cleveland, OH 44121, (800) 321-0595 (in Ohio call [800] 222-CLEO), for around $8.00. Another model, the *Take-Along Back Cushion*, can be ordered for around $17 from Comfortably Yours, 52 West Hunter Ave., Maywood, NJ 07607, (201) 368-0400. Finally, for an amazingly wide selection of back and neck support pillows, get in touch with Accu-Back, Inc., 1475 E. Del Amo Blvd., Carson, CA 90746, (800) 272-8888. They manufacture more than ten different varieties of orthopedic support pillows for the neck, shoulders, and back, including special models made from heat-retaining foam.

5. *Home massage apparatus.* Both electronic and manual varieties are available. A *back massaging body brush* (around $20), a two-intensity *electric hand-held massage machine* (around $17), and a selection of small *hand vibrators* are available from Cleo Inc. (address in number 4). A *portable sonic massager* that relieves deep muscle pain with high-frequency sound waves can be purchased from *The Medical Self-Care Catalog* (address in number 2). A hand-held infrared heating appliance called *Infralux* (around $30) treats muscle spasms with deep electronic infrared heat and is also available from *The Medical Self-Care Catalog.* The *Thermo-Cyclopad* is an elaborate, padded, board-like support that heats and massages the entire back. It costs around $500 from Niagara Therapy Manufacturing Corporation, 98 Highland Ave., Brocton, NY 14716, (716) 792-4161. A similar but cheaper version, the *15-Way Massager/Heater,* is a small padlike device that fits under the back. It has fifteen electric massage and infrared heat settings. You can order it for around $70 from Hammacher Schlemmer, 147 East 57th St., New York, NY 10022, (212) 421-9000. Another electric massage unit, manually operated and specifically designed for massaging the back, is the *Maxi Rub Massager.* It features a contoured orbiting pad that vibrates into the deep muscles; it costs around $100 from Carolina Biological Supply Company (address in number 4). A unique item is the *Backnobber,* an S-shaped rod with a knob at the head, designed to reach those hard-to-get-at areas of the back (like a back scratcher) and to massage specific tension and acupressure points. The small model costs around $13, the large one around $16. It can be ordered from Pressure Positive Company, R.D. 2, Gilbertsville, PA 19525, (215) 754-6204. It comes with a book of instructions.

6. *Manual massage information.* A two-hour VHS video course of instruction in *Shiatsu/Acupressure* costs about $100 and can be ordered from P.A. Shiatsu Associates, 108 E. Maple Ave., Langhorne, PA 19047, (215) 750-0712. Interesting books on Shiatsu/Acupressure include:

The G-Jo Handbook by Michael Blate
David, Florida: Falkynor Books,
1976

Acu-Yoga
Available for $12.95 plus $1.80 shipping from:

Acupressure Workshop
1533 Shattuck Ave.
Berkeley, CA 94709
(415) 845-1059
(The Acupressure Workshop also offers courses
in Shiatsu)

Japanese Finger-Pressure Therapy by Tokujiro Namikoshi
San Francisco: Japan Publications Trading Co.
1972
For those interested in learning the *Feldenkrais system of back, neck, and shoulder manipulation,* six ninety-minute cassette tapes comprising an entire home course are available for $72 from Richard Nisenbaum, P.O. Box 9492, Berkeley, CA 94709. A single *Feldenkrais system tape* costs around $12 and teaches you basic Feldenkrais movements and exercises to improve the back and protect it from further injury. Contact Dr. Frank Wildman, 721 The Alameda, Berkeley, CA 94707, for further information. If you are interested in acquiring a *massage table,* Living Earth Crafts at 429 Olive St., Santa Rosa, CA 95401, (800) 358-8292, offers a variety of models. Ask for their catalog. Another good source for tables is Pisces Productions, P.O. Box 208, Petalunia, CA 94928, (707) 795-8616. If you're interested in learning *massage for infants and children,* a fifty-minute tape can be ordered from The New Age School of Massage, P.O. Box 958, Sebastopol, CA 95472. It costs around $11.

7. *Exercise equipment for backs* can be purchased from HSA, P.O. Box 288, Farmville, NC 27828, (800) 334-1187 (in North Carolina call [800] 672-4214). Their selection includes a *Stride-Setter Motorized Treadmill* with an electronic monitor (around $1,230), a *Cross Country Jogger* (around $270), a *Nautilus Lower Back Machine* to strengthen the back muscles (around $480), several styles of rowing machines, and a *Nautilus Abdominal Machine* to exercise the abdominal muscles (around $490). The Medical Self-Care Catalog (address in number 2) offers a bicycle-type exerciser called the *Bodyguard 955 Exerciser* for around $335 and a *Lifeline Sit-up Bar* (around $17) to steady the legs while doing sit-ups. Most sporting goods and department stores offer a complete line of home exercise equipment.

8. *Heat appliances.* A good one is the old-fashioned *moist heat hydrocollator,* a thick absorbent cloth pack you immerse in hot

water and apply directly to the back. It can be purchased at any good pharmacy. A more up-to-date form of the above, the *Spenco Hot Pack,* is a ribbed pad containing an elastic gel that retains heat for long periods. Order it from Spenco Medical Corporation (address in number 4). An electric version of the hydrocollator, The *Thermo-O-Lax* (around $60) can be ordered from *The Medical Self-Care Catalog* (address in number 2). Regular dry *electric heat pads* can be found at any drugstore, ranging from $15 to $30. Bathtub *hot-water whirlpool units* can be purchased from many pharmacies. A good professional model called the *Jetra 60 Whirlpool* has a one-horsepower motor, built-in timer, and turbulence control mechanism. It costs around $380 from Carolina Biological Supply Company (address in number 2). If you really want to get serious, look into acquiring a *spa steam cabinet* for around $370 from HSA (address in number 7). This home steambath unit has a light, a one-piece molded fiberglass cabinet with thermostatic temperature control, and a heavy-duty steam generator.

9. *General aids for bad back sufferers.* A wide assortment of *canes and walkers* is available from Cleo (address in number 4). Write for their catalog. Cleo also offers items for people who have trouble bending down, such as *an eighteen-inch plastic shoe horn,* a *stocking pulling aid,* and a *bathtub grab bar and safety rail.* For reaching into difficult or potentially back-wrenching places, *an aluminum arm extender* can be handy. It costs around $40 from Carolina Biological Supply Company (address in number 2). A magnetized version of this instrument is obtainable from Walter Drake (address in number 4). Outdoor work can be made easier on the back with a *Backsaver shovel or rake.* The shovel costs $27 plus postage, the rake $16 plus postage from Comfortably Yours (address in number 4). The *Spine-X portable bedboard,* a device designed to fit under the mattress and firm it up for better support, is five feet long and can be folded up into a two-foot-long package for travel. Order it from Nepsco, Inc., 53 Jeffrey Ave., Holliston, MA 01746, (800) 251-2225. If you're looking for *orthopedic back, neck, and shoulder supports,* HSA (address in number 7) offers a wide variety of *cervical collars, adjustable back supports, sacroiliac supports, shoulder immobilizers,* etc.

10. A famous system of back exercise and muscle control taught for years at the YMCA has been put onto a videotape. It is called "Say Goodbye to Back Pain" and costs $39.95 plus shipping from

Impact 2000, 60 Irons Street, Toms River, NJ 08753, (800) 843-9646 (in New Jersey call [201] 370-4422).

11. *Worthwhile books and literature on back problems and massage* include:

The American Medical Association's Book on Back Care by Martin Steinmann
New York: Random House, 1982

Backache Relief by Arthur C. Klein, and Dava Sobel
New York: Times Books, 1985

How to Beat a Bad Back by Shirley Linde
New York: Rawson, Wade, 1980

Goodbye Backache by Dr. David Imrie with Colleen Dimson
New York: Arco Publishing Co., 1983

The Bum Back Book by Michael R. Gach
Berkeley: Acu Press, 1983

Your Guide to Safe Lifting
American Insurance Association
85 John Street
New York, NY 10038
Free

Back to Backs
Krames Communications
312 90th Street
Daly City, CA 94015-1898
Cost: $1.25

Neck Owner's Manual: A Guide to Common Neck Problems
Krames Communications (address above)
Cost: $1.25

Back Exercises for a Healthy Back
Krames Communications (address above)
Cost: $1.25

Back Tips for (People Who Sit)
Krames Communications (address above)
Cost: $1.25

Back Owner's Manual
Krames Communications (address above)
Cost: $1.25

Theory and Practice of Back Massage by Frank Nicolas
New York: Milady Press, 1979

The New Massage by Gordon Inkeles
New York: Putnam, 1980

Psychic Massage by Roberta Millar
New York: Harper and Row, 1979

CHAPTER 18

STRESS

There is little need to expound on the prevalence of stress in modern life. All of us fall victim to it at one time or another, and all of us know that its cumulative effects can be demoralizing if not downright debilitating. It is easy to say that the symptoms of stress arise entirely from psychological causes or entirely from physical causes. The truth is that the mind-body continuum is not divided up so easily. To get to the bottom of the stress dilemma one must consider both.

SELF-DIAGNOSIS OF STRESS

Simply described, stress is a series of psychophysiological tensions that, in total, have a weakening effect on the entire physical organism. Its causes are numerous. Stress can be triggered by money worries, arguments, a divorce, a death in the family, the loss of a job, the purchase of a house—or simply by the anticipation of any of these events. It can be the secondary result of a wide spectrum of diseases ranging from the flu to cancer. It can derive from a deep-seated neurosis, from superficial friction with coworkers, or from continual exposure to environmental hazards such as chemical pollutants or loud noises. Whatever its origins, chronic stress may lead to the development of headaches, ulcers, constipation, heart attacks, strokes, hypertension, and many other serious ailments.

The symptoms of stress vary widely from person to person and from situation to situation. However, certain symptoms are particularly common. These include:

- A general sense of muscular tightness and tension throughout the body, especially in the neck, shoulders, back, and stomach.
- A chronic inability to relax, to slow down, to let go.
- A sense of nameless worry, anxiety, fear, and uneasiness.
- Physical and mental restlessness.
- An inability to concentrate.
- Difficulty getting to sleep or staying asleep.
- Nightmares. Premature awakening.
- A tendency to become easily upset, impatient, or angry.
- Bowel troubles: diarrhea or constipation.

Stress is related to the "fight or flight" mechanism. When a signal of worry or fear is transmitted by the brain the body interprets it as "Danger!" All of its survival support systems are immediately activated: The blood circulation increases, the adrenal glands pour adrenalin into the bloodstream, the muscles tense and tighten, respiration rate speeds up, the heart beats quickly, the mind races to make split-second decisions. The body, in other words, is preparing to fight—or run—for its life.

This metabolic outburst is appropriate to physical threats but not to the psychological threats more common in modern life. Too many of these needless outpourings begin to weaken the body and result in the symptoms of stress: nervousness, tension, insomnia, restlessness, etc. After that come the more severe reactions: headaches, hysteria, ulcers, diarrhea, hypertension, and a host of other woes.

SELF-CARE FOR STRESS

Fortunately, of all the ailments cited in this book, stress is one of the easiest to self-treat and one of the first to respond to personal care. Below you will find a list of really efficient techniques that will reduce stress in your daily life. Not every technique is effective for every person, but you are sure to hit upon several that seem tailor-made.

1. *Exercise.* Regular exercise, either calisthenics or sports, is one of the best and most pleasurable methods for reducing stress. Various exercises that help reduce stress include aerobic exercises, dance classes, Marine Corps calisthenics, the Royal Canadian Air Force exercise plan, yoga, and tai chi. Tennis, basketball, swimming, racquetball, rowing, hiking, canoeing, handball, the

martial arts, and any other sport that stimulates the heart, quickens circulation, increases muscle tone and brings extra oxygen into the system will also have a relaxing effect. Give it a try for a solid month and see why stressed people so treasure their exercise time.

2. *Relaxation techniques.* Even in the midst of noise and confusion it is possible to relax. The trick is remembering to do it. Start by setting aside a few minutes every hour. Take several deep breaths, stretch your arms and legs, walk around, look out the window, think pleasant thoughts; then, if circumstances allow, sit down, close your eyes, and allow your body to relax entirely from head to toe.

The important thing is that you repeat this maneuver three, four, five, six times daily—and that you do it consistently every day. Relaxation efforts are cumulative. Three minutes now, three minutes later, and it all adds up. If you follow this routine carefully, you will find yourself considerably more relaxed at the end of the day.

Several formal relaxation systems are outlined in the chapter on headaches (see pages 39–58). Pay particular attention to the procedures for *Breathing Imagery* and *Self-suggestion.* See the section on technology and resources below for information on relaxation systems available on cassette tapes.

Here is an excellent method for inducing overall relaxation:

• Find a quiet place, away from all distractions. Sit silently for a minute or two, then close your eyes. Relax. Let your muscles unwind. Take ten slow, deep breaths.

• Imagine that your body is filled with water (i.e., tension) and that you intend to drain the water out through imaginary holes in your hands and feet. Start at the top of your head. Make a mental image of the water level as it slowly drains down from your forehead, down to your eyes, to your nose, your chin, your neck, your shoulders. Drain the water down each arm and out the fingers. Picture the water level dropping to your chest, stomach, groin, thighs, calves, and then flowing out through the imaginary holes on the bottoms of your feet. Picture yourself totally empty and utterly relaxed.

• Repeat the process. Notice that certain areas you de-tensed just a moment ago have tightened up again. Relax them. At each repetition you will feel increasingly relaxed and at peace.

3. *Hot and cold water therapy.* A neglected but effective method of reducing tension is to soak in a hot and/or cold tub once a

day for ten to fifteen minutes at a time (five minutes for a really cold bath). Hot water relaxes muscles; cold water stimulates them. Hot baths are an excellent way of winding down at the end of the day and reducing muscular tensions. Cold baths—the colder the better—have an amazingly invigorative effect, not just on the body but on the mind and emotions as well. For this reason they have been used for centuries to combat depression. *Warning:* If you are pregnant or suffer from heart problems or hypertension, consult your physician before using hot and cold water therapy.

4. *Acupressure.* Although acupressure is not a cure-all for tension, it can often be surprisingly helpful. Try stimulating the following acupressure points:

• Make a fist. Press the peak of the mound of flesh formed in the web between the base of the thumb and the knuckle of the index finger for fifteen seconds on each hand.

• Pull the middle and fourth toe on each foot, fifteen seconds each toe.

• Massage your hands, fingers, and wrists.

• Bend your arm toward your chest. Find the point in the crook of the arm where the inner bones of the elbow meet. Stimulate this point for fifteen seconds on each arm.

• Pull your earlobes smartly downward, fifteen seconds each lobe.

• On the palm, draw a line straight from the base of your little finger to the outside edge of your wrist. Stimulate this point for fifteen seconds each wrist.

• Massage the bend of your leg behind the knee.

5. *Vitamins.* Many people claim that vitamins can reduce the effects of stress. The most useful supplement is a B-complex vitamin (vitamin B has been called "the nerve vitamin"). Specific B vitamins for stress include B_1 (thiamine), B_6 (Pyridoxine) and pantothenic acid. Vitamin D, lecithin, and calcium lactate are also said to be helpful.

6. *Avoid caffeine.* Caffeine is a formidable stimulant, capable of producing extreme restlessness and depression in some people.

If you think caffeine may be causing or exacerbating stress, try cutting down slowly. Especially try eliminating it from your breakfast; it's then that the body is most susceptible to its effects. In many instances, a single cup taken in the late afternoon will have the same refreshing effect it has in the morning, but without giving you the heebie-jeebies. Don't forget that many soft drinks, especially colas, contain caffeine. Read the labels. If the drink is caffeine-free it will usually say so. Many prescription drugs and over-the-counter headache remedies (including Anacin and Excedrin) and decongestants (including Dristan) also contain caffeine, so read all labels carefully.

7. *Try natural sedatives.*

• Whenever you are feeling jittery, take a cup of camomile or hops tea. Both have been used for centuries to calm the nerves and to help induce restful sleep.

• An even stronger tea can be made by steeping a teaspoon of crushed valerian root in a cup of boiling water for fifteen minutes. Drink it with a dash of honey. Valerian root extract is sold at natural food stores and can be taken in large doses without side effects.

• Add four ounces of crushed valerian root to a quart of water. Let the mixture stand for a day, then boil it and add it to your bath water while the mixture is still hot. Soak in the tub for fifteen to twenty minutes.

• Make a soothing herbal tea by mixing:

> 1 teaspoon camomile flowers
> 3 teaspoons fennel seeds
> 2 teaspoons crushed valerian root
> 1 teaspoon dried peppermint leaves
> 1 teaspoon dried lavender flowers
> 3 teaspoons crushed milfoil

Steep this mixture in a pint of boiling water for fifteen minutes, sweeten it with a little honey, and drink when needed.

8. *Use biofeedback.* Based on the principle that our minds have the potential to command our involuntary physical functions (such as muscle tension), biofeedback is an extremely effective anti-stress device. (See the headache chapter for details on how biofeedback works and how it can be self-applied.)

9. *Pay attention to psychological needs.*

• Get organized. Postponed phone calls, letters not written, beds not made, materials not purchased, obligations not met, untidy environments, messy desks, all can have a subtle but very real stressful impact on a person's day. Keep checklists, calendars, schedules. Start the morning by reviewing your day's obligations and then methodically set out to fulfill them. Know your limits. Choose your priorities carefully and don't take on more work than you can handle. Guard against procrastination. Don't be afraid to say no.

• When you feel the urge, cry. Crying is a great way to relieve anxiety and to reduce psychological strain. When we hold back tears we hold tension in, too.

• Find a quiet place for yourself and visit it frequently. Tests have shown that stress levels are dramatically reduced when a person regularly schedules time out of the day to simply calm down.

• Develop a hobby. Outside interests are classic stress-reducers. It doesn't matter what they are: model ships, cooking, computers, ceramics, needlepoint, carpentry, poetry, etc. The point is to find an activity that distracts and calms the mind.

• Help other people. The greater our problems, the more self-centered we become. Joining a community-help organization, doing charity or hospital work, simply spending more time helping one's friends, family or neighbors are all excellent specifics against alienation.

• Share your problems. Suffering from symptoms of stress does not mean that you are "sick" or "troubled," only that you are temporarily distracted and that you may need guidance. Such help comes from many different sources. Professional therapists can, of course, be excellent resources as are understanding clergymen, social workers, and counselors. Group therapy sessions are helpful for many people. So are church, civic, and local self-help organizations. And don't forget the value of family and good friends. The important thing is to talk about your problem and to defuse the tension.

Technology, Resources, Aids, and Services

1. *A system of progressive muscle relaxation exercises conjoined with mental imagery* developed by James Lipton, a psychologist at the University of Texas Health Center in Dallas. This system has received a good deal of publicity in the past year. For information on how it works and where you can learn it, contact James Lipton, Ph.D., University of Texas Health Science Center, 5323 Harry Hines Blvd., Dallas, TX 75235.

2. The *cassette tape* "Letting Go of Stress" is available from *The Medical Self-Care Catalog*, P.O. Box 999, Pt. Reyes, CA 94956.

3. *Tapes to aid self-hypnosis* are available from:
Creative Dimensions
P.O. Box 1056-N
Aptos, CA 95001

Tapes
P.O. Box 6414
Santa Barbara, CA 93106
(write for free catalog)

Lifeworks
24A Ohayo Mountain Rd.
Woodstock, NY 12498
4. For information on a doctor-tested *antistress kit* designed to train patients in stress management, send $1.00 (refundable) to:
Healthworks Medical Group
31582 So. Coast Hwy.
South Laguna, CA 92677
5. A remarkably wide line of *materials especially designed to relieve stress* is offered by the Conscious Living Foundation, P.O. Box 9, Drain, OR 97435, (503)836-2358. The Foundation sends out a bimonthly newsmagazine to showcase their latest products.
6. *Relaxation video tapes* that portray peaceful images such as a crackling fire or a tropical fish tank are available in VHS or Beta for around $25 each from Relax Video, 132 West 72nd Street, New York, NY 10025, (212) 496-4400.
7. A company called Day-Timers, Allentown, PA 18001, offers a *free catalog filled with time-saving, time-planning and organizational devices,* all of which can help reduce daily stress at home and at work.
8. A company called New Harbinger Publications, 2200 Adeline, Suite 305, Oakland, CA 94607, specializes in *books and tapes dedicated to relaxation.* Included are *The Relaxation & Stress Reduction Workbook, Relaxation & Stress Reduction Cassette Tapes,* and *Thoughts & Feelings: The Art of Cognitive Stress Intervention.*
9. The *Stressmap* is a self-scoring questionnaire that identifies personal stress factors on twenty-one different scales. Its self-charting system of stress patterns also allows users to pinpoint central sources of tension in their lives. A workbook is included. Available from *The Medical Self-Care Catalog* (address in number 1).
10. The *Ten-Minute Stress Manager* is a cassette tape developed for people in high-pressure social positions (students, executives, etc.) to take at intervals during the day as a quick antidote

to stress. It costs $10.95 plus $1.00 postage from *The Medical Self-Care Catalog* (address in number 1).

11. Valuable *books* and *pamphlets* on dealing with stress include:

Stress Without Distress
by Hans Selye
Philadelphia: Lippincott, 1974

How to Get Control of Your Time and Life
by Alan Lakein
New York: New American Library, 1973

Managing Stress by John Blakenship, Linda Brown, Deborah Hall,
Grace Miller, and Jerry Steinmetz
Palo Alto: Bull Publishing Co., 1980

The Relaxation & Stress Reduction Workbook by
Martha Davis, Elizabeth Eshelman, and Matthew McKay
Richmond, CA: New Harbinger Publications,
1980

Getting Organized by Stephanie Winston
New York: Warner Books, 1978

A Doctor Discusses Learning How to Live
with Nervous Tension
Milex Products, Inc.
5915 Northwest Hwy.
Chicago, IL 60631
$2.50

Tensions—and How to Master Them
Public Affairs Committee, Inc.
381 Park Ave.
New York, NY 10016
$.50

How to Deal with Your Tensions
Mental Health Association National Headquarters
1800 North Kent St.
Arlington, VA 22209
Free

CHAPTER 19

HYPERTENSION (HIGH BLOOD PRESSURE)

High blood pressure, or hypertension, is due to an increase in the pressure of blood as it pulses against the walls of the arteries. Both cause and forerunner of many serious diseases including stroke, kidney disease, and heart attack, hypertension is a troublesome ailment to pinpoint. Its symptoms are often vague, unless blood pressure equipment is used, and sometimes undetectable. Therefore, it is imperative that any man or woman over thirty years old have access to blood pressure monitoring equipment— either at home or on a public machine such as those found in drugstores—and that he or she become familiar with its use. Information on purchasing and operating this equipment is given below.

WHO GETS HIGH BLOOD PRESSURE?

To a certain extent, hypertension sufferers can be picked out before symptoms of the disease begin to manifest themselves. Statistically speaking, you are a low-risk candidate if you answer yes to three or less of the questions in the test below; a moderate risk if you answer yes to four questions or less; and a high risk if you answer yes to six questions or more.

SELF-TEST FOR HYPERTENSION
- Do you smoke?
- Do you drink above the moderation level (one to two drinks per day)?
- Is there a history of hypertension in your family?
- Are you excitable, irritable, and easily angered?
- Are you overweight?
- Are you black?
- Do you suffer from regular symptoms of stress?
- Do you find it difficult to relax?
- Do you drink more than three cups of coffee a day?
- Do you go without exercising for long periods of time?
- Does your diet regularly contain a number of foods high in fat and sugar?
- Do you eat meat at least once a day and sometimes twice?
- Do you use birth control pills?
- Do you have kidney problems?
- Do you regularly take tranquilizers, over-the-counter cold preparations, asthma medications, or acetaminophen?

The so-called Type A Personality is most susceptible to high blood pressure. Although we are all mixtures of sanguine and choleric characteristics, the Type A tends to be especially prone to impatience and stress. He or she can be characterized by a number of traits: restlessness, an insistence on perfectionism in oneself and others, compulsive talking, workaholism, a tendency to become easily angered and upset, a preoccupation with time, an extremely competitive status-conscious nature, a desire to dominate and control all situations, and a tendency to take on too much at once. We all know the type—and we all have a bit of it within us.

The quality of a person's life is generally the decisive factor in the development of hypertension. In some instances, it is true, blood pressure is elevated for no apparent reason, even among those who lead wholesome, quiet lives. More often, however, problems result from poor living habits and carelessness about one's health. At the top of the list of harmful influences are smoking, heavy drinking, overweight, stress, and a family history of high blood pressure. Blacks, particularly men, have a very high incidence of hypertension. Black men who live in urban and suburban environments have an especially high risk. Diabetes sufferers are also extremely prone to blood pressure problems.

Do people with high blood pressure have a greater risk of early death than those with a normal count? The answer is a resounding yes. The largest study ever done on the subject, carried out in Framingham, Massachusetts, revealed that people with high blood pressure (especially a diastolic over 95) are *three times as prone to heart attacks, four times more likely to have heart failure, and seven times more susceptible to stroke than those with normal blood pressure.*

Happily, there is a bright side: In many cases hypertension can be controlled with proper treatment.

How to Take Your Own Blood Pressure

The first step in controlling blood pressure is learning to take your own blood pressure readings.

You will need three tools:

1. A *sphygmomanometer* to measure the actual blood pressure.

2. A *stethoscope* to hear the pulse.

3. A *record chart* (which you can make yourself) to record the results.

The basic sphygmomanometer unit consists of a cloth cuff (encasing an inflatable bladder) to wrap around the arm, a digital read-out device or a mercury gauge with scale markings to measure the pressure, bulb to inflate the cuff, and a control valve to deflate the cuff. The stethoscope can be a cheap model; you won't need anything fancy for this purpose. Some of the more expensive sphygmomanometers come with a battery-operated stethoscope mechanism built in.

As far as your blood pressure record goes, you can keep it yourself: Draw a grid, then mark off areas for the date, the location where the blood pressure was taken, the time of day, the patient's posture (sitting, lying down), the actual pressure measurements, and any other pertinent information (such as medications currently being taken). A typical chart might look like the one on page 214.

1. Sit in a chair or lie flat on your back. Wrap the inflatable cuff around either arm directly above the elbow. Fasten the cuff firmly but not painfully tight.

2. Insert the tips of the stethoscope into your ears and place

Date	Location	Time	Posture	Pressure	Other Pertinent Information

the diaphragm of the stethoscope under the cuff directly over the brachial artery (this major vessel runs down the center of the inner arm and over the inner bend of the elbow). You can locate the pulse under the cuff with your fingers first. Be careful not to tap the diaphragm of the stethoscope with your fingers or knock it against a hard surface while it is in your ears. Even a light tap will be amplified many times and can damage the ears.

3. Inflate the cuff. Listening with the stethoscope, you will notice that as the cuff inflates, the pulse sound continues for some time, then suddenly disappears. Carefully note the point on the measuring gauge at which this cut-off takes place, then inflate the bladder another thirty mmHg. Now, turn off the valve and slowly deflate the cuff, listening carefully for the return sound of the pulse. The instant you hear it, note the reading on the measuring device. This reading indicates your *systolic pressure;* that is, the pressure of your heart during a contraction or beat.

4. Continue to let the air slowly out of the cuff until the sound of the pulse disappears again. Note the reading at this point also. This reading indicates *diastolic pressure,* the pressure of your heart as it rests between beats. When recording blood pressure, the systolic pressure is always written on top of the fraction; the diastolic below, like this:

$$\frac{130}{80} = \frac{\text{SYSTOLIC}}{\text{DIASTOLIC}}$$

5. Release the rest of the air from the cuff and remove it. You might want to take your blood pressure two or three times and then record an average figure. Note that several factors can raise blood pressure reading. These include:

- Heavy drinking
- Sexual arousal
- Emotional arousal (such as watching an exciting movie)
- Heavy smoking
- Use of drugs and medications
- Exercise and busy activities
- Intense nervousness
- Stimulants such as caffeine, cold pills, or amphetamines
- Strong anger or upset
- A recent intake of salt

6. The normal range for systolic pressure is between 100 to 140. The normal range for diastolic pressure is between 60 and 90. Generally speaking, as a person gets older his or her systolic blood pressure rises. It is usual for an infant to register a systolic of around 80, a child to measure around 100, a teenager around 120, and an adult over 40 around 135. For men and women over 40, anything up to 160 is generally considered within the non-dangerous range. As to the diastolic, anything over 90 is usually considered cause for concern.

How to Take Your Pulse

Another method of keeping watch on the cardiac and circulatory system is by monitoring the pulse. A pulse represents the wave of distension that occurs within an artery each time the heart beats. Count it by placing your index and middle finger (never your thumb, which has a pulse of its own) on the crease of the wrist below the thumb. With a stop watch or second hand, count the number of beats in a minute. A normal resting pulse range will vary according to a person's age. Normal pulse range for different age groups includes:

Newborns	90–170
Infants	90–160
Young children	80–115
Older children	70–110
Teenagers	65–100
Adults	60– 90

If your adult resting pulse is below 60 or above 90 to 100, it is best to speak with a doctor. An adult resting pulse that holds steady over 100 qualifies as *tachycardia* (or rapid heart beat) and should receive immediate attention. An increased pulse can be a warning sign of anemia or overactive thyroid and many other illnesses, a decreased pulse a possible indication of kidney trouble or an electrical problem within the heart itself. Other things you should know about your pulse include:

• A fever tends to increase the pulse, sometimes by as much as 10 beats per minute for each degree.

• The pulse can be increased by emotional upset, anger, grief, or exhaustion.

• Both blood pressure and pulse are lowest upon waking in the morning and highest in the late afternoon and evening. A gradual rise during the day is normal.

• A person's pulse is not the same at all times, even if taken under similar circumstances. In fact, the pulse varies from moment to moment, as does blood pressure, and differences in readings are by no means cause for alarm.

• When taking your pulse, look for a steady, regular beat. Skipped beats, intermittent pauses, pounding pulses, a pulse that is difficult to detect, a pulse that beats with irregular intensity (now hard, now soft) may indicate abnormalities and should be called to the attention of a doctor.

THE COLD PRESSOR TEST

Yet another way to monitor the health of your blood pressure is with a simple test called the *cold pressor test*. Take your normal blood pressure and record the count. Then fill a bowl three-quarters full of ice water. Roll up your sleeves, attach a sphygmomanometer to one arm, and immerse the other in the bowl of water. Allow the hand to remain in the water for approximately a minute, then remove it.

Wait several minutes, then take your blood pressure again. If the pressure level rises more than thirty points above the original reading within the first five minutes, this can be an early warning sign of hypertension. Appropriate steps should be taken.

If, after removing your hand from the ice water, the blood pressure has risen *less* than five points in a half hour, if the pressure refuses to return to its normal level, or if the test causes chest discomfort of any kind, there is a possibility of atherosclerosis, and a consultation with a physician is advisable.

Note: If you are being treated for high blood pressure, or if you have real or suspected heart problems, you should consult your physician before taking this test.

SELF-DIAGNOSIS OF HIGH BLOOD PRESSURE

One of the insidious things about high blood pressure is that it is so easy to overlook or misdiagnose. The symptoms, if they do occur, tend to resemble those of lesser ailments. Most of the time *there are simply no symptoms at all,* and for this reason hypertension has been called "the silent killer." However, with alert observation and attention to details, the telltale signs can be spotted when they do occur. Besides a high systolic/diastolic reading, general symptoms of high blood pressure include:

- Headaches (especially when waking up in the morning)
- Ringing in the ears
- Frequent nosebleeds
- Dizziness
- Exhaustion

These symptoms tend to come and go when they appear at all. In the long run, the best diagnostic tool for hypertension is the stethoscope and sphygmomanometer.

SELF-CARE FOR HIGH BLOOD PRESSURE

As with many chronic ailments, there are two routes to improvement, prevention, and therapy. For maximum results, preventive techniques and therapeutic techniques should be used together as part of one overall healing program. Preventive measures are designed for people in the early stages of hypertension and for those who wish to reduce the risk of this ailment by practicing common-sense techniques. Individuals with extremely high blood pressure and/or those with heart conditions of any kind will, of course, profit from these techniques, but such people should invariably be under a doctor's care.

1. *Monitor your diet.* Most experts now believe that a direct link exists between hypertension and diet, and that by eliminating certain foods and adding others, improvements can be made. Important dietary modifications include:

- Cut way down on your use of sodium chloride—salt. There seems to be a direct connection between overuse of salt and increased blood pressure. If you're going to use salt in any quantity, there is some evidence that natural sea salt may be better for you than the commercially processed kind. Note, too, that salt is "hidden" in many over-the-counter medicines, as well as in many commercial food products such as potato chips, pretzels, mustard, most canned soups, soft drinks, most sausages and lunch meats, many canned and frozen vegetables, most fast foods, etc. If you're cutting down on salt, it's a wise idea to cultivate the habit of reading labels before you buy. Note, too, that monosodium glutamate (MSG) acts on the blood pressure in much the same way as salt and that it is often routinely added to the food at Chinese restaurants.

• Cut down on high-fat foods. They promote cholesterol buildup and can make you overweight, two principal causes of hypertension. High-fat foods include oils, lard, dairy products (especially cheese, cream, and butter), all red meats, pork, sausage, fried foods, potato chips, nuts, ice cream, pies and cakes, rich sauces, etc.

• Eliminate caffeine. Foods and beverages containing caffeine have some negative effect on the blood pressure, although just how much varies from person to person. To measure your own reactions, take your blood pressure and pulse, have a cup of coffee (or tea, or a caffeinated soft drink), then measure your pressure and pulse again. Have a second cup several hours later and take another reading. Do this for a week to see how much, if at all, caffeine affects your cardiac system.

• Drink only in moderation. While light drinking (one drink a day) probably has few adverse effects on hypertension, moderate to heavy drinking (more than three drinks a day) wreaks havoc on the blood pressure. Besides contributing empty calories, even two or three drinks can raise the systolic reading several points. Like many factors, alcohol affects people in different ways and you may wish to experiment on your own to establish how much of the substance your blood pressure comfortably tolerates. When you are drinking socially, keep a check on the snacks that invariably accompany cocktails. Peanuts, chips, and pretzels are all loaded with salt.

• Increase your intake of high-fiber foods and natural carbohydrates. Foods combining the two include unrefined wheat, oat and corn products, fresh vegetables (especially beans, lentils, parsnips, peas, potatoes with their skins, yams, sweet potatoes, cabbage, tomatoes, carrots, and beets), and fresh fruits (especially avocados, berries, apples, figs, mangoes, pineapples, and pears). Small amounts of a bran supplement may also help, especially oat bran, which can apparently also reduce cholesterol levels. It is probably not a coincidence that in many countries where the diet includes large amounts of high-fiber foods, hypertension and cardiac problems are rare.

• Increase your intake of foods rich in potassium. People with hypertension are often placed on diuretic medications, which cause substantial potassium loss in some people. This deficiency can be compensated for by taking potassium supplements, but it is better to supply it naturally. Apples, apple juice, asparagus, beans, Brussels sprouts, apricots, bananas, dates, oranges, orange juice, radishes, cabbage, fresh corn, potatoes, prunes, peppers, and peas contain a lot of potassium.

• Cut down on sugar and sweets. There is some laboratory indication—conjectural perhaps—that a high intake of sugar products over a prolonged period increases one's risk of arterial disease.

• Eat more garlic and onions. Garlic is believed to have a dilating effect on the walls of the arteries. Onions contain significant amounts of prostaglandin A1, a hormonelike chemical that helps lower blood pressure. Garlic can be taken as a daily supplement in capsule form available at most natural foods stores.

• Eat less meat. A group of Harvard researchers discovered in 1974 that blood pressure levels for vegetarians were considerably lower than those for meat eaters. When the vegetarians added meat to their diets, blood pressure rates rose accordingly. Experiment with this one on your own and see what happens. If you're going to become a vegetarian, make sure you arm yourself with the proper nutritional information and/or the advice of a nutritionist. You'll have to learn how to balance your carbohydrates, specifically grains and legumes, in order to make up for the loss of certain complete proteins found only in meat. An excellent book on this subject, reprinted many times, is *Diet for a Small Planet* by Frances Moore Lappe (New York: Ballantine Books, 1971).

2. *Exercise.* There are a number of options to choose from, including regular calisthenics, aerobic exercise and dance, walking, jogging, yoga, tai chi, and the martial arts. Rowing, biking, canoeing, tennis, and swimming are also good choices. In general, *isotonic* exercises such as weight lifting are not recommended for high blood pressure sufferers, while *isometric* exercises like biking, swimming, and aerobic exercises are highly recommended. You should supplement a regular exercise program with small helpful activities: walk to work; use the stairs instead of

the elevator; mow the lawn instead of hiring someone; carry the groceries instead of putting them in a cart; try standing instead of sitting.

The minimum amount of exercise needed to make a difference in blood pressure is about thirty minutes to an hour a day three times a week. Far better is an hour a day if you can find the time. Make regular exercise a *positive addiction,* something your very cells yearn for. Exercise benefits the whole body by increasing circulation and lowering cholesterol. It is especially beneficial to the cardiovascular system, which governs blood pressure. Exercise also promotes well being and increases self-esteem. So get yourself a complete checkup, then find an exercise program that suits your age, endurance capacities, time, and temperament—and stick with it.

3. *Slim down.* Overweight is one of the major contributing factors to hypertension, especially for people who are naturally heavy-set (there is some evidence that short, stocky people are more prone to hypertension than tall, thin people). Slim down, but beware of the latest miracle diets and overnight weight-loss plans, and by all means stay away from appetite suppressors and weight-loss pills (most of them will *raise* your blood pressure). Be aware, too, that in many cases proper eating and correct living will result in effortless weight loss. Excess poundage is often produced less by overeating than by poor eating. A diet high in refined carbohydrates, confections, butter fats, sugar, salt, fatty meats, and alcohol is a sure ticket to obesity, while a diet that consists of fresh fruits and vegetables, whole-grain breads and cereals, pure water, and small portions of lean meats practically ensures slimness. A consultation with a nutritional counselor may be helpful.

How much you should weigh depends on your build. The following chart provides representative weights:

MEN

Height	Small Build	Medium	Large
5'1"	112–120	118–129	126–141
5'2"	115–123	121–133	129–144
5'3"	118–126	124–136	132–148
5'4"	121–129	127–139	135–152
5'5"	124–133	130–143	138–156
5'6"	128–137	134–147	142–161
5'7"	132–141	138–152	147–166

5'8"	136–145	142–156	151–170
5'9"	140–150	146–160	155–174
5'10"	144–154	150–165	159–179
5'11"	148–158	154–170	164–184
6'0"	152–162	158–175	168–189
6'1"	156–167	162–180	173–194
6'2"	160–171	167–185	178–199
6'3"	164–175	172–190	182–204

WOMEN

Height	Small Build	Medium	Large
4'8"	92–98	96–107	104–119
4'9"	94–101	98–110	106–122
4'10"	96–104	101–113	109–125
4'11"	99–107	104–116	112–128
5'0"	102–110	107–119	115–131
5'1"	105–113	110–122	118–134
5'2"	108–116	113–126	121–138
5'3"	111–119	116–130	125–142
5'4"	114–123	120–135	129–146
5'5"	118–127	124–139	133–150
5'6"	122–131	128–143	137–154
5'7"	126–135	132–147	141–158
5'8"	130–140	136–151	145–163
5'9"	134–144	140–155	149–168
5'10"	138–148	144–159	153–173

4. *Stop smoking.* Smoking is a major risk factor for both the heart and the lungs, and a one-pack-a-day habit more than *doubles* your chances of developing high blood pressure and *triples* your chances of a heart attack. Smoking interferes with the proper clotting of the blood, slows circulation, disturbs heart rhythms, and is probably a direct cause of hardening of the arteries. Not to mention all the nasty things it does to the lungs. Stop now.

5. *Try biofeedback.* This high-tech healing method has helped thousands of people reduce their blood pressure and gain some control over stress. Many clinics around the country specialize in biofeedback learning procedures, and biofeedback equipment is readily available for home use. It is often used in conjunction with self-hypnosis and/or meditation. For information on how biofeedback works and how you can use it, consult the chapter on headaches.

6. *Nutritional supplements*. It has recently been established that in many instances both lecithin and fish oil are useful in reducing blood pressure. Try taking lecithin capsules in doses of two capsules three times a day (1200 milligrams) along with two capsules, three times a day of the fish oil MaxEPA. Both preparations are available at any good natural foods store, and in some cases they seem to bring astonishingly good results. Note, however, that it takes approximately a month before these results become apparent in the blood pressure rates themselves.

WHEN TO CALL THE DOCTOR

In many instances mild cases of hypertension can be fully controlled by following the suggestions listed above. If these do not work, or if you have any reason to believe that you are suffering from cardiac problems along with high blood pressure, consult a physician immediately.

TECHNOLOGY, RESOURCES, AIDS, AND SERVICES

1. *Home blood pressure monitoring kits* are stocked by many drugstores and electronic gadget shops, and are also available through high-tech mail order houses like The Sharper Image, 680 Davis St., San Francisco, CA 94111, (800) 344-4444. (The Sharper Image Catalog offers one model called the Lumiscope Blood Pressure/Pulse Monitor that automatically takes your blood pressure and, via thermal printer, gives an immediate printout of your systolic and diastolic pressure and pulse rate. It costs about $150.) Blood pressure measurement machines can also be found in drugstores, supermarkets, restaurants, and malls.

2. *A wristwatch pulse counter* comes equipped with an upper and lower limit alarm you can program and a finger tip and earlobe sensor to monitor pulse directly. It also contains a conventional watch and a stop watch. It costs around $40 from Creative Health Products, 10 Saddle Ridge Rd., Plymouth, MI 48170, (800) 742-4478.

3. A number of *antistress mechanisms and devices* are available in retail stores and through the mail. For a thorough listing, consult the technology and resources section in the chapter on stress.

4. *Exercise machines and devices* are useful for hypertension sufferers, especially those whose exercise space is restricted. Consult the technology and resources section in the neck and back chapter for information.

5. *Free blood pressure screening programs* are offered throughout the country by the American Heart Association. For information, request the booklet *Heart Facts* from your local chapter or write to their main office at 7320 Greenville Ave., Dallas, TX 75231. A similar service is offered by Northwestern Mutual Life Insurance Company. Contact local agents or write to their national office at 720 E. Wisconsin, Milwaukee, WI 53202.

6. Useful books and pamphlets on hypertension include:

Special Recipes for Low-Sodium Diets
General Foods Kitchens
250 North St.
White Plains, NY
Free

Understanding High Blood Pressure
Searle Laboratories
Searle Educational Systems
P.O. Box 5110
Chicago, IL 60680
Attn.: Pat Heineman A3W
Free: Booklet #6107

High Blood Pressure: Medicine for the Layman
Office of Clinical Reports and Inquiries
Bldg. 10, Rm. 1A05
National Institutes of Health
Bethesda, MD 20205
Free: Booklet #NIH 79-1803

If You're Black, Here Are Some Facts You Should Know About High Blood Pressure
National High Blood Pressure Education Program
c/o National Heart, Lung and Blood Institute
Public Inquiries and Reports Branch
9000 Rockville Pike
Bethesda, MD 20014
Free: Booklet #NIH 78-1057

High Blood Pressure: A Positive Approach
Boehringer Ingelheim, Ltd.
90 East Ridge
P.O. Box 368
Ridgefield, CT 06877
Free

High Blood Pressure and How to Control It
American Heart Association
7320 Greenville Ave.
Dallas, TX 75231
Free
7. Organizations that will provide information and referrals for hypertension sufferers include:
American Heart Association
(address in number 6.)

Citizens for the Treatment of High Blood Pressure
1101 17th St., N.W.
Suite 608
Washington, DC 20036

Institute of Hypertension Studies
Institute of Hypertension School of Research
7032 Farnsworth
Detroit, MI 48211

CHAPTER 20

ARTHRITIS

Arthritis—the name literally means "inflammation"—is one of the most widespread and painful of all nonfatal degenerative diseases. Primarily a disease of the joints, arthritis is caused by a variety of factors including bacterial infection, endocrine gland secretions, physical wear and tear, and emotional stress. Although predominant among older people, it can strike at any age, from birth onward. While it is painful, and can be disabling and even occasionally disfiguring, early diagnosis and proper care will usually keep its effects under control.

SELF-DIAGNOSIS OF ARTHRITIS

The most common form of arthritis and the one that people over forty-five usually suffer from is *osteoarthritis*. This disorder erodes the cartilage that surrounds and cushions the joints. The cartilage eventually wears so thin that the bones, unprotected, grind against each other, producing pain and swelling. Some erosion occurs in all of us throughout the years, but osteoarthritis speeds up the process and makes it more painful. In effect, it is a kind of premature aging in which the joints age faster than the tissue that surrounds them.

Other common forms of arthritis are gout, bursitis, and rheumatoid arthritis, which attacks the connective tissue *throughout* the body. These conditions are considerably less responsive to self-care than osteoarthritis and usually require intense medical supervision.

The symptoms of osteoarthritis include:

• Pain in the joints, especially the hips, spine, knees, and ankles. Possible swelling of small finger joints.

• Pain when the joints are moving (if the joints do not hurt when they are in motion, then the condition is probably not arthritis).

• Possible worsening of pain in damp weather and during emotional stress.

• Stiffness and redness of the afflicted joints.

• Creaking or cracking of the afflicted joints.

Osteoarthritis does not usually produce constitutional symptoms such as weight loss or high fever. It can occasionally cause joint disability or deformity, and even render a joint entirely immobile. Because arthritis tends to be hereditary, you should be concerned if you have a family history of this problem and suspicious symptoms begin to develop.

SELF-CARE FOR ARTHRITIS

As with many disorders, there are both conventional and unconventional approaches to treatment. Although you should be wary of fantastic claims, a wide range of unorthodox therapies seems to have helped osteoarthritis sufferers through the years. Several of the most highly regarded of these will be included below in the section on conventional therapies.

Conventional Therapies

1. *Aspirin.* Simple aspirin is still the best over-the-counter medication for arthritis pain. For some people it works better than prescription drugs, and in all but the worst cases it reduces swelling and controls pain. Take two tablets every four hours, preferably after meals. (For further information on how aspirin works, its substitutes, and side effects, see the chapter on headaches.)

If your arthritis is especially painful and you find yourself continually digging into the aspirin bottle for relief, consult a health care specialist about its proper dosage and possible side effects.

2. *Heat applications.* Standard heat treatments include:
• Electric heating pad

- Infrared heat lamp
- Hot water bottle
- Contrast baths (alternating hot and cold baths)
- Whirlpool bath
- Hot tub
- Hot compresses

Different techniques work best for different people. Lamps, compresses, and pads are excellent for localized aches; contrast baths for the hands and feet; full body baths for general relief and overall relaxation.

Heat works best as a preventive measure and should never be used when arthritis is acute and severely painful (it may cause the afflicted joint to swell and ache even more). Use heat applications for twenty to thirty minutes per session. If the treatments seem to cause pain, you should try: 1) using less heat, 2) using a different source of heat, or 3) shortening the period of application. Only if all of these suggestions fail should you abandon this method entirely.

Note

If you have diabetes, a weak heart, high blood pressure, or poor circulation, check with a health-care professional before using heat applications for arthritis.

---

3. *Exercise.* Arthritis impedes the mobility of afflicted joints. Exercising the frozen joints and related muscle groups daily will help you regain lost mobility. Aside from moving the joints through what would ordinarily be their full range of motion, you should perform the appropriate exercises given below.

Do these range of motion exercises twice a day at first, in the morning and at night. They may be uncomfortable initially, but unless your reaction is severe (with swelling, muscle tremors, and intense pain), keep trying; in a week or so they will become easier. When you become comfortable with the exercises, you can repeat them up to five times a day. Properly and regularly done, they will help restore mobility, elasticity, and strength. The following are a set of specific movements for the joints most commonly attacked by osteoarthritis.

EXERCISES FOR THE SHOULDERS:

1. Starting with your arms at your sides, swing your arms in wide circles, both clockwise and counterclockwise. Work each day to increase the size of the circles.

2. Let your arms hang loosely at your sides. Swing them forward and then back as far as they will go for several minutes.

3. Move each shoulder in small, comfortable circles.

4. Lie flat on your back, your hands clasped behind your neck. Slowly and carefully, without forcing anything, raise your head, neck, and arms to a comfortable height, keeping your back flat on the floor. Hold for a moment, then release. Repeat several times.

5. Stand straight with both arms hanging loosely at your sides. Raise your arms slowly and clasp them over your head. Release and bring your arms back to your sides. Repeat the movement, this time bringing the *backs* of the hands together over your head. Alternate several times.

EXERCISES FOR THE HIPS:

1. Lie on your back. Keeping your legs straight, raise the right leg as high as it will comfortably go. Lower it, then raise the left leg. Alternate several times.

2. Stand up. Keeping your knees straight, bend forward and try to touch your toes. Remain in this position for several moments, then straighten up slowly, lower back first.

3. Lie on your right side. Carefully raise your left leg as high as it will comfortably go, keeping it straight and pointing your toe forward. Lower the leg and repeat several times. Switch sides.

4. Stand up. Raise your right knee to your chest. Hold it there for a moment, release, then repeat with your left knee. Alternate several times.

EXERCISES FOR THE KNEES:

1. Kneel on your good knee with your arthritic knee carefully bent in front of you, foot flat on the floor. Bend your chest toward the arthritic knee as far as you can comfortably go, then raise it again. Repeat several times. Do not do this exercise if both knees are arthritic.

2. Lie flat on your back. Pull your right knee to your chest, squeeze it carefully, then release. Repeat with the left knee. Alternate several times.

3. Lie flat on your back and do the bicycle exercise until you feel pleasantly tired.

4. Sit in a chair. Raise your right knee as high as it will comfortably go, then lower it slowly. Repeat with the left knee. Alternate several times.

EXERCISES FOR THE WRISTS:

1. Extend your arms in front of you. Revolve both wrists in gentle circles, clockwise and counterclockwise. Repeat several times.

2. Extend your arms in front of you with the palms parallel to the floor. Flex and straighten your wrists several times.

3. Open and close your hands. Repeat several times.

4. Revolve your hand as if you were turning a water faucet on and off. Continue for several minutes.

5. Fan out your fingers, tense them for several moments, then relax and close your fingers. Repeat several times.

6. Shake your hands, allowing them to bob freely on your wrists. Let them go limp. Repeat several times.

EXERCISES FOR THE NECK:

1. Lie on your back. Tightening your neck muscles, bring your head up slowly until your chin touches your chest. Drop your head slowly to the floor. Repeat several times.

2. Stand in a comfortable position. Slowly turn your head to the left as far as you can. Return to center and move it to the right. Repeat several times.

3. Stand in a comfortable position. Slowly revolve your head in a circle, letting the weight of your head carry your neck through its full revolution. Repeat for several minutes.

4. Imagine that you have a pencil attached to your chin. Draw small circles, clockwise and counterclockwise, on an imaginary pad in front of you. Repeat several times.

EXERCISES FOR THE FINGERS:

1. Crumple a large piece of newspaper into a ball. Repeat several times using fresh newspaper.

2. Place your hand flat on a table. Raise and lower each finger, one at a time. Repeat several times.

3. Move each finger in small circles, both directions.

4. With your fingers straight and together bend them up and down at the knuckles as if waving good-bye.

5. Squeeze a rubber ball whenever you can.

A few pointers on arthritis exercises:

- Don't strain or push yourself. You are not training for an athletic event. Do *not* go for the burn!
- Be regular. Sudden and extreme exercise interspersed with periods of inactivity is almost useless, and may even be harmful. Do your exercises faithfully every day.
- Apply heat to the afflicted area before you do your exercises.
- General exercise can be helpful, too. Jogging or aerobics are obviously inappropriate for arthritic ankles or hips, but swimming, rowing, calisthenics, yoga, and other exercise can help. A good form of exercise can usually be found for practically any arthritic condition. Finally, a note of caution: If you already dislike making the effort to exercise, don't let arthritis become an excuse for dropping it completely. Exercise is too important a part of anyone's preventive health regimen to neglect.

4. *Massage.* Massage is another old standby for arthritis. It can be self-applied to accessible areas like the arms, legs, and neck. For unreachable areas like the back, you will have to recruit another person's services. Because massage relaxes the afflicted joints, brings fresh, healing blood to relieve stiffness, and makes tissues more elastic and pliable, it helps restore some of the joint's mobility.

In general, it is best to apply heat to the arthritic joint immediately before massage. Do *not* rub the joint itself. Knead and rub the surrounding area with a gentle, rhythmic motion. Use the thumbs and fingers to knead, the heels of the hands to press and stroke. If the massage becomes painful, do not continue. Use massage oil, talcum powder, or peanut oil (peanut oil is reputed to have a therapeutic effect on arthritic joints) to reduce friction. A ten-minute session every day or every other day should produce marked results. *Under no circumstances* massage a joint that is swollen, inflamed, or acutely painful. Massage is a preventive technique and should be used *only* when arthritis is quiescent.

5. *Rest.* Get plenty of rest *and* rest the afflicted joint. Take as many breaks as you can during the day and avoid stressing the painful joint. Rest does not necessarily mean complete immobility. Although severely arthritic persons are sometimes confined to bed, most people with osteoarthritis should take short breaks and more or less continue about their business.

6. *Other aids:*
• Keep all arthritic joints warm and well protected from cold and dampness, which are sure to exacerbate arthritis.
• Keep your weight down. Excess weight adds to the burden on the joints. Losing a few pounds will help, especially if the arthritis afflicts a weight-bearing joint such as the ankle or knee.
• Swimming and water exercises in general are excellent for people with arthritis.
• Use mechanical supports and aids whenever possible. There is an entire industry devoted to self-help products for arthritis sufferers, and you might as well take advantage of it. Special scissors, easy-grip doorknobs, slicing aids, pillows, back supports, long-handled dustpans, hand exercisers, dressing sticks, and a lot more are available on special order from most health product supply houses. Addresses are listed below in the technology and resources section.
• Properly distributing pressure on arthritic joints is a prerequisite to their healing and well-being. Do not place too much weight on a single joint—learn to distribute the weight over as wide an area as possible.
• Maintain good posture. Poor posture leads to fatigue, which worsens arthritis. Sleep flat on your back, and use no more than a thin pillow under your head. Again, it's better for the back to raise the knees slightly. When you reach down to pick something up, bend your knees. Walk with your back straight, push off from the balls of your feet. Don't slump. When reading or watching television, sit in a firm chair and keep your back straight. Avoid crossing your legs. Plant your feet on the floor. Avoid recliners and overstuffed furniture.
• Tension, worry, and depression seem to worsen arthritis. See the chapter on stress for practical methods of reducing tension.

Unconventional Therapies

More quackery has been associated with arthritis than perhaps any other medical disorder. Nevertheless, so-called unorthodox healing techniques have been used for centuries, and many of them form the very backbone of alternate healing systems. Below are a few of the more popular methods.
1. *Diet.* Few medical issues are so hotly debated as the effect of diet on arthritis. Although nothing has yet been proved in the laboratory, innumerable arthritic patients claim to have been

helped, if not cured, by dietary means. Try the following suggestions for several weeks. At worst, you will lose weight, which is helpful in itself.

• Avoid sugar, sweets of all kinds, soda, citrus fruits, pork, roast beef, chocolate, pepper, cigarettes, alcohol, coffee, tea, stimulants, and narcotics. Reduce intake of dairy products and eggs.

• Eat as many raw fruits (except citrus) and vegetables as possible. Especially good are avocados, cherries, bananas, and pineapples. Have salad at every meal. Drink fresh-squeezed fruit and vegetable juices. Eat cottage cheese and limited amounts of chicken or turkey several times a week.

• Eat whole-grain breads and cereals and sourdough breads as frequently as possible.

• If possible, avoid foods containing preservatives and additives. Avoid canned and frozen foods.

• Try not to eat too much at one sitting. Drink plenty of water. Get a lot of exercise.

2. *Vitamin and mineral supplements.* Certain supplements apparently help certain people. They include:

• Vitamin C—1000 milligrams a day
• Calcium—250 milligrams a day
• Cod-liver oil—1 teaspoon after each meal
• A good vitamin-B complex, strong on vitamins B_6, pantothenic acid, and B_{12}—twice a day
• Potassium—250 milligrams a day

Cod-liver oil is said to be particularly helpful for arthritis, especially if it is mixed in a glass of warm milk (one teaspoon per glass) and taken twice a day before meals. There is some laboratory evidence that this mixture reduces tissue inflammation and helps improve overall stamina and strength.

3. *Sea water.* Arthritics have often found that swimming in the ocean for prolonged periods has an astonishingly therapeutic effect. Several teaspoons of sea water taken after the swim and following each meal supposedly complements the healing force of the water. Two swims a day, each at least twenty minutes long, are recommended. It should be noted, however, that some cases of arthritis respond *negatively* to saltwater swims. Discontinue the swims immediately if this occurs.

4. *Copper bracelet.* These have been worn for centuries on the hands and feet as an arthritis remedy. The copper treatment works

rapidly for a few people, slowly for others, not at all for most. If you try this method, give it six months before passing judgment.

5. *Apple cider vinegar.* An old New England remedy used by thousands of arthritis sufferers calls for one teaspoon of honey mixed with one teaspoon of apple cider vinegar (be *sure* it is made from apple cider) to be drunk once in the morning and once at night. Take faithfully for at least two months.

WHEN TO CALL THE DOCTOR

Arthritis should be treated by a physician if:
- The arthritis does not respond to any of the conventional or unconventional treatments.
- The pain is localized in one or two severely aching joints (it may be gout).
- There is a progressive inability to move and to use the afflicted joints.
- There are signs of disfigurement of the afflicted joints.
- There is severe pain (especially if aspirin provides no relief or produces side effects).
- The afflicted joints become warm, red, and very swollen.
- There is fever, fatigue, and malaise traceable to the arthritis.

TECHNOLOGY, RESOURCES, AIDS, AND SERVICES

1. The *Arthritis Information Clearinghouse* (P.O. Box 34427, Bethesda, MD 20034) publishes booklets, bibliographies of arthritis materials, information bulletins, audiovisual materials, and educational supports.

2. The *Stanford Arthritis Center* (Medical Center S-102, Stanford, CA 94305) will provide information on how to establish arthritis self-care educational courses in your area.

3. An incredibly wide range of *mechanical and electronic aids* are available for arthritis sufferers. From the Sears Catalog (contact your nearest Sears or call [800] 323-3274 for ordering information) you can, for instance, purchase special jar openers, cervical neck supports, dressing and bath aids, magnet-tipped extension grips, cervical collars, vacuum feeding cups, and a variety of electronic massage aids. From the catalog *Arthritis Self-help Products* issued by *Aids for Arthritis,* 3 Little Knoll Ct., Medford, NJ 08055, you can buy buttoning instruments for arthritic fingers, pen and pencil grips, long-handled scrubbers, card shufflers, key holders, and boxtop removers. From Cleo, Inc., 3957 Mayfield Rd.,

Cleveland, OH 44121, you can obtain special eating utensils such as bent spoons, one-hand cutlery sets, and no-tip glasses as well as giant push-button telephone adapters, light-switch extension handles, zipper pulls, and "no-stoop" hardware shears. Most health-product supply houses feature their own line of arthritis products.

4. Helpful *books on arthritis* include:
Arthritis: A Comprehensive Guide by James F. Fries, M.D.
Reading, Mass.: Addison-Wesley Publishing Co., 1979

The Arthritis Helpbook by Kate Lorig, R.N., and James Fries, M.D.
Reading, Mass.: Addison-Wesley Publishing Co., 1980

The Arthritis Book: A Guide for Patients and Their Families by Ephraim Engleman and Milton Sherman
New York: Dutton, 1979

The Copper Bracelet and Arthritis by Helmar Dollwet
New York: Vantage, 1981

Natural Relief for Arthritis by Carol Keough and *Prevention Magazine* editors
Emmaus, Pa.: Rodale, Press, 1983

The Arthritis Exercise Book by Semyon Krewer
New York: Cornerstone, 1981
5. Also see *Chapters 3, 17,* and *18* of this book.

CHAPTER 21

FIRST AID
SELF-CARE

Why first aid is such a little-known skill in this country and why it is not taught as a mandatory subject in schools and colleges along with history and geography is anyone's guess. The fact is that most people's knowledge of the subject, despite the heroic efforts to teach emergency medicine by such organizations as the Red Cross, is woefully inadequate, and worse, filled with inaccuracies and misconceptions.

One reason for this sad state of affairs is that like most unpleasant things, first aid is a subject we want to think about only when the need arises. An understandable sentiment, perhaps, but a dangerous one. With a little attention to a few details, however, the basics of the art can be learned without on-the-spot training, enabling one to face the physical uncertainties of life with more assurance. This chapter describes some of the most important first aid techniques for both normal injuries and emergencies. Treatments are divided into two categories: *emergency treatment* and *nonemergency treatment.* Emergency treatment requires speedy and confident action, sometimes of a lifesaving nature. Nonemergency treatment is for routine injuries that occur around the house or at work and that may or may not require a doctor's attention. Needless to say, the emergency treatments are designed only to keep symptoms under control until medical help is obtainable.

WHEN TO APPLY EMERGENCY FIRST AID MEASURES

When exactly is emergency first aid required? Answer: Anytime a person is badly injured or taken seriously ill and a doctor's help is not immediately available. These illnesses and injuries include uncontrolled bleeding, major cuts and lacerations, breathing problems, convulsions, unconsciousness, burns, heart attacks, strokes, severe pain, and broken bones. Since we know that accidents are the leading cause of death among persons one to thirty-eight years old in the United States, and that certain injuries, if not given swift and appropriate attention, can be life-threatening, the name of the game is to be quick and prepared.

How to Assess an Emergency Situation

Before the first-aider can help a victim of a crisis, he or she must rapidly and logically evaluate the seriousness of the situation and decide on appropriate action. The following is a checklist of what to look for in times of emergency and how to determine your priorities quickly.

1. Appraise the general situation. Is the injury serious or mild? Can you take care of it alone or will you need help?

2. If help is necessary, get it as quickly as possible. If you are the injured person, shout, call, wave, do whatever is necessary to get the help of bystanders. If you are in the helping role, delegate authority, sending one bystander to call for aid on the phone, another to get a local doctor, etc.

3. Take a moment to determine the best method of rescue, relief, medication, bleeding control, whatever. Make a fast review in your head of everything you know about treating the specific problem before you. Then do it. Pay special attention to the following:

• Keep the victim's airways open, especially if he or she is unconscious (see page 237). Give mouth-to-mouth resuscitation if necessary (see page 238).

• Stop all serious bleeding (see page 238).

• Check the pulse (see page 241).

• Check for shock and if necessary, treat for shock (see page 242).

• Be extremely careful when you handle or lift the accident victim. Be absolutely certain there are no breaks, no spinal, head, or lung injuries before attempting to move or elevate him or her. Do not let the victim walk around unnecessarily if there is evidence of head or back injury. When in doubt, do *not* move the victim.

• Treat all life-threatening situations *immediately*. Do not wait for medical help. Each accident or injury will have to be assessed individually, of course, but in general, life-threatening situations such as poisoning, heart attack, heat stroke, choking, drowning, smoke inhalation, dehydration, frostbite, severe bleeding, and allergic reactions to insect bites all require on-the-spot attention.

• The golden rule of first aid is: *Always treat the most serious symptoms first.* In other words, you would attend to unconsciousness before nausea, a blocked airway before a laceration, uncontrolled bleeding before broken bones, and so forth. Always set your priorities before you begin.

4. Remain calm. An essential part of the rescue process is providing victims with psychological support. Most victims will be upset and may demonstrate reaction symptoms such as diarrhea, frequent urination, shaking and chills, nausea, and disorientation. These symptoms are to be expected and will usually pass quickly. Speak soothingly to the victim. Present a calm front. Encourage the victim to talk freely, describing, if possible, the circumstances of the accident. Let the victim eat or drink (if appropriate), and encourage him or her to relax. Let the victim know you are there, that you care, and that help is on the way.

Fundamental Methods of Emergency First Aid

Key emergency first aid measures are designed to provide temporary treatment of breathing difficulties, bleeding, shock, and broken bones.

CHECK THE BREATHING AND AIRWAYS

An open airway is a prerequisite for survival in times of accident. Is the victim's throat clear? Is he or she having trouble breathing? Can he or she speak? Is there an obstruction of any kind in the mouth or breathing tube? Are the victim's tongue, fingernail beds, or lips turning blue? If breathing problems develop, artificial respiration may be necessary. The most effective form is mouth-to-mouth resuscitation. Instructions on how to perform it are as follows:

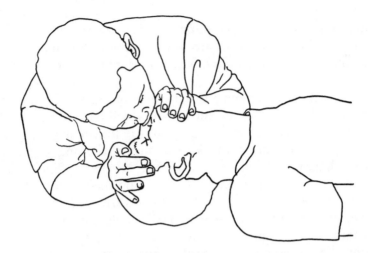

1. Place the victim on his or her back. If there is any sign of severe head, neck, or back injury, do *not* move victim but perform mouth-to-mouth in place.

2. Using the index and middle fingers, clean the victim's mouth of any foreign matter.

3. Open the victim's mouth (making sure his or her tongue is not blocking the airways) by tilting the head back, supporting the neck with your hand. Pinch both nostrils tightly closed with your thumb and index finger. Open the mouth, take a breath, place your mouth tightly against the victim's mouth so that an airtight seal is made, and exhale forcefully. Remove your mouth, take another breath, replace your mouth, and exhale again. Repeat breaths approximately once every five seconds (twelve breaths a minute).

4. Continue until the victim starts to breathe again.

5. For infants and very young children, the operation is similar, but with the following exceptions:

• Do not tilt the child's head as far back as you would for an adult.

• Puff into the mouth every three seconds (as opposed to every five for an adult).

• Puff with less force than you would for an adult. Short, gentle breaths are adequate.

STOP THE BLEEDING

Loss of more than a quart of blood can threaten survival. Therefore, in times of serious accident, all efforts must be made to conserve the victim's blood supply and to stem blood loss *as quickly as possible*. In general, you will know there is an external bleeding emergency when:

- Blood spurts from the wound.
- The bleeding will not stop no matter what is done to control it.
- An artery is severed.

Several emergency methods are available for stopping uncontrolled blood flow. These include, in order of increasing efficiency:

1. *Elevation*

Elevate the wound above the level of the victim's heart. If, for example, the bleeding is on the victim's hand, raise it over the head. If it is on the victim's leg, have him or her lie down and elevate the leg. Then apply direct pressure (see below) to the bleeding. The force of gravity will work with you this way, reducing blood pressure and slowing blood loss. Be careful, though—if there is any sign that the wound is located on a fracture or break, you may have to forego this technique.

2. *Direct Pressure*

The bleeding from most wounds, even the most serious, can usually be controlled by the direct pressure method. This involves placing firm pressure over the wound until the bleeding slows and the clotting process begins. You will need a gauze pad or a piece of wadded cloth. A sterile gauze pad is best, but in a pinch a shirt, a handkerchief, or any absorbent material will do. (When no material is available use your bare hand.) With the flat of your hand, press the pad or cloth firmly against the wound, pushing steadily down on the hemorrhaging vessel until it shows signs of clotting. Even if the cloth becomes a bloody mess do not remove it—lack of pressure may cause the bleeding to begin again. Instead, continue to push, adding extra pieces of absorbent cloth as they are needed. Once blood flow has been staunched, bandage the wound with a clean linen dressing and get help.

3. *Pressure on a major artery*

If an arm is injured and bleeding, apply pressure to the *brachial artery* at a point located halfway between the armpit and the elbow (see picture). Grip this spot tightly with your fingers and thumb, and squeeze with some force. Because pressure here will slow circulation throughout the entire arm, this method should be practiced only as long as the bleeding continues.

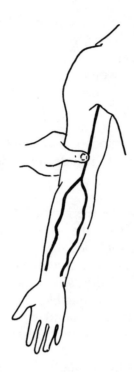

For wounds of the leg, constriction of the *femoral artery,* located at the crease of the groin (see page 241), will provide similar relief. Place your palm on the indicated spot and push
downward, into the hip bone, letting your body weight help—
the harder you push the better. Again, discontinue pressure as
soon as the bleeding has slowed.

4. *Tourniquet*

As a last-ditch effort, and *only* as a last-ditch effort, apply a
tourniquet. It must be stressed very strongly that a tourniquet
cuts off blood entirely to the damaged arm or leg, and often causes
loss of the injured limb. According to the American Red Cross,
"The decision to apply a tourniquet is in reality a decision to risk
sacrifice of a limb in order to save a life." This method is used,
therefore, if part of a limb is severed and/or if several arteries are
bleeding at once.

With these facts in mind, the way to apply a tourniquet is as
follows:

• Find any strip of material (or in a pinch, any piece of rope
or string) and wrap it immediately above the wound.

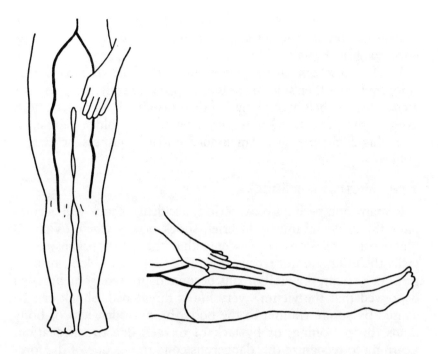

• Place a stick or any hard, straight object through the wrapping. Knot it in place, if possible. Then twist the stick and tighten it until the bleeding stops. Do not cover the wound.

• Secure the stick onto the tourniquet. Treat for shock (see page 242). Get help as quickly as possible.

CHECK THE PULSE

In many emergency situations the pulse rate will provide a good index of your own or a victim's condition. A pulse is taken as follows:

1. Place the tips of your fingers (never your thumb, which has its own pulse) on the thumb side of the patient's wrist, your third finger resting on the crease of the wrist.

2. Using a watch (if possible, a stop watch), count the number of beats in a minute.

3. A normal rate is between sixty and ninety beats a minute. Anything over one hundred is considered a rapid pulse rate. Anything over 120 is very rapid. Anything over 140 is dangerously rapid.

4. Note the strength of the pulse. A very weak pulse can be a sign of shock. It may also indicate that a dangerous amount of

blood has been lost. A very rapid pulse can signal fever (as in heat stroke) or, in some instances, brain injury. An irregular, jumpy pulse suggests heart problems.

5. The pulse can also be taken along the cartoid artery. This is located on either side of the neck approximately three to four inches directly below the hinge of the jawbone. Never check both sides at the same time, however, especially on older people, as even this slight pressure can induce unconsciousness or even a stroke.

TREAT VICTIMS FOR SHOCK

In many and perhaps most serious accidents, shock will accompany the principal injury. In brief, shock occurs when a victim's blood pressure drops so suddenly that the major organs, especially the brain, do not receive adequate supplies of blood or oxygen. As a result, the vital organs become depressed, sometimes so depressed that the victim's very life is threatened. Shock can be caused by severe trauma to the body, by a sudden loss of body fluids, by poisoning, or by lack of oxygen due to suffocation. Learning to recognize this dangerous condition is one of the foremost requirements of good first aid.

1. In the early stages, the shock victim seems weak, pale, listless, cold, and clammy to the touch. The pulse may be quick (over one hundred), but it will be difficult to locate. The skin may be bluish. The victim may complain of thirst.

2. As the condition worsens, breathing turns shallow or irregular. The victim becomes increasingly apathetic and dulled, sunken-eyed and unresponsive, sometimes to the point of wishing only for sleep—a bad sign.

3. In the last stages, the victim's pupils become widely dilated, the cheeks become mottled, and the victim loses consciousness. Death may follow.

The main objectives in treating shock are: 1) to restore proper blood circulation, 2) to regain a sufficient oxygen supply, 3) to return the dropped blood pressure to an acceptable level, and 4) to get help. The following procedures should be applied:

1. Keep the victim calm, and lying down if possible. Loosen all clothing. Elevate the victim's legs ten or twelve inches if the injury permits. If there is vomiting or bleeding from the face or mouth, turn the victim on his or her side to avoid aspiration of fluids.

2. Keep the victim warm. If possible, wrap in blankets and protect against strong winds, chills, dampness, etc.

3. If medical help is not immediately available, give the victim small sips of lukewarm water mixed with salt and baking soda (one half teaspoon of soda and one teaspoon of salt to a gallon of water). A half glass of this mixture every half hour is adequate. Do *not* administer liquids if the victim is vomiting or if he or she shows signs of convulsions, abdominal pain, unconsciousness, or brain injury.

4. Get help.

MAKING SPLINTS FOR BROKEN LIMBS

For breaks or bad sprains, a temporary splint can be improvised using practically any hard, straight material that is available in the vicinity: a branch, a metal rod, a rolled-up blanket or newspaper. The purpose of the splint is to immobilize the injury and keep it as rigid as possible until help is found.

To make a splint, take a board or whatever splint material you are using and place it carefully against the broken arm or leg. Two thin boards, one on either side of the break, are ideal for splinting broken arms and legs. With strips of tape, string, or material secure the boards in place, being careful not to wrap them too tightly (numbness is a sure sign that the splint is binding). When applying the splint *never* attempt to straighten the broken arm or leg past the point of comfort. Apply ice to the break. Get help immediately.

Keeping and Stocking a Home First Aid Kit

Every home should have one. This doesn't mean you must run out and buy a really expensive $150 first aid kit, although if you can afford it, it's not a bad idea. It does mean that there should always be a stock of first aid items somewhere in your house just in case. A well-supplied family first aid kit contains the following items:

Bandages and sterile gauze pads
Tourniquet stick and wrappings
Roll of adhesive tape
Elastic Ace-type bandages
Cotton
Cotton swabs
Razor blades

Knife
Needle and thread
Matches
A candle
Tweezers
Safety pins
Scissors
Cough syrup
An antihistamine
Aspirin and/or aspirin substitutes
Calamine lotion
Baby oil and/or mineral oil
Petroleum jelly and any favorite salves and ointments
Epsom salts
Smelling salts or ammonia (for treating unconscious persons)
Antacids
Iodine
Rubbing alcohol
Hydrogen peroxide
Eye drops
Diarrhea medication
An emetic (such as syrup of ipecac)
Hot and cold packs
Oral or rectal thermometer
Stethoscope
Sphygmomanometer
Otoscope
A pen, paper, and small flashlight
Important phone numbers (doctor, dentist, hospital, your local
    Poison Control Center, police, fire department, ambulance,
    the address of the nearest emergency room, etc.) (Some peo-
    ple tape important emergency phone numbers on every phone
    in the house.)
A good book on the application of first aid

Although you need not keep all these supplies together in one
enormous box, it's good practice to have them close together—
in a medicine chest, say, or in a bathroom closet—so that if the
need arises, you won't trip all over yourself looking for the proper
items. Make sure everyone in the household knows where they
are. Be aware, moreover, that certain first aid supplies spoil after
some time, especially medications. If you do keep a first aid kit

on hand, check it now and then, and replace any supplies that have become suspiciously dried, fragile, or brownish.

How to Deal with Emergency First Aid Situations

NECK AND BACK INJURIES

Persons who suffer a fall, are hit by a car, or experience any type of major physical trauma should be quickly immobilized on the chance that spinal or neck damage has occurred. If you yourself are the victim, lie still and wait for help, especially if you feel pain in your back or neck, numbness, or immobility of the limbs. If administering to another person, gauge the extent of the damage, keep the victim still, and get help immediately. The following steps can be taken while waiting for help:

1. Make sure the victim's airways are clear. Do not move the victim unless it is absolutely necessary.

2. Check for shock. Treat for shock if necessary. Keep the victim warm and comfortable.

3. Immobilize the victim by surrounding his or her body with pillows, blankets, bedding, wadded clothing. If soft items are not available, stones, cinder blocks, or pieces of wood can be used.

4. If the victim is conscious, question him or her about the particulars of the accident. Indications that there is neck or spine damage include:
- Intense pain in the neck or back.
- Paralysis in any part of the body. An inability to move the arms, legs, neck, torso, etc.
- Numbness and/or tingling over various parts of the body.

5. If the victim's life is endangered by imminent fire, flooding, fumes, etc., and he or she must be moved immediately, grip the shoulders or feet and drag the victim away from the source of danger. This should be done *only* in emergency situations.

6. Get help immediately.

EMERGENCY BURNS

Burns are divided into three categories: first-, second-, and third-degree burns.

- *First-degree burns* produce mild redness, swelling, and pain, and usually respond to simple self-care. They are caused by ordinary household accidents such as contact with a hot lightbulb, a pan on the stove, etc.

• *Second-degree burns* are far deeper and more serious than first. They quickly show heavy blistering and redness, and assume a swollen, mottled appearance. Due to plasma loss, the wound develops a weeping, watery surface and is highly painful. Second-degree burns may occur from deep sunburn, scalding, touching a flame, hot metal, or stove.

• *Third-degree burns* appear black and white and charred. Sometimes the flesh is literally seared to the bone. Since these wounds tend to destroy nerve endings, less pain may be felt than with second- or even first-degree burns. Third-degree burns usually come from electric shocks, severe gasoline fires, burning clothing, or severe scalding. They are *always* a medical emergency, even when very small.

Following are steps to follow in treating second-degree, third-degree, and chemical burns.

1. *Second-degree burns.* Wet the wound thoroughly with cool water or, if possible, immerse the burned part in cool water (no ice water). Wet cloth compresses may also be used. Keep the burned area wet for at least five minutes until all the heat has been drawn out. Then carefully pat the wound dry, cover it with clean linen or sterile gauze, and get help. Do not attempt to break the blisters. *Never* put butter or first aid ointments on a burn; they will seal the heat inside the wound and cause greater tissue damage. Aspirin will deaden the pain until help comes.

2. *Third-degree burns.* Remove all tight clothing or jewelry on the victim's body right away (generalized swelling may soon occur, which will make removal more difficult). Do not, however, attempt to remove any burned or charred clothing. Soothe the burned parts with cool water and cover them with wet compresses, making certain the compresses are clean (deep burns are extremely vulnerable to infection). Burned hands and feet should be elevated. Keep the airways open and treat for shock, if necessary. Aspirin may be given for pain. Get medical assistance *immediately.*

3. *Chemical burns.* Sudden dowsings with harsh acidic or alkaline chemicals can burn the skin in exactly the same way as a flame. First aid procedure calls for the immediate adulteration and neutralization of these substances on the skin by means of flushing or washing the burned area, preferably with a hose, shower, or bucket of water. Continue to spray or wash for at least five minutes. Remove all clothing covering the burned area.

To treat alkaline substances, a weak solution of vinegar and water may be washed on as a final rinse, but only after all the chemical has been removed. Baking soda (a teaspoonful dissolved in a quart of water) can be used in the same way after washing for acid burns. Following removal of the chemical, treat the wound as you would any second- or third-degree burn (see above), and get help immediately.

CHOKING

First aid for choking should be applied only if the victim cannot breathe. Violent coughing and sputtering, if accompanied by a clear airway, will usually pass and should not be forced with slaps on the back, drinks of water, etc. If, however, it is clear that the victim is not getting air and his or her throat is blocked, do not wait for medical help—*take first aid steps for choking immediately.* (A good rule to apply is: If the victim can speak, the airway is clear, and he or she most likely does not need emergency first aid. If the victim cannot speak, he or she most likely requires immediate aid.) Here's what to do in a choking emergency:

1. Determine whether or not the person is actually choking, that is, whether his or her airway is blocked by a foreign object. A choking victim may do any of the following:

• Silently clutch or point at the throat (this is the universal distress sign for choking).
• Cough and gag uncontrollably.
• Gesture wildly.
• Become incapable of speaking.
• Turn blue in the face.
• Suddenly collapse or lose consciousness.

2. Apply three or four sharp blows to the choking person's back with the heel of the hand while placing your other arm around his or her chest. Wait a moment, then repeat.

3. If the step above fails, apply the Heimlich Maneuver. This is done as follows:

• Stand behind the choking person and wrap your arms around his or her midsection, hands located over the solar plexus. Make a fist with one hand and grip the fist with the other, keeping the arms locked in place.

• Make a hard, sudden inward and upward thrust with the clutched hands, directly into the victim's solar plexus, as if trying to force out air. Repeat this movement four times in a row.

• If the Heimlich Maneuver does not work the first time, give several more blows to the victim's back, then repeat the maneuver again.

• The Heimlich Maneuver can also be self-applied. Make a clutched fist with both hands as described above, place it over your solar plexus, and pull it in sharply toward your stomach four times in a row. Don't be afraid to do this with some force. You can also lean your upper stomach against an object such as a chair or the edge of a table and push in the same way.

4. If the person has come close to suffocating, treat for shock (see page 242).

POISONING

A serious yet common household and on-the-job emergency, poisoning must be treated according to the type of toxic substance that has been swallowed. Follow these steps:

1. Ask the victim:
• What type of poison was swallowed
• How long ago it was taken
• How much was ingested
• What the symptoms are
• Whether or not he or she has vomited
• His or her age
• What type of first aid, if any, was administered

2. Call both a physician and your local Poison Control Center (the operator can connect you directly to the latter) and ask for help. If there is any question about the poisonousness of a substance, the Poison Control Center will know. If any suspicious empty containers are in evidence, keep them to show the doctor. A sample of the vomitus will also help.

3. If you cannot get help right away, take the following steps, and don't panic—even the worst ordinary poisons need time to take effect. With quick and careful action, poison victims can almost always be helped.

• If the victim is unconscious, keep his or her airway open. Use artificial respiration, if necessary.

• Induce vomiting *only* if the victim has taken or overdosed on the following substances:

Rat poison

Ant and roach poison

Medicinal drugs
Narcotic drugs
Camphor
Poison berries
Poison bark or leaves
Household soaps or detergents
Rubbing soaps or detergents
Rubbing alcohol
Nail polish remover
Cosmetics, perfumes, and toiletries
Sulphur

Vomiting can be induced by inserting a finger, spoon, or pen into the back of the victim's throat. If an emetic such as syrup of ipecac is available, give it according to directions on the label (usually one tablespoonful per dose). Avoid the risk of choking by making sure the victim is seated upright. Victims who may have taken an overdose of narcotics or sleeping medications can be given coffee and tea if they are awake. While waiting for help, keep the victim warm and calm. Treat for shock, if necessary. If an emetic does not produce vomiting within twenty-five minutes, give another dose, but no more after this. Always withhold emetics from anyone who is not alert enough to swallow them; otherwise, you may have an even larger problem if the victim aspirates the emetic into his or her lungs.

• Do *not* induce vomiting if the victim has swallowed:

Strong acids: car battery fluid, sulphuric acid, iodine, styptic pencil, toilet bowl cleaner, etc.

Strong alkalis: ammonia, lye, detergent, bleach, etc.

Petroleum products: gasoline, kerosene, lighter fluid, paint thinner, turpentine, rust remover, paint, floor polish, etc.

If the victim is conscious and has taken any of the above poisons, give several glasses of milk, followed by egg whites in water or in cooking oil. If *strong alkali* substances are swallowed, give water with vinegar or lemon juice added. If *strong acids* have been taken, milk of magnesia may be given after the milk and egg. If *petroleum distillates* have been swallowed, give four ounces of mineral oil instead of the milk and egg. Treat for shock (see page 242). Get help.

When storing poisons around the house, keep them out of children's reach, preferably on a high shelf or in a locked cabinet. Make sure they are all well labeled. Some people teach their chil-

dren that any bottle that displays a frowning face drawn on it
(by you) is dangerous. Keep a poison control kit on hand and
within easy access (see the technology and resources section for
information on obtaining a poison control kit).

Toxic Fumes

Although we think of toxic fumes as emanating exclusively from
industrial sites, they may be found just about anywhere. Think,
for example, of refrigeration gases, cooking smoke, carbon mon-
oxide from the car, carbon dioxide from wells and sewers, cleaning solvents like carbon tetrachloride, and natural gas from stoves
and heating units. Take the following steps for victims of such
fumes:

1. Remove the victim as quickly as possible from the source of
the toxic gas.

2. Loosen all clothing, check the airway, and treat for shock.
If the victim has stopped breathing, administer artificial respiration.

3. If possible, give oxygen.

4. Arrange for the victim to be transported to the hospital as
soon as possible.

A Few DON'TS for Dealing with Poison Victims

• Don't use saltwater or epsom salt solution as an emetic.

• Don't try to wrestle with or subdue a poisoned person who
is in convulsions.

• Don't place any type of restraining device in the mouth of a
person with convulsions.

• Don't remain in the room if poison fumes are present. Drag
the victim to safety *before* administering first aid.

• Don't induce vomiting if the substance is a strong acid, alkali, or petroleum product.

• Don't panic when treating the victim. It will communicate
itself to the victim and intensify the effects of the poison.

• Don't attempt to induce vomiting in an unconscious poison
victim. If the person is lying down leave them in this position,
but do tilt their head to the side if that person is vomiting.

• Don't assume that a poison must have been swallowed immediately before the reaction. The symptoms of aspirin poisoning, for instance, can in some cases take more than a day to appear.

HEATSTROKE AND HEAT EXHAUSTION

Although heatstroke and heat exhaustion are frequently spoken of as the same ailment, there are significant differences between them. *Heatstroke* occurs when the body temperature is raised to a potentially dangerous level and the sweating mechanism no longer functions properly. *Heat exhaustion* is characterized by fatigue, lassitude, confusion, and dehydration, although the body temperature is only slightly elevated or even normal. Heatstroke is considerably more dangerous than heat exhaustion. Here is a detailed breakdown to help you distinguish between the two:

Body Function	Heatstroke	Heat Exhaustion
Temperature	Sometimes as high as 106°F	Slightly elevated, never above 102°F
Skin	Red, dry, and hot	Pale and clammy
Pulse	Strong and disturbed	Normal or slightly fast
Pupils	Constricted	Dilated
Perspiration	No sweating	Heavy sweating
General	Convulsions, loss of consciousness, confusion, severe dehydration	Dizziness, weakness, nausea, cramps, confusion, fatigue

Treating Heatstroke

Emergency treatment for heatstroke consists of the following:

1. Remove the victim from the heat and transport him or her to a cool place, preferably to a spot where a fan or air conditioner is available. Remove all clothes down to the undergarments. Call for help immediately. While you're waiting, go on to Step Two.

2. Sponge patient's body with cool, wet compresses, ice packs, or rubbing alcohol, and if available, apply ice packs to the person's head, chest, stomach, neck, and wrists. The victim can also be immersed in a tub of cold water (no ice). The goal is to bring the body temperature down as quickly as possible before brain damage results.

3. When the victim's temperature has gone below 102°F, the immediate danger can be considered past. If the victim's temperature shoots up again, repeat the above treatment. Otherwise, dry the victim, keep him or her in a cool place, and massage the arms and legs while talking in a calm and reassuring manner.

4. Treat for shock if necessary (see page 242). Get the victim to a doctor as quickly as possible.

Treating Heat Exhaustion

Take the following steps:

1. Remove the victim from the heat. Transport to a cool place, preferably near a fan or air conditioner.

2. Elevate victim's legs.

3. Loosen victim's clothing and cool his or her body with wet compresses or ice packs If cramping occurs, massage the victim's arms and legs.

4. Give the victim frequent sips from a glass of lukewarm saltwater (approximately a tablespoonful of salt per twelve ounces). If victim vomits, stop all fluids.

5. Even if the victim feels better after several hours, he or she should be checked by a doctor and should not be allowed to perform strenuous activities for a day or so following the emergency.

Treating Hypothermia (Lowered Body Temperature)

Prolonged exposure to cold can cause an overall drop in the body temperature with attendant slowing of circulation, constriction of blood vessels, and decreased flow of blood to the brain and nervous system. Hypothermia is potentially life-threatening. Symptoms include:

• A drop in body temperature (sometimes so low it does not register on a thermometer).

• Shaking and chills, followed by general numbness and lack of all sensation.

• Pale swollen skin, which sometimes turns a bluish pink color.

• Intense muscular weakness.

• Disorientation, drowsiness, dizziness, slurred speech, impairment of judgment and coordination, failed eyesight, muscular rigidity.

In the absence of immediate medical help, this true medical emergency can be treated in the following way:

1. Remove the victim from the cold. Bring person into a heated environment. Treat for shock, if necessary (see page 242).

2. Take off all cold, wet clothes and replace them with warm clothes and ample blankets.

3. If there is no sign of frostbite (see below) on particular parts of the arms and legs, massage the victim's limbs to restore circulation.

4. Give victim *nonalcoholic* drinks. Try to prevent the victim from losing consciousness. If the emergency takes place in the wilderness, close body contact with one or more persons will help restore body heat. Transport the victim to a hospital as quickly as possible.

FROSTBITE

Frostbite occurs when the deeper layers of the skin freeze. Ice crystals actually form below the epidermis. Exposed parts of the body such as the hands, nose, and cheeks are most vulnerable to frostbite, but even well-covered areas can be affected after prolonged exposure. Symptoms include:

• Change of skin color in the area from pink to mottled white or grayish yellow.

• Pain at the site, later replaced by numbness.

• Possible blisters on the frozen area.

Note: Victims are commonly unaware of frostbite until it is observed and pointed out by another person. Do not rely on pain alone to reveal this condition.

The key to emergency treatment for frostbite is gentle but immediate rewarming of the exposed area. Follow these steps if medical assistance is not available:

1. Quickly remove the victim from the cold and bring into a warm environment.

2. Warm the frozen part as quickly as possible by immersing it in lukewarm (*not hot*) water. If warm water is not available, cover the wound with blankets or any material that retains heat. Do *not* attempt to thaw the wound with a heating lamp or electric heating pad. If the wound is located on the feet, do *not* allow victim to walk or otherwise put pressure on the feet.

3. Elevate the frostbitten area.

4. Give the victim a warm *nonalcoholic* drink. Obtain medical assistance as quickly as possible.

Eye Injuries

Irritating Chemicals in the Eye

1. Wash chemicals off the victim's face. Hold the victim's eye(s) open and flush them with large quantities of cool water. Continue to flush for at least ten to fifteen minutes.

2. Cover both eyes with a sterile dressing and take victim to a doctor or hospital immediately. Bring the chemical container, if possible, to help the doctor determine which poison was involved in the accident.

Cuts, Lacerations, Bruises to the Eye

1. Clean the area surrounding the eye carefully if blood is present.

2. Cover both eyes with a sterile dressing and tape gauze *loosely* in place. Keep the victim in a lying position. Transport him or her to the nearest medical facility.

Objects Embedded in the Eye

1. Cover both eyes with a sterile dressing and tape dressing down loosely. Do *not* attempt to remove the object no matter how easy this operation may appear. Transport victim to a medical facility immediately.

2. If the embedded object is large or protruding, cover the wounded eye with a plastic or paper cup and tape the cup securely in place. Cover the other eye with a taped sterile dressing and get help immediately.

For further information on eye injuries, see chapter on Eye Problems (pages 90–98).

Heart Attack

Statistically speaking, at least three quarters of heart attack scares turn out to be indigestion, stress, lung infections, or one of many other nonemergencies. Occasionally, though, pains in the chest do indeed indicate that an obstruction is present in one of the vessels supplying blood and oxygen to the heart muscles, and at such times knowledge of first aid may save a life. First on the list of priorities is learning correctly to identify the symptoms.

Although none of the following symptoms guarantee that a heart attack is taking place, when two or more occur simultaneously or in sequence, your suspicions should be aroused. The following are listed in order of decreasing importance and in the sequence in which they *usually* occur:

1. Continuous gripping pains in the center of the chest. Be especially concerned if the pain tends to radiate up the arms, to the shoulders, and into the neck and jaw. Also, look for numbness of the arms and/or fingers, usually of the left extremity.

2. Shortness of breath and possible gasping that tends to improve when the victim is seated, to become worse when he or she is lying down.

3. Profuse sweating.

4. Nausea and vomiting (this sometimes confuses victims, making them believe they are simply having stomach trouble).

5. Pallor and a bluish cast to the lips and fingernail beds.

6. Extreme fatigue and prostration.

7. An irregular pulse.

8. Disorientation and confusion.

Emergency First Aid for a Heart Attack

1. Call for an ambulance immediately, preferably one equipped with oxygen. Victims of a heart attack can die at any moment. It is *absolutely imperative* that you rush the victim to an emergency room as quickly as possible. Don't let the victim talk you out of taking him or her to the hospital.

2. If the victim is unconscious and not breathing, administer artificial respiration. (If the victim is still breathing, artificial respiration is not necessary.) If the victim's heart has stopped and if you know the technique, apply CPR (cardiopulmonary resuscitation).

3. If an emergency oxygen supply happens to be nearby, administer it to the patient. Do *not* give liquids or food. *Never* put the stricken person in a hot tub. Have the victim sit up in a comfortable position. Loosen all tight clothing. Keep the person warm. Speak soothingly and give assurances that help is on the way.

4. If the victim is carrying nitroglycerine, it is almost always appropriate to give it even before he or she is brought to the hospital. Most other heart medicines are contraindicated during heart attacks, however, and can cause large problems—*unless* the victim is carrying a medicine prescribed specifically by his or her physician for acute chest pain.

Sudden High Fever

In adults, any fever above 102°F is cause for alarm. Children tend to run much higher temperatures, especially when suffering from standard childhood maladies such as measles, mumps, etc. Such fevers should always be watched and should never be taken for granted. If allowed to climb too high, they can cause convulsions, both in adults and especially in children. If a person's fever shoots up suddenly and inexplicably, you will need to seek medical help immediately. While waiting, an emergency situation may exist and the temperature must be kept from rising too severely. The following steps will help:

1. Take the child's temperature frequently. Use a rectal thermometer for small children. Oral thermometers are fine for all others unless the person has mouth injuries. Remember that rectal temperatures run at least one degree higher than oral temperatures.

2. If the person's temperature is exceedingly high, remove excess blankets and clothing. For adults, give aspirin or an aspirin substitute immediately. For children suffering from a viral disease, seek a doctor's advice before giving aspirin (there may be a connection between the use of aspirin in children with high fevers and development of the dangerous Reye's Syndrome). Give the child plenty of liquids to avoid dehydration.

3. If the temperature is above 103°F in an adult, sponge him or her down with cool water. If the temperature is above 105°F in a child, place him or her in a tub of cool water. Continue the cooling process for approximately a half hour, then briskly towel the patient dry. Repeat the process frequently until the fever shows signs of abating. Call a doctor for advice.

Unconsciousness

Many emergency situations can cause loss of consciousness. When this condition occurs, the task of the rescuer becomes doubly difficult, as the victim is not able to participate in the helping process. When dealing with an unconscious victim, approach the situation in the following way, making allowances, of course, for individual needs:

1. Check the victim's airways. If breathing has stopped, apply artificial respiration, after first checking for obstructions in the mouth and throat.

2. Keep the victim lying down. Loosen all tight clothing. If the victim has been vomiting, and if there are no signs of neck injury, turn his or her head to the side to prevent aspiration of the vomitus.

3. If there are no signs of back injury, elevate the victim's legs.

4. Keep the victim warm until help comes. If necessary, treat for shock (see page 242).

5. Do *not* do any of the following for a person who has lost consciousness:
- Throw water in his or her face.
- Give smelling salts.
- Give liquids.
- Slap the victim on the face or back.
- Shake to awaken.
- Move the victim unnecessarily.

6. Get help as quickly as possible.

CONVULSIONS

Although a convulsion rarely causes physiological harm, the danger lies in the damage the victim may inflict on him or herself or others in the process. Choking during seizure is a real possibility. So are head injuries and broken bones—the types of injury one might expect when a human body flails and writhes without control. Often, though not invariably, convulsions are caused by epilepsy, especially in children. They may also result from a high fever, electric shock, allergic reaction to an insect bite, heatstroke, a head injury, or various infectious diseases. Since no home-care methods can stop a seizure, the only thing you can do when a convulsion occurs is to protect the victim from harming him or herself. Get the victim to a doctor unless he or she is an epileptic and the seizure is a typical one.

You will recognize convulsions from the following indications:
- Sudden loss of consciousness. The victim falls to the ground, develops a dazed, vacant look in the eyes, and is unable to respond to external contact. The muscles over the entire body begin to twitch and jerk. (Certain forms of convulsions are characterized by jerking movements localized to one part or side of the body only.)
- Lack of bowel and bladder control.
- Irregular respiration accompanied by bluish lips, face, and nailbeds.

- Drooling, foaming at the mouth.
- Bleeding from the mouth if the tongue or lips have been bitten during the convulsion.

Convulsions last from a few seconds to half a minute or more. They then subside quickly, leaving the victim utterly depleted, disoriented, and sleepy.

First Aid for Convulsions

1. If the person collapses into unconsciousness, do your best to break or catch the fall. Keep the area around the victim free from all dangerous pointed or sharp objects. For example, if the victim has a seizure inside the house, keep him or her away from all furniture, hot stoves, glass, and sharp corners. If it occurs outside the house, keep the victim away from trees, rocks, and bodies of water. If the victim's breathing stops, administer artificial respiration.

2. Keep victim under careful watch. Do not move him or her unless absolutely necessary. Loosen all tight clothing.

Do *not*:

- Restrain victims with ropes, ties, etc.
- Stuff anything into victim's mouth to prevent him or her from biting the tongue.
- Slap or throw water in the victim's face.
- Give victim smelling salts.
- Argue, scream at, or otherwise try to "talk sense" to the victim.
- Give victim anything to eat or drink.

3. If the attack lasts longer than a minute, get help as quickly as possible. Otherwise, when the attack subsides, keep the victim still and quiet. Sleep is safe after an attack; don't discourage it. Check the person for broken bones, tongue lacerations and head or neck injuries. If there are signs of regurgitation or blood in the mouth, turn the victim's head to one side to prevent aspiration of blood or vomitus.

4. If convulsions take place in a child due to high fever, sponge the child's entire body down with cool water until the fever is lowered.

5. If the victim is epileptic and this seizure is a typical one, medical help will probably not be required. (A call to the person's physician is, however, not a bad idea.) If the origin of the convulsion is unknown, or if it continues longer than a minute, seek medical help immediately.

Minor Pains and Injuries

The following injuries fall more or less within the realm of self-care. Unless extreme, they rarely require hospitalization or even a doctor's attention. Use your discretion in judging such matters, of course, and if you are uncertain as to the seriousness of any injury, opt on the side of conservatism and seek professional help.

Bruises

1. As soon as the bruise occurs, elevate the injured area and cover it with an ice pack. Keep pack in place for at least thirty minutes to control swelling. Do *not* apply heat to a bruise in the early stages.

2. Twenty-four hours after the bruise has appeared, apply hot compresses to increase circulation and to speed up healing.

Cuts and Incisions

1. Clean the cut and the area around it with mild soap and water. Any debris or dirt that clings to the wound can be flushed off with warm water or hydrogen peroxide. Rinse and blot dry.

2. If the bleeding continues, apply pressure to the injured area with a sterile gauze pad.

3. Disinfect the wound with first aid cream, hydrogen peroxide, a topical antibacterial spray, or an antibiotic ointment. Any of the three will do.

4. When bleeding stops, cover the wound with a bandage or gauze pad. For a small cut, a prepackaged adhesive will be fine. Large incisions require a gauze pad. Keep the wound covered the entire time it is healing—covering speeds the process. Apply a fresh dressing whenever necessary.

5. If the wound turns red, swells, and shows signs of oozing, this means an infection has set in. Get medical help.

Puncture Wounds

1. Let the wound bleed freely to remove all foreign material. Wash thoroughly and disinfect with hydrogen peroxide. Make certain that no part of the object that caused the puncture remains in the wound.

2. Bandage and check for infection. If the object that caused the puncture is rusty or has been near waste, manure, or garbage,

see your doctor about getting a tetanus shot (if you have not had one in the past five years). If the wound shows any indication of redness, swelling, or oozing after the first twenty-four hours, this is a sign of infection. Medical help may be required.

Mild Sprains

Most sprains occur in the knee and ankle joints. As a rule they are minor, involving a stretching or slight tearing of the ligaments around the joint. Usually they will swell a bit, become quite sore, and sometimes turn black and blue. Minor sprains can be treated at home in the following way:

1. Keep the sprained joints elevated as much as possible, especially for the first twenty-four hours after the injury.

2. Apply ice packs to the hurt area for at least thirty minutes after the injury occurs.

3. Wrap the sprained joint in an elastic bandage.

4. A day after the sprain has occurred apply frequent moist heat treatments. Hot water from the tap or in a compress is best.

5. Keep the sprained area firmly but not tightly wrapped in a bandage until healing takes place. Rest and elevate the sprained area wherever possible.

Muscle Cramps

Muscle cramps are painful muscular contractions that may affect almost any muscle in the body. Especially prone to cramping are muscles in the feet, legs, arms, and abdomen. Cramps tend to come and go relatively swiftly. The following measures should help speed them along:

1. *Swimmer's cramps.* A contraction of the muscles due to over-exertion or sudden exposure to cold water. They are best treated by avoiding the conditions that cause it—do not exert yourself in the water beyond natural limits. Do not swim or shower in very cold water. Do not stay in cold water for too long a period of time. Do not swim, exercise, or exert yourself immediately after eating a meal.

2. *Leg cramps.* As soon as the leg cramps begin, stretch your leg out straight and keep it extended until the cramp passes. For cramps in the calf or on the bottom of the feet, stand and lean forward with the feet fixed flat on the floor. Massaging the cramped area will sometimes help. So will applied moist or dry heat.

3. *Heat cramps.* These come from prolonged exposure to heat

and excessive sweating. They can be avoided by taking salt pills and drinking plenty of water when exposed to heat.

TECHNOLOGY, RESOURCES, AIDS, AND SERVICES

1. *The Spenco first aid burn kit* includes adhesive knit tape, cold compresses, roll gauze, antiseptic cream, etc., and is available for around $8.50 plus postage from: HSA, P.O. Box 288, Farmville, NC 27828, (800) 334-1187 (in North Carolina call [800] 672-4214).

2. *A poison antidote kit* containing charcoal, ipecac, and other anti-poison substances is available from Bowman Pharmaceuticals, Canton, OH 44702. Another *poison safeguard kit* is available for around $6.95 plus postage from Marshall Electronics, 7440 North Long Avenue, Skokie, IL 60077.

3. For information on putting together *a home black bag medicine kit,* see the chapter on medical self-examination.

4. *A poison antidote slidewheel* which, slide rule-wise, allows you to turn wheels within wheels and match antidote to poison costs around $3.50 plus $.65 postage from Dunn & Reidman, Box 241, Pacific Palisades, CA 90272.

5. *The Hip Pocket Emergency Survival Handbook* is a unique emergency guide that not only gives you hard-core information on survival in the great out-of-doors, but also comes packaged with a mylar mirror for signaling in times of danger, staples that can be bent into fishhooks, and covers impregnated with a wax chemical for quick fire starts in the wilderness. Get it from Recreational Equipment, Inc. P.O. Box C-88125, Seattle, WA 98118.

6. *A series of audiovisual self-teaching cassettes on the subject of first aid* from Medcom Film Library, Box 16, Garden Grove, CA 92642, (800) 854-2485 (in California call [800] 472-2479). Send for their catalog and peruse the selections yourself. A random sampling of first aid-type films includes *Dealing with Snakebites and Other Emergencies* (#900090), *First Aid, Second Nature* (#000047), *Poison!* (#900051), *For Those Who Live Outdoors* (#900034—emergency measures for survival), *State of Seizure* (#900042—on epilepsy), *Disaster Drill* (#900021—emergency disaster first aid measures), *This Is An Emergency* (#900028—follows a paramedic through a first emergency). Especially good for classroom situations.

For more information see sections on:
For fevers: Colds and Flu (page 99)

For eye injuries: Eye Problems (page 90)
For dizziness and ear first aid: Ear Problems (page 98)
For rashes: Skin Problems (page 123)
For insect bites: Insect Bites and Stings (page 33)
For sudden headaches: Headaches (page 39)
For dizziness and motion sickness: Motion Sickness (page 59)
For dental emergencies: Mouth, Teeth, and Gum Problems (page 148)

FURTHER ASPECTS OF SELF-CARE

CHAPTER 22

PERFORMING A HOME MEDICAL SELF-EXAMINATION

The more familiar you become with the workings of your own body the better your skills will be in times of illness. An excellent way of acquiring these skills is to give yourself or members of your family a home medical examination. Not meant to replace the doctor, of course, these techniques are intended to make you a more active participant in your own health care. They will provide you with enough information to recognize early warning signals of dangerous ailments and hence to describe them accurately to a physician.

The insistence of some physicians that laymen are incapable of learning to assess the state of their own bodies is simply not true. Most basic examination techniques are relatively easy to learn. Thousands of graduates of medical self-care courses across the country have mastered them. Ideally, simple self-examination procedures should be taught in elementary schools and should become an integral part of health care, like brushing our teeth or taking a bath.

Below you will find a series of instructions for conducting a medical self-examination and for translating your findings into practical self-care information. Since the examination is painless, inexpensive, and relatively quick, it is good practice to do it once a year—twice a year if you are over forty. Older people may want to examine themselves more frequently.

A few pieces of equipment, such as a stethoscope and a blood pressure meter, will make the examination more efficient. (Your physician may be willing to lend you these instruments for the short time it takes to perform the exam.) A resource list below tells you how to stock your own medical black bag.

Assuming that your doctor is friendly to self-care—and more and more doctors are—he or she can help you in the following ways:

• By instructing you in the use of medical instruments such as the otoscope, stethoscope, etc., and by supplementing the information and instructions provided in the text below.

• By helping you to procure the medical instruments necessary for self-examination.

• By referring you to pertinent medical literature and materials.

Stocking Your Black Bag

More or less basic to your black bag are:

1. *Stethoscope*—You can buy third-rate models for $15 or less, but for $20 or $30 more you can purchase an instrument that will last for many years. Cheap stethoscopes have a domed plastic chestpiece; better models have a flat metal diaphragm chestpiece surrounded by a corrugated holder.

2. *Thermometer*—The old-fashioned mercury thermometer is quite adequate, and either the oral or the rectal model will do. Because they're inexpensive, it's probably wise to keep both varieties on hand (oral thermometers are easier to use, rectal ones are a bit more accurate). The new digital thermometers are extremely fast and accurate. They cost from $10 to $50.

3. *Blood pressure measurement device (sphygmomanometer)*—A sphygmomanometer consists of an inflatable bladder wrapped in a cloth cuff (for winding around the arm), a pressure measurement device (either mercury or digital), a pressure-control valve, and an inflation bulb or hand pump (see the chapter on hypertension). Prices range from $20 to $1,500. Many of the newer models are equipped with a mechanism in the cuff that reads the blood pressure, rendering a stethoscope unnecessary.

4. *Otoscope (earscope)*—An instrument for examining the ears that costs from $20 to $500.

5. *Vaginal speculum*—This small tool allows women, with the help of a hand mirror, to perform a vaginal self-examination.

Although you can pick up pointers on the correct use of this device from books, it won't hurt to go over the instructions with a gynecologist. Vaginal specula cost only a few dollars.

6. *Other instruments*:
- Tongue depressors
- Reflex hammer
- Peak flow meter (see page 271)
- Hand mirror
- Dental mirror
- Tweezers
- Scale
- Height measuring device
- Flashlight
- Scissors
- Surgical forceps
- Carrying case or bag for all of the above

You can buy either the basic tools (thermometer, stethoscope, and sphygmomanometer) or a black bag kit containing the works. Kits are available from:

The Medical Self-Care Catalog
P.O. Box 999
Pt. Reyes, CA 94956
(415)663-8462
Around $85 including postage.

Health Activation Network
P.O. Box 923
Arlington, VA 22180
(703)938-4447.

Marshall Electronics
7440 North Long Ave.
Skokie, IL 60076
Around $125.

Performing the Medical Self-Examination

A self-examination can be performed alone or with the help of a friend. You should keep a record of your medical history on file for future reference.

The following facts should be recorded:
- Age and date of birth

- Height and weight
- Family doctor (name, address, and phone)
- Blood type
- Allergies
- Foods not tolerated
- Medications not tolerated
- Medications being taken (if any)
- Chronic illnesses (past and present)
- Family history (see chart below):

Family Member	Ailment	Years Suffered
Father	asthma	since childhood
Mother	none	
Maternal grandmother	diabetes	developed age 52 cancer 1962–1964 (died)
Maternal grandfather	arthritis angina emphysema	developed in late 30's developed in late 60's developed in late 60's
Etc.		

- Major ailments for which you have been treated in the past year (record medications and duration of ailments)
- Minor ailments for which you have been treated in the past year (record medications and duration of ailments)
- Hospitalizations during the past year
- Dental visits and treatments
- Childhood ailments (check):
    ___ Measles   ___ Tonsillitis
    ___ Whooping cough   ___ Chicken pox
    ___ Heart murmurs   ___ Appendicitis
    ___ Mumps   ___ Other ___
    ___ Scarlet fever
- Present state of health (excellent, good, fair, poor)
- Present symptoms (name undiagnosed symptoms, if any, that have been bothering you recently)
- Lifestyle:
    ___ Exercise habits
    ___ Type of diet (high or low in fats, etc.)
    ___ Smoking habits

_____ Alcohol consumption

_____ Environment (polluted, unpolluted)

EXAMINING THE CARDIOVASCULAR SYSTEM

To assess the heart and circulatory system you will need:

• A stethoscope

• A sphygmomanometer

• A stop watch or timer with second hand

1. *Take your blood pressure.* Consult the chapter on high blood pressure for a detailed description of how to take and evaluate your blood pressure.

2. *Take your pulse.* A detailed description of how to take and evaluate a pulse is also featured in the chapter on high blood pressure.

3. *Listen to your heart.* It takes a lot of experience to become proficient at using a stethoscope, but most laymen can learn to distinguish the sound of a healthy heart from the sound of one that is obviously weakened or diseased. You should seek instruction from a trained health-care professional and practice using the stethoscope on friends and family members. Once you have learned to identify the rhythm of a healthy heart, the sounds of an unhealthy heart should be apparent.

Place the diaphragm of the stethoscope over the left side of the chest just below the nipple and listen for a beat. It may take several tries before you hear it. Any thunderous, fuzzy, rumbling sounds are most likely an echo in the stethoscope, *not* the heartbeat. What you're looking for is a deep, loud, resonant pumping sound. Check for the following:

• The beat should be deep, rhythmic, and regular.

• A normal heartbeat has a two-part sound—ka-plúm, ka-plúm. Note any irregular beats, skips, jumps, or periods of rapid irregular beats.

• A hissing or "windy" sound may indicate the presence of a heart murmur.

If you know anyone who has a heart condition, listen to his or her chest carefully and note how the sound differs from a normal heartbeat.

4. *Check for symptoms of potential cardiac problems.*

If you answer yes to several of the following questions, consider getting a cardiovascular checkup.

• Have you recently had any of the following symptoms?

Palpitations and general heartbeat irregularities
Sudden nosebleeds
Lightheadedness, dizziness, fainting spells
Undiagnosed chest pains or discomfort
Rapid breathing
- Are you severely winded after climbing two flights of stairs?
- Do you find it particularly difficult to breathe when you are lying down? Does breathing improve when you sit up?
- When you become angered, excited, or stressed, do you experience a feeling of heaviness in your chest?
- Do you frequently have discomfort in your chest after brisk activity? Is the pain *not* relieved by belching but only by rest?

EXAMINING THE LUNGS

For this part of the exam you will need:
- A stethoscope
- A stop watch or a timer with a second hand
- Paper matches
- Peak flow meter (optional) (see page 271)

1. *Assess your breathing rhythms.* Breathing should be slow and steady. It should originate from low in the chest and under the rib cage, not from high in the chest. Note any shortness of breath and/or rapid breathing.

2. *Listen to your lungs with a stethoscope.* The breath should make a clear, steady, windlike noise during inhalation and exhalation. Be on the alert for wheezing, rasping, or foaming sounds, possible signs of asthma, bronchitis, or emphysema. People with chronic bronchitis or asthma usually wheeze when they breathe out. Crackling sounds in the lungs can indicate the presence of fluids, a sign of pneumonia or heart disease. Take the stethoscope off the chest wall, cough, and then listen again. A crackling sound that clears immediately after the cough is a possible indication of bronchitis.

3. *Palpate your chest.* Feel across the full width of your chest for lumps, tender spots, and tender muscles. Press on the rib cage. Intense pain here may indicate inflammation of the cartilages attaching ribs to the breast and back.

4. *Check your respiration rate.* Clock the number of breaths per minute, counting each inhalation-exhalation cycle as a single breath. A normal adult, at rest, usually draws between fourteen and twenty breaths per minute. However, the rate is affected by age and level of activity.

RESPIRATION RATE NORMS

Age	Breaths Per Minute
Newborn	30 = 80
1 through 12	12 = 30
12 through adult	15 = 20
65 on	15 = 25 and up

5. *Test your lung power.* Use these simple tests:

• *The match test*—Light a match and hold it approximately six inches from your mouth. Open your mouth wide and exhale. Using the power of your lungs and diaphragm only—that is, without puckering your lips—try to blow out the match. If you succeed several times in a row, your lungs are probably strong and healthy.

• *The forced expiratory time test*—Get a stop watch or timer with a second hand. Open your mouth wide and fill your lungs to capacity. Exhale forcefully. Using your stop watch, mark the time it takes to exhale all the air. Exhale with plenty of gusto— the idea is to get all of the air out as quickly as possible. Repeat this test several times. A person with normal lungs should finish exhaling in two or three seconds. A person with lung trouble may take from five to seven seconds, and perhaps even longer (people with asthma, for instance, will make a prolonged exhalation that lasts for many seconds and sounds like one continuous wheeze).

• A valuable and affordable tool for testing lung function is the *peak flow meter*, a simple device designed to measure lung capacity and force. It is easy to use, and all necessary charts and directions are included. You can purchase a peak flow meter from *The Medical Self-Care Catalog*, P.O. Box 999, Pt. Reyes, CA 94956, (415)663-8462. It is called the Vitalograph Pulmonary Monitor and costs around $25 plus postage. A better-quality model, the Mini-Wright Peak Flow Meter, can be ordered for around $65 from Armstrong Industries, Inc., P.O. Box 7, North-brook, IL 60062. Armstrong also sells a professional-quality peak flow meter for around $450—not a bad idea if you suffer from chronic lung problems. A really inexpensive model (around $7) can be ordered from Biotrine Corporation, Woburn, MA 01801.

EXAMINING THE EYES

For this part of the examination you will need:
• Snellen eye chart
• Mirror

- Flashlight
- Astigmatism chart (optional)

1. *Check the general appearance of your eyes.* Look into a mirror. The whites of the eyes should be relatively free of scratches, red spots, and pigmentation. A yellow cast may indicate liver problems. Bloodshot eyes (due to the breakage of capillaries in the eye) suggest infection, hypertension, eyestrain, general fatigue, or heavy drinking. Chronic puffiness can signal kidney problems, heart disease, or low thyroid function. Bulging of the eyes may suggest a hyperthyroid condition. Eyes that feel spongy and soft beneath the lid may indicate a vitamin A deficiency. Bulging in only one eye may indicate the presence of a tumor in the socket behind the eye. Droopiness in only one eye, especially in women, can signal *myasthenia gravis,* a condition characterized by a weakness of certain voluntary skeletal muscles. A pallid rather than healthy pink color on the inside of the eyelids may indicate anemia.

Allergic children are likely to demonstrate heavy dark circles under the eyes called "allergic shiners." These markings, although perfectly harmless, serve as a good indication that an allergic condition is present. Examine the pupils of the eyes. Pupils that are unnaturally constricted may indicate a concussion, a stroke, damage to the central nervous system, or recent use of narcotics. Extremely dilated pupils can result from shock, fear, glaucoma, or stimulant drugs such as cocaine.

Shine a flashlight into the eyes. The pupils should constrict with uniform speed and consistency. If one pupil constricts and the other does not, or if there is a marked difference in the size of the pupils when exposed to equal light, there could be a serious problem with the nervous system. In a person who has just been in an accident, pupils of markedly uneven size may indicate brain or nervous system damage. Call a doctor right away.

2. *Test your vision.* You can determine the acuity of your eyesight by using the familiar Snellen Eye Chart. This chart contains rows of letters graded from ³⁄₁₆ to 3½ inches in height. It is available free from the National Society to Prevent Blindness, 79 Madison Ave., New York, NY 10016, and, for several dollars, from Graham-Field Surgical Company, 415 Second Ave., New Hyde Park, NY 11040. You might also ask your local optometrist.

Attach the chart to a wall, stand back twenty feet, cover one eye, and read off each line. Start with the large letters at the top

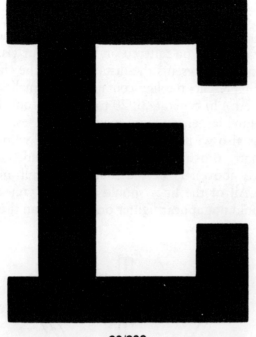

20/200

ECFDP

20/40

PODEFTEC

20/20

and read down until you can no longer read half the letters on a single line. Cover the other eye and repeat.

If you faltered on line twenty, as marked on the chart, you have 20/20 vision. If you faltered on line 40 your vision is 20/40. (The top number represents the distance from the chart; the bottom number represents the line containing the smallest figure your eyes can discern.) In general, 20/20 to 20/40 is considered normal vision. Anything larger, and you may need glasses.

You might also wish to test for astigmatism with an astigmatism star chart (procurable from Graham-Field Surgical Company, address above). Place the chart on a wall and step back twenty feet. All of the lines should have the same appearance. One line should not appear lighter or darker than the others. Any

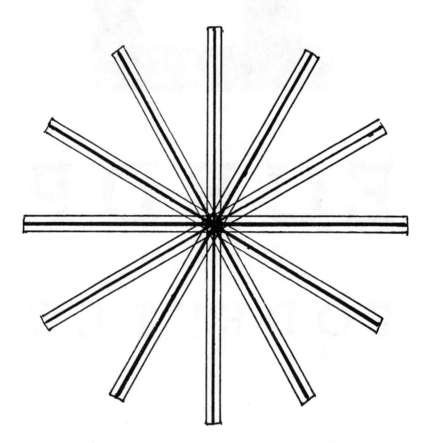

Figure 20. A sample astigmatism test chart (the lines should be 12 inches long and 1/8 inch thick).

discrepancies may indicate an astigmatism. You can use the astigmatism chart reproduced below if you hold it three feet away from your eyes. Professional astigmatism charts are, however, a good deal more accurate.

(Astigmatism chart)

3. *Test your eye muscle strength and coordination.* It is best if someone helps you perform this part of the examination. Have your partner move his or her finger up, down, and to either side at a moderate speed. Follow this movement with your eyes. If you have difficulty keeping your eyes on the finger or if your eyes tend to oscillate during the test, you could have a visual disorder or inner ear problem.

Have your partner sit facing you about three feet away. Cover your left eye and have your partner cover his or her right eye. Take a small object, such as a pen or a spoon, and move it slowly in circles of increasing size. You should both see the object at the same time in your peripheral vision. Repeat with the other eye. If you do *not* see the object when your partner sees it—assuming your partner's eyesight is normal—you may have a defect in your peripheral vision.

EXAMINING THE EARS

For this part of the exam you will need:
- Otoscope
- Partner

1. *Examine the outer ear.* Is it a healthy pinkish color? Do you see any lumps, indentations, cuts, or bruises on the ear shell or around the ear hole? Are there signs of excess wax? Is any part of the ear especially warm, red, or painful to the touch?

2. *Examine the inner ear with an otoscope.* An otoscope is a hand-held instrument that comes equipped with a built-in light, a lens, and a funnel-shaped viewing tip known as a speculum. An otoscope is a handy item to have in your medical tool kit. You can purchase a reasonably priced model from *The Medical Self-Care Catalog,* P.O. Box 999, Pt. Reyes, CA 94956 (around $22 plus postage). Otoscopes in different price ranges ($49.00, $89.00, $174.93) are available from Health Supplies of America, P.O. Box 288, Farmville, NC 27828, (800)334-1187 (in North Carolina call [800] 672-4214).

An otoscope is a relatively tricky instrument to master. Your first few attempts to observe the topography of the outer ear and eardrum may end in frustration. As with the stethoscope, it is a good idea to get some pointers from a health-care professional.

To use the otoscope:

• Disinfect the speculum. Sit next to the person, brace you arm on a steady surface, and bring the otoscope up to the ear. Grasp the shell of the person's ear and gently pull it out and up to create a straight view into the ear canal. Have the person incline his or her head to increase visibility further. Carefully insert the speculum into the earhole and look through the lens. You may wish to turn the otoscope upside down to get a better angle. If you encounter any obstruction (such as earwax accretions) do *not* force the speculum. Clean the ear out (see the chapter on ear self-care for information on removing earwax) before continuing.

• Once the speculum is inserted, set it at different angles to get a full view of the canal walls and the tympanic membrane (eardrum). The inside of the ear canal should be a healthy pink; the walls should be slightly shiny. Some wax should be present but not abnormally large amounts. Signs of infection in the ear canal include redness, swelling, and mucous or pus accumulations. The eardrum itself should be a whitish gray or pearlescent color with a muted, almost metallic surface. Perforations of the eardrum, swelling, bulging, red or blue coloration, or fluid buildup are indications of possible infection

EXAMINING THE NOSE, MOUTH, AND THROAT

For this part of the examination you will need:

• Tongue depressors
• Flashlight

1. *Look into your nose.* Using a flashlight, examine the inside walls of the nostrils. The surfaces should be moist, light pink, and devoid of lumps, swelling, redness, or polyps. There should be no dilated blood vessels or blood deposits of any sort. Check the corners of the nose for redness or sores. Infections here can be serious because this area is drained by veins that connect directly to the brain. A bad infection can be fatal. You can tell whether nasal congestion is caused by an allergy or by a cold by consulting the following chart:

Cold	Allergy
Nasal membrane is dark red	Nasal membrane is pale
Mucus secretions are brown and/or greenish	Mucus secretions are clear, loose, and watery

| Mucus secretions irritate the nose and lips | Mucus secretions do not irritate the nose and lips |
| Nose does not itch | Nose itches |

2. *Examine your mouth.* Put out your tongue. A healthy tongue should be moist, smooth, and a healthy shade of pink. Move it around in a wide circle—there should be no pain or immobility. Furrows on the tongue may indicate dehydration or a tendency toward mouth breathing. A red, swollen tongue can indicate vitamin B and C deficiencies. A fuzzy, coated tongue may suggest excessive drinking. Note any lumps, fissures, or plaques (flat white patches). The latter may be an early sign of cancer of the tongue, especially if you are a pipe smoker. When you take antibiotics, look for white patches, "hairiness," or a general blackening of the tongue. Note the breath, too. Fruity, sweet-smelling breath can indicate diabetes. A smell of urine or ammonia may be associated with kidney problems or diarrhea. Ordinary halitosis is a sign of poor oral hygiene or stomach upset. Bad breath coupled with greenish-yellow sputum may signal sinus problems.

Examine the lips. They should be smooth, pink, and moist. Cracking at the corners of the mouth may be due to a vitamin C or D deficiency. Dryness of the lips can be due to mouth breathing or exposure to harsh weather.

Using a flashlight and tongue depressor, examine the front and back of the throat. Red spots or patches can be a sign of infection, cold, or flu. Look for lumps, sores, or discoloration. Are the tonsils enlarged? Test the gag reflex by sticking your finger or a tongue depressor partway down your throat. Gagging is an unpleasant sensation, but a lack of this reflex may suggest several serious nerve disorders. Now feel your neck for lumps and swollen glands. Swelling under the chin may mean you have a virus infection or an infection of the mouth or tongue.

EXAMINING THE STOMACH

1. *Palpate your stomach.* Although you can perform this maneuver yourself, it is better to have someone do it for you. Lie flat on your back and remove all garments covering the stomach. Beginning at the upper right side of the abdomen just below the rib cage and moving clockwise, palpate the entire abdominal area from the solar plexus to below the navel. Move the hands slowly in a wide circle, pushing and kneading carefully. Note all sore areas. Note any unusual lumps, soft spots, tenderness, or swell-

ing. A navel that bulges prominently may indicate a hernia of the abdominal wall. A distended abdomen may indicate constipation, bowel obstructions, or in rare cases, cancer. Any rigidity or sharp, unexplained pains in this area should be called to the attention of a physician. Also, consider a consultation with a physician if you answer yes to any of the following questions:

• Have you recently gone ten days or more without a bowel movement?

• Have your bowel habits changed dramatically over the past several weeks or months?

• Do you ever find blood, pus, or mucus in your stool?

• Have you recently lost your appetite?

• Are you abnormally hungry all the time?

• Have you recently (and inexplicably) gained or lost a good deal of weight?

• Have your stools been consistently thinner than normal?

EXAMINING THE BREASTS

The importance of a breast self-examination for women, and to a lesser extent for men, is now fully recognized as one of the best early detection methods for cancer. The procedure is fast, easy, and painless, and most doctors recommend that women over twenty perform it at least once a month.

1. Lie flat on your back with a pillow or rolled towel beneath your head. Place your right hand behind your head and raise your head just enough so that you have a clear view of your breasts.

2. Cup the fingers of your left hand over your right breast and gently push inward toward the breastbone until you feel the muscle beneath the skin.

3. Maintaining the pressure, slowly move the fingertips clockwise around the breast, feeling for suspicious lumps, hard spots, dimples, or depressions. Start with one very wide circle (making sure you palpate the area between the edge of the breast and the armpit as well as under the armpit itself), work toward the nipple with increasingly smaller circles. If you find any lumps, thickening, spongy masses, or changes in skin color or texture, consult your doctor immediately.

4. Palpate the nipple, then squeeze it firmly. If any discharge appears, or if the nipple has recently become inverted, see your doctor.

5. Switch hands and repeat the same procedure on the opposite breast.

6. Now stand with breasts bared in front of a large mirror. Place your hands at your sides, behind your head with elbows pulled back, over your head, on your hips with the breastbone pressed in, and behind your back, with the breastbone thrust out. With every shift of body position, study the breasts for evidence of dimpling, lumps, or marked unevenness between the two breasts. Any irregularities should be brought to the attention of a physician.

Several things you should know about breast self-examination:

• Men can and should perform periodic breast self-examinations simply by palpating their breast areas and looking for lumps, dimplings, or irregularities.

• Many women find that breast exams are best carried out in the shower when their breasts are wet and soapy. Under these conditions the hands can move freely over the skin without friction or resistance.

• Most lumps in the breast are *not* malignant. If you find one, do not panic. The odds are greatly in your favor that the lump will be a benign fibrocyst (one woman out of four develops at least one fibrocyst between age fifteen and menopause).

• The best time to examine the breasts is several days to a week after the end of the menstrual period. Avoid breast examinations immediately before the period—the breasts will be especially sensitive and swollen at this time.

• If you do find a lump in your breast, keep in mind that benign cysts are usually tender or painful to the touch, and seem to "roll" or move about when fingered. They sometimes come in groups. Cancerous lumps are usually painless, and feel as if they are rooted to the breastbone. They usually come alone.

If you are prone to fibrocysts, several preventive measures known to be beneficial include:

• Eliminating all caffeine. A direct link has been established between this substance and the formation of fibrocysts.

• Losing weight. Statistically speaking, the heavier a woman is, the greater her chances are of developing fibrocysts.

• Quitting smoking. Nicotine encourages the formation of cyst-producing chemicals.

• Eliminating sugar. Like nicotine and caffeine, sweets encourage cyst growth.

• Cutting down on fats. A link has been established between cyst formation and high-fat foods. Foods that seem to help *prevent* cysts and (possibly cancer as well) include high-fiber foods, fruits (especially bananas, apples, oranges, and grapefruits), foods with high vitamin E and B$_6$ content, soybeans, pumpkin and sunflower seeds, and Brewers yeast.

A new and highly praised method of breast self-examination has been developed by an organization called the MammaCare Center. This method trains the subject to seek out lumps on the breasts using horizontal and vertical movements rather than the standard circular motions. Studies indicate the practitioners of the MammaCare method detect more lumps and smaller lumps than those who practice the conventional examination technique. Presently there are over twenty MammaCare Centers in the United States. For information on one near you, contact Mammatech Corp., 930 N.W. 8th Ave., Gainesville, FL 32601, (800) MAM-CARE.

A free breast self-examination guide, complete with illustrated instructions and reminder stickers for monthly exams, can be obtained from Cancer Action Now Headquarters, 110 East Warren Ave., Detroit, MI 48201. A free booklet called *If You've Thought About Breast Cancer . . .* by Rose Kushner is available from Women's Breast Cancer Advisory Center, P.O. Box 224, Kensington, MD 20895.

Home Diagnostic Test for Breast Cancer

A self-care kit known as the Breast Cancer Screening Indicator is currently available for home use. It consists of specially treated pads that are worn over the breasts for about fifteen minutes and change color to signal any suspicious irregularities of skin temperature along the breast surfaces—a possible sign of tumor or growth. The kit is available for around $15 from many pharmacies or directly from the manufacturer: Faberge Incorporated, 1345 Avenue of the Americas, New York, NY 10019.

EXAMINING THE NERVOUS SYSTEM

To test your reflexes you will need:

• A rubber percussion hammer (or any small rubber-headed mallet)

• Ice bag

Reflex testing is a method of gauging your body's reaction to external stimulation of its nerve and muscle systems. Both an exaggerated response and a complete lack of response may indicate some type of spinal cord or nervous system damage.

1. *Knee.* Sit comfortably on a stool or high chair with your legs dangling freely. With a rubber percussion hammer (or any small rubber-headed mallet), tap lightly on the tendon located directly below the kneecap. The leg should kick out spontaneously each time this point is tapped. Practice on several people to get the hang of it.

2. *Ankle jerk.* Pull the foot up gently. Then with a rubber percussion hammer, lightly tap the Achilles tendon, located on the web of skin directly above the heel. The tap should cause the top of the foot to point downward. Marked slowness or lack of this reflex may indicate thyroid problems or a nervous system defect.

3. *Babinski test.* Grasp the ankle. Take a blunt instrument (a pen, a ruler, a wooden dowel with a rounded tip) and stroke the sole of your foot from the heel up to the ball of the foot, across the base of the toes toward the big toe. Your toes should curl and contract. If your toes spread out rather than flex, nerve or brain damage may be indicated.

4. *Cold face reflex.* Fill an ice bag with ice and hold it against your cheek or forehead for one minute, taking your pulse as you do. A temporary slowing of the pulse is a normal reaction.

CHECKING THE URINE AND FECES

1. *Feces.* Check your feces after each bowel movement. The stools should be long, approximately an inch to an inch-and-a-half thick, and have a pumpkin or dark brown color. They should smell but not too strongly (the stools of meat eaters tend to smell more than those of vegetarians, and to be firmer). Extremely strong stool odor can indicate pancreas problems, digestive disorders, or parasites, among other things.

Examine the stool for blood or mucus. Pencil-thin or ribbon-like stools may indicate an obstruction in the bowel. Black or tarry stools may suggest internal bleeding or intestinal problems. Gray stools may mean gall bladder difficulties. Unexplained diarrhea that continues for more than several days should be brought to the attention of a physician. There are several stool diagnostic tests that can be performed at home. Consult the chapter on self-diagnostic tests for more information.

2. *Urine.* Check your urine every day. Look for unusual color-ations. Healthy urine ranges from dark yellow to pale yellow. A dark tea- or mahogany-colored urine may indicate the presence of bile. Watery, colorless urine is occasionally a warning sign of diabetes. Consistently cloudy urine may be a result of infection. Blood in the urine (dark brown or pink) is *always* a danger sign and should be reported to a doctor right away. Note, however, that certain drugs—especially antibiotics, tranquilizers, antide-pressants, and laxatives—can turn the urine strange colors in-cluding red, blue, or brown. Exercise tends to make urine a dark yellow color, but so do anemia and kidney problems. If you take large quantities of vitamin B, don't be surprised to see your urine turn a lurid orange-yellow.

Whenever there is a dramatic change in the color or pattern of your urination (including consistently painful urination) that lasts for several days, it's time to see a doctor. Become accustomed to looking into the toilet bowl after every urination (and after every bowel movement). Although it is not a very aesthetic habit, it may save you a good deal of grief. At the same time, remember that certain food colorings and foods such as beets and licorice will turn your urine odd colors, and that it is not necessarily a danger sign if your urine is a shade of shocking pink or green.

There are several urine diagnostic tests you can do at home. Consult Chapter 23 for more information.

EXAMINING THE GENITALS

For a vaginal examination you will need:
• Mirror
• Strong source of light
• Vaginal speculum
If you are using a metal speculum, it is best to warm it before insertion. Plastic specula do not need to be warmed (they are also transparent for better viewing and usually inexpensive).

1. Wash the speculum carefully, then lie on your back with your knees drawn up and a mirror positioned close by.

2. Aim a bright light directly at the vaginal opening.

3. Separate your legs, spread the labia, and insert the specu-lum, making sure to lock the speculum's blades carefully in place after insertion. (You can rub a little lubricating jelly on the spec-ulum to ease insertion.) Position the mirror so that you can see directly into the vagina.

4. Examine the outside of the vagina for lumps, irritation, or unusual markings.

5. Then open the speculum and look into the vagina itself. It should be a healthy pink color without any cuts, blood deposits, sores, or deep red spots. The walls will almost always exhibit small amounts of milky white or clear discharge. This is natural.

Be suspicious if you see:

• Thick white discharge that resembles cottage cheese, has a "yeasty" smell, and causes severe itching (possible *candida* [yeast] infection).

• Creamy white or gray discharge with a strong odor (possible *haemophilus vaginalis*).

• Thick yellow discharge with cloudy, frequent, and painful urination (possible gonorrhea).

• Greenish and frothy yellowish-white discharge with an acrid odor (possible *trichomona*).

• Watery gray discharge with a fishy smell (possible bacterial infection).

• Red fluid-filled blisters within the vagina that itch, cause pain, and produce excessive discharge (possible herpes). Small craters along the vaginal wall, labia, or cervix may be herpes sores that have already ripened and burst.

For an examination of the male genitals you will need:

• A strong source of light

1. Examine the shaft of your penis under a focused source of light. Look for sores, swelling, craters, lumps, or moles that have changed shape or size.

2. Check the head of the penis. Examine it for reddening or signs of infection in the crease between the shaft and head.

3. Check the urethral opening; it should be free of redness and dribbling secretions.

4. Any weeping blisters may be due to venereal herpes. Blood in the sperm during ejaculation, although frightening, usually stems from congestion of the veins of the seminal vesicles and is not necessarily cause for great worry. Have it checked only if it continues. Any indication that you are suffering from *priapism*, a state of chronic erection, should be called to the attention of a doctor immediately. It is a potential symptom of neurological damage.

5. Now the testicles. When rolled between your fingers they should feel firm yet spongy. Palpate both testicles for lumps,

bulging, varicose veins, cysts, swelling, sores, or signs of skin infection. Next, stand in front of a mirror and observe the way the testicles hang. Ordinarily, the left testicle will hang a bit lower than the right. If there is a large discrepancy between the two, or if there is a noticeable difference in their sizes, consult your doctor.

ASSESSING YOUR GENERAL HEALTH

Finally, a few techniques for determining your overall health. For this section of the examination you will need:
• Scale
• Height measuring device
• Thermometer

1. *Weigh yourself.* Check your weight frequently and note any dramatic gains or losses. For a table of recommended weights per size see page 220–221.

2. *Measure your height.* Use either a tape measure or height measuring device available at most pharmacies or health supply stores.

3. *Take your temperature.* Along with blood pressure, pulse, and respiration rate, internal temperature is one of the best indications of a person's health and metabolism. Each of us has subtle changes of body temperature throughout the day, sometimes as much as a whole degree, so it is a good idea to take your temperature at different times during one day for the purpose of this exam. Normal temperature of 98.6°F, but one degree above or below is within the normal range. In adults, any fever over 102°–103°F can be dangerous and should be referred to a physician. Anything above 103°F in a child is cause for concern.

The standard oral or rectal mercury thermometer is perfectly adequate for home use. Rectal temperature tends to run a point higher than oral. Also useful is the digital thermometer, which presents readings on a liquid crystal display and is generally faster than the mercury thermometer. Another type is the *plastic strip thermometer,* a heat-sensitive swatch that is taped to the forehead and can be left in place for long periods to allow for continuous monitoring of temperature. Plastic strip thermometers are available from most pharmacies. Strip thermometers are less accurate than either the digital or mercury variations.

4. *Check your hair.* The hair is a prime indicator of the state of one's health. Pull at it—it should not come out easily. A healthy

head of hair is elastic and springy with a vital sheen. Dry, dull hair with many split ends or excessively oily hair with a matted, gummy texture can indicate nutritional deficiencies or a poor state of general health.

5. *Check your fingernails.* Your nails should be a healthy pink with a pleasant matte shine and well-defined whitish half-moons. Nails that chip and break easily may be a sign of poor nutrition. Blue or purplish coloration of the nail beds can be a sign of inadequate oxygen intake, anemia, disease of the heart or lungs. Troughlike depressions down the center of the nails can be a sign of iron-deficiency anemia.

6. *Check your skin color and tone.* A pallid complexion can be a sign of general debility or anemia. A yellowish cast to the skin may signal liver problems or pernicious anemia. Extremely dry skin may be due to a deficiency of vitamin A or to thyroid problems.

TECHNOLOGY, RESOURCES, AIDS, AND SERVICES

1. The *Wellness Inventory* by John Travis, M.D., is a one-hundred-item questionnaire designed to determine the strong and weak points in your life-style. It costs $.50. Mail a self-addressed, stamped envelope to Wellness Resource Center, 42 Miller Ave., Mill Valley, CA 94941. The same outfit offers a *Wellness Workbook*, also by Dr. Travis, which explains how to give yourself a thorough medical exam and how to do a complete evaluation of your present state of health. The layman edition costs $25.00, the professional edition $60.00.

2. Two excellent books on the subject of medical exams are *A Guide to Physical Examination* by Barbara Bates, M.D. (Philadelphia: J. P. Lippincott, 1974), and *The Complete Medical Exam* by Isadore Rosenfeld, M.D. (New York: Simon & Schuster, 1978).

CHAPTER 23

MEDICAL TESTS
YOU CAN
PERFORM AT HOME

The high cost of laboratory tests has caused many consumers to turn to over-the-counter home medical tests. Although many doctors approve of this trend, they stipulate that the tests be used not as diagnostic tools, but as methods of self-assessment. They warn that if a test indicates potential trouble, the results should be called to the attention of a health-care professional.

Manufacturers of home medical tests are understandably enthusiastic about their products, but at times they can become unrealistic in their assessment of how well these products really work. Be aware that no matter what glowing statistics they may dangle before you, no matter how sweeping the claims may be on the box, most home medical tests are still far from 100 percent, and many have a rather wide margin of error. Seventy percent accuracy, for instance, is considered a good accuracy rate for any do-it-yourself test, and no doubt it is. But 70 percent of cases accurately diagnosed means that almost *one third* of cases are *inaccurately* diagnosed. This means one out of three is a miss—a record far from perfect, to say the least.

Do-it-yourself medical tests are often a good deal less sensitive than their laboratory counterparts. They may show incorrect abnormal results and send you to the doctor's office unnecessarily, or they may show incorrect normal results and lull you into a false sense of security about a condition that requires swift medical attention. If a test shows negative results but the symptoms continue, it's best to see a physician anyway and get the matter cleared up once and for all.

The drawbacks notwithstanding, however, do-it-yourself medical tests are among the finest self-help tools ever placed in the hands of the medical consumer. Many lives have already been saved using these tests, especially tests designed for the early detection of cancer, and countless dollars have been conserved that would otherwise have been spent on costly trips to the doctor's office.

Below is a list of the most effective home test kits now available. The home test business is in its infancy, and the list below will no doubt be upgraded, expanded, and improved drastically within the next few years. Prices for these kits change frequently, and new products are constantly appearing.

Since the field of home testing is still a new one, the chances of coming upon a test that fails to live up to its claims is always a possibility. To help you, the FDA maintains a toll-free number you can use to report any problems. The number is (800) 638-6725.

COLON SCREENING TESTS

Purpose: To test for occult blood (hidden blood) in the stool. Occult blood can be an early warning of colon cancer. It can also indicate colitis, diverticulitis, ulcers, and several other gastrointestinal ailments.

Form and procedure: Colon screening test kits come in several forms. One is a toilet paper that turns bluish green if blood is present in the stool. Another is a pad, designed to be dropped into the toilet after a bowel movement, that turns orange in the presence of blood. Still another requires testing the stool itself.

Availability: Colon screening tests can be purchased at most pharmacies. You can also order the ColoScreen self-test from *The Medical Self-Care Catalog,* P.O. Box 999, Pt. Reyes, CA 94956. The Hema-Chek Fecal Occult Blood Test is available from HSA, P.O. Box 288, Farmville, NC 27828, (800)334-1187 (in North Carolina call [800] 672-4214).

Cost: From $8.00 to $12.00. The Hema-Chek Fecal Occult Blood Test includes enough materials for one hundred tests and costs around $37.00 plus postage.

Breast Cancer Screening Indicator

Purpose: To detect early symptoms of breast cancer.

Form and procedure: Specially treated heat-sensitive pads to be inserted into the bra and left there about fifteen minutes. If there are any "hot spots" on the breasts—possible indications of tumors under the skin—color changes register on the pads.

Availability: You can order a Breast Cancer Screening Indicator kit from Faberge Incorporated, 1345 Ave. of the Americas, New York, NY 10019. Some pharmacies also stock this item.

Cost: From $10 to $15.

Blood Glucose Tests

Purpose: To measure the amount of glucose in the blood. This test and the electronic equipment that comes with the more expensive kits is designed to allow diabetics (and, to a lesser extent, hypoglycemics) to monitor their blood sugar levels.

Form and procedure: Less expensive kits contain a supply of reagent strips and a master color chart. A drop of blood is placed on the strip and any color changes are matched against the chart to determine the concentration of glucose in the blood. CHEM-STRIP bG, VISIDEX, and Dextrostix are popular brands. The more expensive type includes a glucose meter to make testing easier and more accurate. A sample of blood is wiped onto a test strip, and the strip is fed into the meter, which immediately provides a highly accurate printed readout of the glucose level. Accu-Check, Glucoscan II, and Glucochek II are popular models.

Availability: VISIDEX and Dextrostix can be found at pharmacies. CHEMSTRIP bG is available at many pharmacies or from *The Medical Self-Care Catalog,* P.O. Box 999, Pt. Reyes, CA 94956. The Accu-Check glucose monitor is also obtainable from the *Self-Care Catalog.* The Glucoscan II is available from Lifescan, Inc., 1025 Terra Bella Ave., Mountain View, CA 94043, (800)227-8862. The Glucochek II is available from Larken Industries, 8397 Melrose, Lenexa, Kansas 66214, (800)452-7536.

Cost: Reagent strips cost around $40 for one hundred strips. Glucose meters range in price from $150 to $200; they usually come with a large supply of reagent strips.

Hemoglobin Test

Purpose: To determine the hemoglobin level in the blood. A low hemoglobin count can indicate anemia, thyroid problems, or certain types of cancer. High hemoglobin levels may point to an increased risk of stroke.

Form and procedure: The Tallquist Haemoglobin Scale consists of a series of absorbent papers. Blood samples are placed on the papers and any color changes are matched against a master chart.

Availability: The Tallquist Haemoglobin Scale is available from Graham-Field Surgical Company, 415 Second Ave., New Hyde Park, NY 11040.

Cost: From $3.50 to $5.00 for a large supply of papers, a color chart, and instructions.

MONOSTICON-DRI-DOT TEST FOR MONONUCLEOSIS

Purpose: To determine if the mononucleosis virus is present in the bloodstream.

Form and procedure: The Monosticon-DRI-DOT test kit contains pretreated slides. A drop of blood is placed on the slide and instructions are followed.

Availability: The Monosticon-DRI-DOT test can be purchased from most pharmacies or directly from the manufacturer, Organon.

BLOOD TYPE TESTING KITS

Purpose: To determine the blood type.

Form and procedure: The kit includes a set of pretreated cards, lancets for taking blood, pipets, and a mixing comb.

Availability: You can order the kit from HSA, P.O. Box 288, Farmville, NC 27828, (800)334-1187 (in North Carolina call [800] 672-4214).

Cost: A kit that can determine the blood types of four people costs $3.60 plus postage. A test for ten people costs $8.95 plus postage.

BLOOD SAMPLE EQUIPMENT

Purpose: To take blood sample for any purpose including the blood tests mentioned above.

Availability and cost: Fingersticking lancets can be purchased at $10.00 per hundred from Sherwood Medical, 831 Olive St., St. Louis, MI 63103. A permanent lancet model called the Autoclix (around $19.00) is available from *The Medical Self-Care Catalog,* P.O. Box 999, Pt. Reyes, CA 94956. A wide array of lancet devices and kits is available from HSA, P.O. Box 288,

Farmville, NC 27828, (800)334-1187 (in North Carolina call [800] 672-4214). The prices range from $5.00 to $25.00.

PREGNANCY TEST KITS

Purpose: To determine pregnancy.

Form and procedure: All brands use the same basic method: A urine sample taken first thing in the morning is mixed with a test solution or reagent and color changes are interpreted according to the instructions. Depending on the brand, test results are available fifteen minutes to two hours after testing.

Availability: Home pregnancy tests are available today in practically every drugstore in the country. The better-known brands include e.p.t., ACU-TEST, Predictor, Fact, and Daisy 2, and most usually work within twenty-four hours.

Cost: From $10.00 to $15.00, depending on how many tests are contained in the package.

Note: When pregnancy tests err, they tend to err on the negative side, i.e., negative results are not necessarily conclusive. On the other hand, positive results are generally accurate. Tranquilizers, antibiotics, pain killers, and certain other medications tend to interfere with test results. Be sure to read all instructions carefully.

URINALYSIS

Purpose: To monitor the progress of certain ailments, such as diabetes; to test for infections; to test for preliminary signs of kidney or bladder disease; and to judge the values of certain medications. Home urinalysis kits can be used to test for the following properties:

• pH (acidity or alkalinity) of the urine (The pH level indicates the balance between acids and alkalines in the urine. Irregularities can indicate blood, nerve or hormone disorders.)

• Ketones (Ketones are acids and acetones, the appearance of which can indicate diabetes or faulty carbohydrate metabolism.)

• Traces of blood in the urine (Blood in the urine can indicate anemia, kidney stones, urinary tract infections, kidney tumors, bladder tumors, or parasites.)

• Glucose level (sugar level in urine) (Positive tests can indicate diabetes and several other metabolism problems.)

• Nitrite (Nitrites caused by urinary bacteria can be a sign of infection in the body.)

• Specific gravity (Specific gravity refers to the amount of solid materials present in urine. Imbalance of specific gravity can indicate kidney problems.)

• Vitamin C levels (Low levels can indicate anemia, infection and digestive problems.)

• Leukocytes (white blood cells) (An increase can indicate that infection is present.)

• Bilirubin (A by-product of hemoglobin breakdown which can turn urine dark yellow and which, can indicate anemia, liver ailments and presence of medicinal drugs like antibiotics.)

• Protein (Excess protein in urine can indicate kidney, liver, and nerve disorders.)

• Urobilinogen (absence or excess of the bile pigment) (Urobilinogen in the urine can indicate liver diseases, or blood diseases such as anemia.)

Form and procedure: A specially treated reagent strip is dipped into a urine sample. All color changes (and/or discolorations) on the strip are checked against a master color chart. The less expensive strips are designed to test for two or three items only, generally glucose, ketones, and vitamin C. More expensive strips test for many or most of the items mentioned above.

Availability: Several major manufacturers of urine tests are listed below.

1. BioDynamics:

Chemstrip LN—Leukocytes and nitrite

Chemstrip uGK—Glucose and ketones

Chemstrip 9—All items mentioned above except specific gravity

Chemstrip 4—Blood, pH, glucose, protein

2. Ames:

Albustix Strips—Protein

Diastix Strips—Glucose

Hema-Combistix Strips—Glucose, pH, blood, protein

N-Multistix-C Strips—All items mentioned above except specific gravity and luekocytes

3. Curtin Matheson Scientific:

Uri-TRAK 7AN—All items mentioned above except specific gravity and leukocytes

Uri-TRAK 6A—All items mentioned above except specific gravity, urobilinogen, nitrite, leukocytes

Uri-TRAK 4A—Vitamin C, pH, blood, glucose, protein

Most of the strips listed can be purchased from a pharmacy or from a medical supply house such as HSA, P.O. Box 288, Farmville, NC 27828, (800)334-1187 (in North Carolina call [800] 672-4214). You can also write directly to the manufacturers for ordering information:

BioDynamics
9115 Hague Rd.
Indianapolis, IN 46250

Miles Laboratories, Inc., Ames Division
P.O. Box 70
Elkhart, IN 46515

Curtin Matheson Scientific, Inc.
P.O. Box 1546
Houston, TX 77251

Cost: Urinalysis kits usually contain one hundred strips; prices vary according to the number of tests each brand is capable of performing. Strips that test only for protein and glucose cost from $8 to $10 per hundred. Tests that measure a number of variables (including specific gravity) all in one strip cost from $35 to $45 per hundred.

Note: A useful booklet, *How to Perform Your Own Urinalysis without a Doctor for under $.50* by Richard Anthony, is available for $10 from P.I. Industries, P.O. Box 949, Loveland, CO 80537.

BREATH ALCOHOL

Purpose: To determine whether the amount of alcohol in the bloodstream is high enough to affect judgment and coordination.

Form and procedure: The test is performed either by breathing into an electronic breath monitoring apparatus (AlcoCheck and Biotron Alcohol Tester are two popular brands) or by using a disposable balloon and test tube device called the Drink-O-Meter. A blood alcohol level of .10 percent (one tenth of one percent) is the legal definition of drunkenness in many parts of the country, although the figure varies from state to state. Some bars and taverns are now providing breath detection devices for their customers' use. If the customer is driving, they base the number of drinks they will serve on the results of these tests.

Availability: The Drink-O-Meter can be purchased at many pharmacies or directly from the manufacturers, Luckey Laboratories, Inc., 725ʌ Osbun Rd., San Bernadino, CA 92404. The AlcoCheck is manufactured by National Draeger, Inc., P.O. Box 120, Pittsburgh, PA 15230. The Biotron Alcohol Tester is made by Edmund Scientific, 101 E. Gloucester Pike, Barrington, NJ 08007.

Cost: Disposable alcohol breath tests cost several dollars per kit. Electronic breath measuring devices cost from $40 to $100.

TEST FOR GONORRHEA

Purpose: To determine if the gonorrhea infection is present. (This test works only for men.)

Form and procedure: A drop of discharge from the penis is tested and observed for certain color changes according to instructions.

Availability: The Gonodecten test is available from United States Packaging Corporation, 506 Clay St., La Porte, IN 46350. It is currently available only with a doctor's prescription, but several detection kits for venereal disease are expected to be marketed over-the-counter in the near future.

Cost: Around $5.00.

CHAPTER 24

THE HOME-CARE ALTERNATIVE

Home care is similar enough to self-care to be considered here. A once ignored and even discouraged alternative to hospitalization, it has become a high-growth industry over the past several years, and its growing popularity is based on a number of sound reasons that will be discussed below. It is, however, important to stress that anyone considering home care should master the basics of self-care. They complement each other and both will be playing an increasingly important role in the future of American health care.

WHAT IS HOME CARE?

Although the term has become familiar, it still causes a good deal of confusion and misunderstanding. Simply stated, a person who has home care has chosen to be diagnosed, treated, cared for, and rehabilitated by a team of health-care professionals *at home rather than in a hospital*. Home care does *not* mean that a patient has rejected conventional medical therapies or decided to take medical matters into his or her own hands. On the contrary, a good program is a cooperative effort involving the patient, the physician, the nurse, the family, and any other professionals on the home-care team. Patients treated by home-care professionals almost always remain under the supervision of a regular doctor.

Home care is not a substitute for a doctor's care. It provides most, if not all, of the same medications, therapies, and care that a patient would receive in the hospital.

WHY USE IT?

The obvious advantage of home care is that being nursed back to health—or waiting out the terrible process of a terminal illness—in one's home, surrounded by loved ones and living as normal a life as possible, is more conducive to convalescence and comfort than confinement to a hospital ward. Many studies have indicated that patients tend to recuperate faster at home than in an institution. Furthermore, home care enables the patient to feel more in control of the healing process, less the victim of impersonal forces.

Another advantage of home care is that it is generally less expensive than hospitalization. While it is true that some people have private and federal health insurance that covers up to 80 percent of their hospital bills, at around $700 a day for a hospital room, plus doctors' fees (which are not included in all insurance policies), plus the deductible, plus the dozens of hidden costs that magically crop up on the final bill, a major illness can devastate a patient's savings.

Home care, though certainly not cheap, is almost always a better deal. Home-care agencies usually charge a single daily rate based on all services provided. Because you do not pay the hospital's overhead as well as your own medical bills, there are no hidden costs. Agency prices for tests, therapies, rental equipment, nursing services, etc., tend to be considerably less expensive than those charged in hospitals. In hospitals, just about everything from medications to Kleenex is automatically marked up, but with home care you purchase your own drugs and sundries, sometimes at half of hospital prices. The best news is that Medicare and most medical insurance policies now cover part or all of home-care costs. Insurance companies are highly supportive of anyone who chooses this option because it saves them money, too. Home-care expenses are also tax deductible.

Finally, home care benefits hospitals. There is an escalating hospital space crisis, and home care frees more beds and rooms for patients in immediate need. Hospitals were designed to be acute care institutions, not places for the chronically ill patient or long-term convalescent.

Who Needs It?

Anyone who is seriously ill but not in medical crisis is a candidate for home care: patients recovering from accidents, patients with chronic diseases, patients in need of rehabilitation (most good home-care agencies offer home orthopedic and rehabilitative therapy services), patients recovering from surgery, patients on kidney dialysis, and patients who are disabled. Candidates also include patients with terminal illnesses (almost all the medical services that can be offered the dying person can be provided at home or in a hospice).

How Does It Work?

The person who has decided to use home care must first discuss the matter with a doctor. Although the medical community has traditionally resisted the idea of home care, an increasing number of physicians now support it, and some are pleased to take an active part in the process. A few go so far as to make house calls when necessary and give out their private phone numbers for emergencies.

The next step is to have the doctor write out an order for home care and recommend an agency suited to the patient's needs. There are many types of agencies. A number of hospitals and nursing homes maintain their own home-care departments, which is especially useful if a patient has already received acute care from the same institute. There are visiting nurse services, unaffiliated with hospitals, that send qualified nurses into a patient's home on either a part-time, full-time, or live-in basis. Also useful are community service organizations, professional home-care agencies that provide a full spectrum of home-care and homemaker facilities, and home health-aid services that provide special skills such as speech therapy or respiratory therapy.

Be aware, however, that since home care is a booming industry, it is impossible to be too careful in choosing the proper agency. Fly-by-night companies are becoming an increasingly common sight in the Yellow Pages, and many of these organizations consist of nothing more than a one-room office, a telephone answering machine, and a desire to get rich quick. Be certain that the agency is at least "certified," which means that it is authorized to receive payment from Medicare (and sometimes Medicaid) and that it meets minimum federal standards for patient care. Even better is an agency that is "accredited," which means the agency has voluntarily allowed its staff and facilities to be studied by a consumer-protection organization such as the National HomeCaring Council or the Joint Commission on the Accreditation of Hospitals and has been found to meet all professional standards.

Once the doctor has been consulted and the home-care agency chosen, the home-care team is assembled. The basic members are the patient, the doctor, and the in-home nurse. The help and support of the patient's family is absolutely necessary. The program is generally supervised by both a home-care coordinator and a clinical coordinator. They will process your application, make out schedules, and assign workers. They will also coordinate with the supervising physician and visit the patient's home to assess his or her particular needs. The coordinators will also provide dietitians, social.workers, physical therapists, or homemakers if required. Respirators, X-ray machines, intravenous therapy equipment, orthopedic equipment, and other special apparatus can be rented through agencies or, in some cases, purchased directly from the manufacturer.

Next, the agency presents the patient with a home-care plan that outlines the treatment: therapy schedules, required equipment, dietary plans, personnel assignments, and treatment goals. Ideally, this plan is tailored to the patient's needs and conforms to the financial and psychological needs of the family. Once approved by the doctor, the program is put into operation, and the agency oversees it until completion.

FINDING HOME-CARE AGENCIES

Any doctor who supports home care will probably know of the best local organizations. Even hospitals that do not maintain their own home-care affiliates can provide you with the names of reputable agencies and services, as can social workers and discharge administrators associated with the hospital. Don't forget the value of personal referrals and word-of-mouth. You can, of course, also try the Yellow Pages. If you do, be sure to ask the following questions:

• What services are available from the agency and how much do they cost? How long has the agency been in business? Does it have other offices? Is it independent or part of a chain?

• How is the billing handled? Is the agency covered by insurance plans and Medicare? Does the agency maintain a sliding scale or part-pay program based on the client's income?

- Is the agency certified or accredited? If not, why? Is it profit or nonprofit? Can it provide references from doctors or administrators at community organizations and hospitals? Ask for specific names and organizations, and call these people directly.
- How large is its staff and what specialists is it capable of providing? What kind of training, experience, and credentials are required of the staff? Are the homemakers and health-care aides screened?
- How does it handle providing medical machinery to the home? What machinery is it capable of providing? What machinery is it *not* capable of providing? How does the billing work for machinery rental?
- During what hours does the agency provide services? Twenty-four hours a day, or just eight to eight? Are services available on weekends? On holidays? Are fees higher for services during off-hours? How much higher? Must you pay for a minimum number of hours even if you do not use them?
- What type of relationship does the agency maintain with the supervising physician?
- Who provides general supervision and coordination of the in-home program?
- Does the agency provide a contract or service agreement stipulating its rates, services, specialists provided, hidden costs, hours of care, etc.?
- Does the agency provide you with a complete home assessment before treatment begins? How thorough is it? Who conducts it? Does it provide a complete home-care program *in writing*, tailored to your needs?
- What type of emergency response system does the agency offer?

If you have difficulty finding a home-care organization that suits your needs, try consulting your phone book for the name of the closest home-care association or contact any of the organizations listed below for more information. Keep in mind that it is wiser to pay the extra dollar for quality service than to hunt around for cheaper but less efficient alternatives.

American Affiliation of Visiting Nurse
    Associations and Services
21 Maryland Plaza
Ste. 300
St. Louis, MO 63108

American Federation of Home Health Agencies
429 N St. SW
Ste. S-605
Washington, DC 20024

Home Health Care Medical Directors Association
P.O. Box 16626
Mobile, AL 36616

National Association for Home Care
519 C St. NE
Washington, DC 20002

National HomeCaring Council
235 Park Ave. South
11th Floor
New York, NY 10003

National Institution on Adult Daycare
600 Maryland Avenue SW
West Wing 100
Washington, DC 20024

American Association for Continuity of Care
1101 Connecticut Ave. NW
Suite 700
Washington, DC 20036

CHAPTER 25

STAYING HEALTHY: SOME BASIC RULES OF THE GAME

In ancient China it was said that the worst doctor saves the lives of the sick. The better doctor cures people before their lives are endangered. And the perfect doctor, the best of the three, keeps patients so healthy that they never need a physician in the first place. In short, prevention is the best medicine.

Yet, ask the person on the street to define health and most will say: "To be healthy means not to be sick." Most of us have been brought up to believe that if we are not ailing, this automatically means we are the very picture of wellness. Such a notion has been ingrained in us since childhood, starting at school, with parents and in the doctor's office where the physician smiled at us and announced: "Your pneumonia is cured; you are well now." So the message is clear; we have been sold the bill of goods that health means eliminating sickness through medical treatment.

Now, ask the person who believes in prevention to define the same term. "Health," this person will say, "is achieving *a high level of wellness.*" Health, he or she will assure us, does not mean the simple absence of disease; it means the presence of extra energy, a sense of well-being and clear mindedness, organs that function at their full capacity, and a psyche that is harmoniously adjusted to the mental and emotional components of daily life. In short, wellness is:

- A total body-mind event.
- A deliberate *choice* to move toward optimal health.
- A *process*. . . a developing awareness that there is no end point, that health and happiness are possible at every given moment.
- A way of life . . . a life-style that you design, to achieve your highest potential for well-being.
- A reaching out for the *best* that you can be.
- Wellness is not an individual's right—it is each person's responsibility.

How does one achieve high levels of wellness? Principally, by cultivating a set of preventive living habits that keep us protected from the destructive elements of modern living.

Specifically, this means becoming aware of small things as well as large: that we can make better and healthier choices when we eat at a restaurant; that we can prepare gourmet meals at home that are low in fat and calories; that we can take time out each day to exercise without disturbing our regular living routine; that we can cut down on our coffee and junk foods, get more sleep, stop smoking, drink purer water, drive more carefully, reduce stress, avoid drugs, and generally reprogram ourselves to learn a new set of habits. Interestingly, researchers now believe that twenty-one repetitions of a particular act turn that act into a habit; and once locked in, these new habits then become the stuff of permanent change.

We *can* change our life-style. We *can* achieve high levels of wellness. To understand that it is possible, and feasible, and practical, and practicable, is the first step toward life-style modification.

Prevention and Longevity

What then, it might be asked, is preventive medicine? In short, it is:

The intentional practice of specific physical and mental life modification activities which, when used together in a consistently applied program, produce a statistical increase in a person's chances of remaining healthy and living longer.

Through the extensive research that has recently been done on health maintenance, we now know precisely what many of these preventive do's and don'ts are, and in many cases we can calculate the number of statistical years their addition or subtraction to our lives will bring. Below is a self-test based on such figures.

Take it right now, before learning about specific preventive measures below, to get some sense of how your present life-style is effecting your potential longevity.

A Self-Test for Longevity

The life expectancy test featured here is based on statistical averages. Its self-assessed scores will help you to estimate your life expectancy and to get a scientific look at your physio-psychological weaknesses and strengths. To take this test, mark your score for each item in the appropriate column, leaving entries blank when they do not pertain, or when you do not know the answer. At the end of the test, follow the directions given for calculating your score and for figuring your life expectancy quotient.

Note: People under twenty-five or who have heart disease, cancer, cirrhosis of the liver, emphysema, or other chronic diseases will not get valid results from this test.

CHART A: LIFE-STYLE	+	−
1. PERSONALITY. Exceptionally good-natured, easygoing (+3); average (0); extremely anxious, tense most of the time (−6).	___	___
2. ACTIVITY LEVELS. Physically active employment or sedentary job with well-planned exercise program (+12); sedentary with moderate, regular exercise (0); sedentary work, no exercise program (−12).	___	___
3. HOME LIFE. Unusually pleasant, better than average (+6); average (0); unusually tense, family strife common (−9).	___	___
4. JOB. Above average satisfaction (+3); Average (0); discontented (−6).	___	___
5. AIR POLLUTION. Substantial exposure (−9).	___	___
6. SMOKING. Nonsmoker (+6); occasional smoker (0); moderate, regular smoker —20 cigarettes per day, 5 cigars or 5 pipefuls daily (−12); heavy smoker — 40 or more cigarettes daily (−24); daily marijuana smoker (−24).	___	___
7. ALCOHOL CONSUMPTION. None or seldom (+6); moderate with fewer than 2 beers or 8 oz. wine or 2 oz. whiskey or hard liquor daily (−6); heavy, with more than above (−24).	___	___

8. FOOD CONSUMPTION. Drink skim or low-fat milk only (+3); eat much roughage (+3); heavy meat, eaten 3 times daily (−6); over 2 pats butter daily (−6); over 4 cups coffee/tea/cola daily (−6); usually adds salt at table (−6). Enter total.   _____ _____

9. AUTO DRIVING. Regularly less than 20,000 miles annually and always wears seat belt (+3); regularly less than 20,000 but belt not always worn (0); more than 20,000 (−12).   _____ _____

10. DRUG USE. Use of street drugs other than marijuana (−36).   _____ _____

Subtotals   _____ _____

Chart A Total (+ or −)   _____ _____

CHART B: PHYSICAL CONDITION   +   −

1. WEIGHT. "Ideal weight at age 20 was _____. If current weight is more than 20 pounds over that, score (−6) for each 20 pounds. If same as age 20, or gain less than 10 pounds (+3).   _____ _____

2. BLOOD PRESSURE. Under 40 years, if above 130/80 (−12); over 40 years, if above 140/90 (−12).   _____ _____

3. CHOLESTEROL. Under 40 years, if above 185 (−6); over 40 years, if above 200 (−6).   _____ _____

4. HEART MURMUR. Not an "innocent" type (−24).   _____ _____

5. HEART MURMUR WITH HISTORY OF RHEUMATIC FEVER (−48).   _____ _____

6. PNEUMONIA. If bacterial pneumonia more than three times in life (−6).   _____ _____

7. ASTHMA (−6).   _____ _____

8. RECTAL POLYPS (−6).   _____ _____

9. DIABETES. Adult onset type (−18).   _____ _____

10. DEPRESSIONS. Severe, frequent (−12).   _____ _____

11. REGULAR MEDICAL CHECKUP Complete (+12); partial (+6).   _____ _____

12. REGULAR DENTAL CHECKUP (+3).   _____ _____

Subtotals   _____ _____

Chart B Total (+ or −)   _____ _____

CHART C: FAMILY AND SOCIAL HISTORY   +   −

1. FATHER. If alive and over 70 years, for each 5 years above 70 (+3); if alive and under 70 (0); if dead of medical causes (not accident) before 70 (−3).   ____ ____

2. MOTHER. If alive and over 78 years, for each 5 years above 78 (+3); if alive and under 78 or dead after age 78 (0); if dead of medical causes (not accident) before 78 (−3).   ____ ____

3. MARITAL STATUS. If married (0); unmarried and over 40 (−6).   ____ ____

4. HOME LOCATION. Farm or small town (+3); suburb (0); large city (−6).   ____ ____

                           Subtotals   ____ ____

             Chart C Total (+ or −)   ____ ____

CHART D: FOR WOMEN ONLY   +   −

1. FAMILY HISTORY OF BREAST CANCER IN MOTHER OR SISTERS (−6).   ____ ____

2. MONTHLY BREAST SELF-EXAM (+6).   ____ ____

3. YEARLY BREAST EXAM BY PHYSICIAN (+6).   ____ ____

4. PAP SMEAR YEARLY (+6).   ____ ____

                           Subtotals   ____ ____

             Chart D Total (+ or −)   ____ ____

CALCULATIONS   +   −

                     Total from Chart A   ____ ____

                     Total from Chart B   ____ ____

                     Total from Chart C   ____ ____

                     Total from Chart D   ____ ____

                        Chart Subtotals   ____ ____

                          Chart Total

(sum of the two Chart Subtotals, positive or negative)1   ____ ____

                   Life Expectancy Score

             (Chart total divided by twelve)   ____ ____

ANALYSIS

IF YOUR LIFE EXPECTANCY IS GREATER THAN ZERO, you stand a good chance of living that many years longer than the U.S. norm of 78 (for women) or 70 (for men).

IF YOUR LIFE EXPECTANCY SCORE IS LESS THAN ZERO, you stand a good chance of dying that many years earlier than the U.S. norm would predict for you. However, by improving your personal health habits and life-style you can "buy time" and increase your life expectancy.* The information in this chapter (and throughout the book) will get you started.

*This chart is reprinted from Keith Sehnert, M.D., *The Family Doctor's Health Tips* (Deephaven, Minnesota: Meadowbrook Press, 1981).

Preventive Do's and Don'ts

What exactly are the DO'S and DON'TS upon which this life-expectancy test is based? Below is a comprehensive list of the most important ones. Many entries on this list are physical measures, you will notice, and require actual changes in your physical life-style. At the same time, doctors are beginning to realize that health is more than a matter of heart beat and good elimination, and that emotional, mental, and spiritual concerns are as crucial to disease prevention as somatic ones. Thus, psychological do's and don'ts take their place on the list, too.

Although naturally it is impossible to quantitatively measure each of the many factors featured on this list, and to say that one factor is more important than another, there is a general consensus among health-care professionals that certain preventive measures are, generally speaking, especially significant. The list below is thus prioritized, starting with the most necessary preventive methods and proceeding to the least. Remember, however, that these priorities are not written in stone and that for different people different measures work best.

Finally, mention should be made of the fact that for some people it may simply not be practical to put all of the procedures listed here into immediate use. In such cases, all that can be done is to proceed slowly and build from there. It is a good idea, in fact, to take the measures mentioned below as informed suggestions, pieces of sound advice that have helped other people feel good and which will probably help you, too, even if the circumstances of your life allow you to follow only a few of them Do your best, remembering always that a little bit of prevention is worth a good deal more than a lot of cure. Here's the list:

Preventive Measures that May Save Your Life:
A Comprehensive Program

1. *Stop Smoking*

Doctors know for certain that smoking shortens longevity, that each cigarette you smoke contains at least five cancer-causing ingredients, and that tobacco smoke is a proven trigger for a wide spectrum of fatal disorders ranging from heart disease to cancer. To what extent smoking decreases the length of each life, and how dangerous cigarettes really are is difficult to know precisely, of course, as tolerances vary widely among members of the smoking population. One statistic, based on studies of several thousand subjects, shows that each cigarette smoked shortens a person's lifetime by ten minutes.

If you do smoke, and if you *must* continue, be aware that smoking seriously depletes the body of vitamin C and folic acid. Vitamin supplements will help, but better are vitamin C-bearing foods (citrus fruits, green peppers, kale, spinach, turnip-green tops) and folic acid-bearing foods (most leafy vegetables). A good deal of evidence has also been gathered to indicate that vitamin A in the form of carotene (carrots, sweet potatoes, parsley, kale) has protective value against lung cancer. Best of all is to stop completely—that's true prevention.

2. *Drink in Moderation—If At All*

Alcoholism kills more people each year than most other diseases combined (notice that cirrhosis of the liver is high on the list of death-causing diseases, not far behind cancer and heart disease). If you do drink, it's best to do so after you have eaten, as alcohol has a particularly destructive effect on the lining of an empty stomach. Also, like cigarettes, alcohol depletes the body of folic acid (see above) along with most other vitamin B–related vitamins (this is true even if you are moderate in your cocktail habits). So, get into the habit of taking regular B-supplements and eating vitamin B-rich foods if you are a steady drinker.

3. *Keep Your Seat Belt Fastened*

Statistically speaking, you have approximately a 30 to 50 percent greater chance of surviving a motor accident if your seat belt is fastened. Buckling your belt costs nothing and in some states it is law. Why take chances, especially when the price is so great and the remedy so small? Buckle up.

4. *Drive Safely*

As you probably know, more people die from traffic accidents than from cancer. Safe driving means alert driving—watching the other guy and not taking anything for granted. Think how often you yourself make foolish driving errors, then realize that other drivers are no less fallible. Don't speed: even 20 percent over the limit increases your chances of an accident by a third. If you are driving long distances, keep the window open, the radio going, and pause frequently along the road (in protected places) for stretching exercises and short catnaps. The most dangerous times on the road are during evening rush hour from 4:30 to 6 P.M., especially in the dark winter months, and from 12 P.M. to 3 A.M.—when the bars close.

5. *Reduce Stress*

The following tips, taken from an article called "Plain Talk About Handling Stress" by Louis E. Kopolow and made available by the American Health and Wellness Association, says it all about this dangerous and ubiquitous killer:

When stress does occur, it is important to recognize and deal with it. Here are some suggestions for ways to handle stress. As you begin to understand more about how stress affects you as an individual you will come up with your own ideas of helping to ease the tensions.

• Try physical activity. When you are nervous, angry, or upset, release the pressures through exercise or physical activity. Running, walking, playing tennis, or working in your garden are just some of the activities you might try. Physical exercise will relieve that 'uptight' feeling, relax you, and turn the frowns into smiles. Remember, your body and your mind work together.

• Share your stress. It helps to talk to someone about your concerns and worries. Perhaps a friend, family member, teacher, or counselor can help you see your problem in a different light. If you feel your problem is serious, you might seek professional help from a psychologist, psychiatrist, or social worker. Knowing when to ask for help may avoid more serious problems later.

• Know your limits. If a problem is beyond your control and cannot be changed at the moment, don't fight the situation. Learn to accept what is—for now—until such time when you can change it.

• Take care of yourself. You are special. Get enough rest and eat well. If you are irritable and tense from lack of sleep or if you are not eating correctly, you will have less ability to deal with stressful situations. If stress repeatedly keeps you from sleeping, you should ask your doctor for help.

• Make time for fun. Schedule time for both work and recreation. Play can be just as important to your well-being as work; you need a break from your daily routine to just relax and have fun.

• Be a participant. One way to keep from getting bored, sad, and lonely is to go where it's all happening. Sitting alone can make you feel frustrated. Instead of feeling sorry for yourself, get involved and become a participant. Offer your services in neighborhood or volunteer organizations. Help yourself by helping other people. Get involved in the world and the people around you. You're on your way to making new friends and enjoying new activities.

• Check off your tasks. Trying to take care of everything at once can seem overwhelming, and, as a result, you may not accomplish anything. Instead, make a list of what tasks you have to do, then do one at a time, checking them off as they're completed. Give priority to the most important ones and do those first.

• Must you always be right? Do other people upset you—particularly when they don't do things your way? Try cooperation instead of confrontation: it's better than fighting and always being "right." A little give-and-take on both sides will reduce the strain and make you both feel more comfortable.

• It's OK to cry. A good cry can be a healthy way to bring relief to your anxiety, and it might even prevent a headache or other physical consequence. Take some deep breaths; they also release tension.

• Create a quiet scene. You can't always run away, but you can "dream the impossible dream." A quiet country scene painted mentally, or on canvas, can take you out of the turmoil of a stressful situation. Change the scene by reading a good book or playing beautiful music to create a sense of peace and tranquility.

• Avoid self-medication. Although you can use drugs to relieve stress temporarily, drugs do not remove the conditions that caused the stress in the first place. Drugs, in fact, may be habit-forming and create more stress than they take away. They should be taken only on the advice of your doctor.

6. *Maintain Proper Weight*

Several prevalent deteriorative diseases such as heart disease, stroke, artheriosclerosis, and hypertension are made worse by overweight, and estimates have it that morbidly obese people have a life expectancy approximately 40 percent lower than those who maintain a weight proper to their size. What exactly is proper weight? This varies from person to person, depending on build, bone structure, and height. Check the weight charts on page 220–221 Generally speaking, the following rules apply:

• If you are more than 30 percent overweight, as based on the percents given in these charts, statistically speaking you can expect to die five to twenty years before persons who maintain normal weight.

• If you are 20 percent overweight, you are a prime candidate for heart problems, high blood pressure, and other weight-related ailments.

7. *Exercise*

Doing it adds to your life; not doing it takes away. It's as simple as that. Why? Because the human machine is built to get plenty of movement, even strenuous movement, every day it is on this earth. To deny the body its invigorating birthright is to invite atrophy of the muscular, joint, and cardiovascular systems, which keep one alive and vital. This omission, in turn, lowers physical resistance, reduces energy, and invites disease.

Of course, in the modern world where desk jobs are prevalent and where most of our movement is done by our brains and our voices rather than our bodies, strenuous movement is not always easy to put into practice. And so, the activity must be artificially duplicated—through exercise.

Which exercise? This depends on the person. Today a smorgasbord of possible programs is presented to just about everyone and you can more or less take your pick: aerobic exercise, Marine calisthenics, school exercise programs, weight lifting, jumping rope, walking, swimming, yoga, tai chi, martial arts, jogging, rowing, Nautilis equipment, tennis, handball, gymnastics, dancing, cycling, hiking, basketball, and lots more. Whichever method you prefer, be sure it fulfills the following requirements:

• Exercise should cause some sweating.

• Exercise should last at least a half hour per session.

• Exercise should give your respiratory system a workout and should make you at least a little breathless.

- Exercise should put most of the major joints of the body through their full range of motion.
- Exercise should thoroughly stretch the major muscles and ligaments.
- Exercise should build strength, stamina, and endurance.
- Exercise should *always* feel good.

When you exercise, the first rule is to start slowly and warm up thoroughly. Exercise at least three times a week—anything less is not going to do you a lot of good. Be regular about it, too; exercising at the same time each day is a good habit to cultivate. Most important, find your own pace and stick to it. Don't always "go for the burn"; sometimes pushing it can be worse than not exercising at all. On the other hand, don't be too self-indulgent. In all, find the rhythm and the speed that makes you feel best and follow it faithfully, making sure to note your improvements and to take pride in your progress—self-satisfaction is one of exercise's benefits, too.

8. *Eat Properly*

There are twelve basic rules here:

First: Avoid all junk foods.

Second: Cut down on—or eliminate completely—all sugar and confections from your diet.

Third: Eat whole grains. Stay away from processed grains. Many people believe that at least 50 percent of our diet should consist of whole-grain foods—bread, cereal, rice, millet, barley, etc.

Fourth: Eat a wide variety of *fresh* fruits and vegetables. Stay away from the canned and frozen varieties. At least 20 percent of our diet should include these foods. Plenty of fiber here—that's crucial.

Fifth: Eat lots of legumes—peas, beans, lentils, etc. Mix them with grains for a complete protein. Approximately 10 percent of our diet should include these foods. Plenty of fiber here, too.

Sixth: Eat meat sparingly. Three times a week is more than enough. Poultry and fish are better for you than fatty meats such as pork and beef. Especially avoid the fatty parts of the animal. If you are cooking steak, slice the fat off it before putting it in the fire. If you are cooking chicken, remove the skin.

Seventh: Cut down on your butterfat intake. Eat products made of skim milk rather than whole.

Eighth: Special foods deserve special attention. The following should find their way into everyone's menu at one time or another They're *all* good for you:

bean sprouts	miso	bean curd
tahini	homemade sauerkraut	dandelion greens
couscous	buckwheat	sesame seeds
whole-wheat kasha	pumpkin seeds	sunflower seeds
garlic	ginger	yams
Jerusalem artichokes	chick-peas	Tamari sauce
hummus	daikon radish	mustard greens
yogurt	alfalfa tea	soba noodles
wheat germ	buttermilk	chia seeds
bok choy	papayas	kale

Ninth: Avoid fried foods and cook with high-quality vegetable oils. The cold-pressed, unrefined varieties are best. In general, don't eat too much oil of any kind. Avoid animal oils entirely, if possible.

Tenth: Whenever possible, stay away from highly processed, refined and chemicalized foods.

Eleventh: Eat certain foods infrequently and even then in moderation. Coffee is on this list. So is tea. Be especially sparing on the salt and pepper, and go light on hot, spicy dishes.

Twelfth: Make as many of your own foods as you can. Bake your own bread; don't buy it. Put up your own pickles. Culture your own yogurt. Grow your own vegetables and fruits. Grind your own peanut butter. Sprout your own seeds. And so forth.

9. *Get Adequate Amounts of Sleep*

Though everyone's requirements differ in this department, it's sound policy to get a minimum of seven hours' sleep a night. If your body tells you it needs more, give it more; if less, give it less. Burning the midnight oil now and then isn't going to hurt you, but prolonged sleep deprivation can have cumulatively negative effects on mind and body alike. If you find you are constantly irritable and out of sorts, go to bed an hour earlier and see if it helps. Generally speaking, it's best to establish regular bedtime and rising hours and stick to them. The body loves, and needs, routine.

10. *Develop Good Health Habits*

There are many pleasant things you can do along these lines. Wear clothes that fit well and that do not bind or cut off circulation. Sleep in a well-aired, comfortable room. Use blankets made of natural materials such as cotton, wool, or down. Take frequent steam baths, either the wet or dry varieties; both will get you really clean. Wash your hands frequently and take a shower every day. If you live in a large city or in a highly polluted area, avoid the tap water and drink bottled spring water instead.

11. *Take Advantage of Early Detection Tests*

The chapter on medical self-tests features a number of commercial kits you can use to test for such problems as bowel cancer, breast cancer, venereal disease, blood sugar disease, blood pressure, and many more. Modern technology has given us these wonderful early detection tools and they really work. To not take advantage of them is to throw away a powerful aid both for better health and for increased longevity. If you haven't made use of these tests already, start now.

12. *Develop an Inner Life*

When all is said and done, we have only our bodies and our hearts to get us through this long and difficult life. Our bodies will more or less serve us at the task even if we abuse them, at least while we are young. But our psychic parts, our secret selves, are more delicate and vulnerable; they must be handled with special sensitivity if we are to experience a full range of joy, awareness, and transcendence. Though each person is different, many believe that beneath all human exteriors lies a single common longing for what is best in this life—harmony, contentment, and a yearning for something beyond the physical world.

Thus, while each person must seek his or her own spiritual path, each person *should* seek. Without an aspiration for something beyond the trivialities of the television set and the marketplace, we grow cynical and weary, and the health of the body alone is not enough to sustain us. If our goal is indeed health, true health, then we must find what benefits the whole man, the whole woman. And as humankind has known from time beginning, the search for this particular kind of self-care begins—and ends—within.

USEFUL SELF-CARE TECHNOLOGY, RESOURCES, AIDS, AND SERVICES

CHAPTER 26

MEDICAL SELF-HELP OVER THE TELEPHONE

Most people are not aware of the many self-care services now available over the telephone. This chapter will introduce you to some of the most important and efficient ones.

MEDICAL SELF-CARE HOTLINES

Hotlines for a variety of physical and mental problems are among the most useful telephone services. Most of these are crisis oriented and many are toll-free. The following hotlines provide advice, diagnostic information, and referrals.

AIDS Hotline (800) 342-AIDS

This organization provides diagnostic information, addresses of local AIDS self-help groups, and physician referrals for patients suffering from Acquired Immune Deficiency Syndrome (AIDS). Open 24 hours a day, 7 days a week.

Alcohol Abuse Hotline (800) ALCOHOL

This organization counsels on drinking problems and helps callers find local treatment centers. It also provides help and advice for drug problems. Open 24 hours a day, 7 days a week.

Amputation Information (718) 767-0596

Call the National Amputation Foundation for information on local self-help programs for recent amputees. Open 10 A.M. to 4 P.M., EST, Monday through Friday.

Bulimia and Anorexia Nervosa Hotline (312) 831-3438

Provides counseling and referrals for those who suffer from eating disorders. Open 9 A.M. to 5 P.M., CST, Monday through Friday.

Cancer Hotline (800) 525-3777

Provides free information and advice on cancer-related problems. Open 8:30 A.M. to 5 P.M., MT, Monday through Friday.

Cancer Information Service (800) 4-CANCER; in Alaska, (800) 638-6070; in Hawaii, (800) 524-1234

An organization funded by the National Cancer Institute that provides information on cancer detection, diagnostic data, suggestions for therapy, and referrals to local medical help and support groups. Open 9 A.M. to 10 P.M., EST, Monday through Friday.

Child Abuse Hotline (800) 422-4453

A hotline to help parents control child abuse. Counselors from Parents Anonymous are available twenty-four hours a day to advise you during crises and to refer you to local self-help groups. Open 24 hours a day, 7 days a week.

Childbirth (Information on the Lamaze method of natural childbirth) (800) 365-4404; in Virginia, (703) 524-7802

Information is provided on the Lamaze method, and referrals are made to local certified instructors and trained physicians. Open from 9 A.M. to 5 P.M., EST, Monday through Friday.

Drug Addiction (800) 548-3008; in Arizona, (800) 551-4141

A self-help clearinghouse for people addicted to cocaine, heroin, alcohol, or prescription drugs. This group puts callers in touch with professional counselors at Sedona Villa, a nonprofit chemical-dependency center in Arizona. Open 24 hours a day, 7 days a week.

Gastrointestinal Problems Hotline (GUTLINE) (301) 652-9293

Provides information, advice, diagnostic data, and referrals for problems of the gut. Open 7:30 A.M. to 9 P.M., EST, Tuesdays only.

Grief Hotline (312) 990-0010

An organization called The Compassionate Friends provides support and referrals for those who have recently lost a loved one. Open 9 A.M. to 3 P.M., CST, Monday through Friday.

Handicapped Women Support Group (704) 376-4735

A source of information and referrals to self-help programs for handicapped women. Open 9:00 A.M. to 5:00 P.M., Monday through Friday.

Headache Hotline (800) 843-2256; in Illinois, (800) 523-8858

Provides information and referrals for chronic headache sufferers. Open 9 A.M. to 5 P.M., EST, Monday through Friday.

Home-Care Hotline (202) 547-7424

The National Association for Home Care serves as both a telephone and mail clearinghouse for referrals concerning medical home care in your area. Open 9 A.M. to 6 P.M., EST, Monday through Friday.

Infertility Hotline (617) 484-2424

Provides information on the latest therapies and referrals to physicians and self-help groups for infertile men and women. Open 9 A.M. to 12 P.M. and 1 P.M. to 4 P.M., EST, Monday through Friday.

Medical Self-Help Hotline (312) 328-0470

Provides information on where to find medical self-help groups in your area. Open 9 A.M. to 5 P.M., Monday through Friday.

Pain-Control Hotline (703) 368-7357

Answers all questions pertaining to pain control. Open 24 hours a day, 7 days a week. (If no one is there, calls will be taken on an answering machine and volunteers will call you back *collect*.)

Panic and Phobia Hotline (215) 667-6490

A college-based organization that provides referrals for people who suffer from phobias and anxiety attacks. Open 9 A.M. to 5 P.M., EST, Monday through Friday.

Poison Control Center (Ask operator to connect you)

Almost all areas of the United States have a local chapter of the Poison Control Center. Consultants are available 24 hours a day. They have access to an enormous data bank describing which substances are poisonous, which are not, how to identify them, and how to treat the victim. Although best reached directly through an operator, the local Poison Control Center should also be listed in the phone book under "Poison."

Premenstrual Syndrome Hotline (800) 327-8456; in Florida, (800) 432-2382

Provides diagnostic and therapeutic information for women who suffer from PMS. Also features a referral service to clinics that deal with PMS. Open 24 hours a day, 7 days a week.

Rape Victims' Hotline (202) 333-RAPE

Provides emergency crisis counseling for rape victims plus medical information and referral services. Open 24 hours a day, 7 days a week.

Sexual Problems Hotline (415) 621-7300

A San Francisco–based staff of trained volunteers will answer your questions on all aspects of sexuality and sexual health: contraception, homosexuality, pregnancy, venereal disease. They will also provide referrals if therapy or medical help is needed. Open 3 P.M. to 9 P.M., Monday through Friday.

Suicide Hotline (213) 381-5111

Provides immediate telephone counseling for people contemplating suicide. Also offers referrals to suicide-prevention clinics. Open 24 hours a day, 7 days a week.

Surgery (Hysterectomy Hotline) (215) 667-7757

A hotline for people who need information concerning the advisability of undergoing a hysterectomy, who are looking for a second opinion, or who need a referral. Also puts people in touch with postoperative support groups, which are especially useful for those who have had operations such as mastectomies and colostomies. Open 24 hours a day, 7 days a week.

Surgical Second-Opinion Hotline (800) 638-6833

A government-sponsored service that provides information on where to get a second opinion on a specific operation. Open 8 A.M. to midnight, 7 days a week.

Venereal Disease Hotline (800) 227-8922; in California, (800) 982-5883

A service that provides callers with information and referrals for sexually-transmitted diseases. Open 8 A.M. to 8 P.M., Monday through Friday.

TOLL-FREE DIRECTORY

A telephone book featuring over 3,000 toll-free numbers, many of them related to health-care services, is available for $3.95 from Dial 800 Publishing Company, P.O. Box 995, Radio City Station, New York, NY 10019.

THE TEL-MED LIBRARY

Another medical telephone service worth knowing about, the Tel-Med Library is a nonprofit self-care line that provides access to a large library of tape-recorded health messages. Designed to help callers recognize early symptoms of specific diseases, the tapes furnish local referrals, home-care information when appropriate, and preventive methods. A local number connects the caller with an operator who puts on whatever tape is requested. The service is free.

Messages are from three to five minutes long. Although they are not a substitute for professional diagnosis, they provide a lot of valuable information, both for those who suspect they have a certain ailment and for those already suffering from it. To find the number nearest you, dial Tel-Med's central California office at (714) 825-6034. Local Tel-Med numbers are sometimes listed in the white pages of the telephone book.

Because there are about 400 tapes now available from Tel-Med, space does not allow us to list them all. Here is a sampling to give you some idea of the depth and scope of the subject matter covered on these tapes:

Alcohol Problems

570 Cirrhosis of the Liver
942 Alcoholism: The Scope of the Problem
943 Is Drinking a Problem?
944 To Drink or Not to Drink
945 So You Love an Alcoholic?
946 How A.A. Can Help the Problem Drinker
947 Fetal Alcohol Syndrome

Animal/Insect

163 Rabies
195 Bee Sting—It Can Cause Death
1165 Bite Injuries to Your Dog or Cat
1166 Your New Puppy
1167 Insect Bites
1172 Spider Bites

Cancer

6 Breast Cancer—How Can I Be Sure?
176 Cancer of the Prostate Gland
177 Cancer Patient Services and Rehabilitation
178 Rehabilitation of the Breast Cancer Patient
179 Lung Cancer
180 Cancer of the Colon and Rectum
181 Cancer—The Preventable or Curable Disease
182 What Is a PAP Test?
183 Cancer's Seven Warning Signals
184 Hodgkin's Disease
185 Cancer of the Skin
186 Uterine Cancer

Kidney/Urinary Tract

77 What Can Be Done about Kidney Stones?
1140 Blood in the Urine
1141 Kidney and Urinary Tract Infections
1142 Kidney Transplants

Patient Home Care

CHAPTER 28

OTHER SELF-CARE PHONE RESOURCES

1. *Information and Referral on Community Health Resources.*
Several hundred cities in the United States currently maintain a telephone number you can dial to learn which government, state, public, and private health and social services are available in your community. Information on these services is not always easy to come by, especially if you do not know the exact names of the desired organizations. Fortunately, consultants from the Information and Referral Service are experts at finding the right organization for your needs. To track down the local Information and Referral Service in your area, try the white pages of the phone book under *Information and Referral on Community Health Resources.* If it is not listed, call their main office in Phoenix at (602)263-8856. You can also write for this information to Alliance of Information and Referral Services, P.O. Box 10705, Phoenix, AZ 85064.

2. *Free telephone crisis intervention service.* An organization called CONTACT offers free telephone counseling and crisis intervention for just about any type of crisis: family problems, suicide, drugs, and more. Although they are a church-based organization, they make a point of being nondenominational. They really can help in times of personal difficulty, both by providing

advice and by lending a sympathetic ear. To get their number in your area, call or write to the national headquarters at CONTACT Teleministries USA, Inc., 900 S. Arlington Ave., Harrisburg, PA 17109, (717)652-3410. CONTACT maintains hundreds of offices throughout the country.

3. *Telephone reassurance service.* This is an organized volunteer program whose members call people at designated hours of the day or night to check on their mental and/or physical health. If the client does not answer the phone at the scheduled time or if something is wrong when he or she does, the volunteer caller then goes to the person's home to check. You can organize your own telephone reassurance service with the help of a booklet on the subject from the Administration on Aging. Write for catalog #OHD 75-20200, USGPO, Washington, DC 20402.

4. *Early Alert Program.* Another aid for shut-ins or convalescents is the Early Alert Program. Members of the program mark their mailboxes with a small red dot. The local mail carrier, who has been alerted to the fact that the Early Alert Program is being used, checks the person's box each day. If the mail carrier notices that a red-dotted box has not been emptied in several days, he notifies his supervisor, who contacts Early Alert. The organization immediately notifies a designated friend or relative of the member. For more information, write Mrs. Friedhielm Milburn, Director, Early Alert, 250 Broadway, New York, NY 10006.

5. *Phone Care signaling alarm.* A rather expensive but potentially life-saving device for the sick and convalescent is Phone Care. Installed in the convalescent's home, it sends out a beeping sound at regular intervals. If the signal is not switched off in a designated amount of time, the Phone Care alarm automatically triggers a prerecorded emergency phone call to several people including the patient's doctor, family members, or friends. The device comes with a pocket unit that allows the patient to transmit the same message when away from home. Phone Care costs around $750 from National Phone Care, Inc., 3109 Hennepin Ave., Minneapolis, MN 55408.

6. *Phone help for persons with pacemakers.* The international Association of Pacemaker Patients provides an inexpensive service that allows members to test their pacemakers for performance and function from a home phone. For more information, contact International Association of Pacemaker Patients, 610 Equitable Bldg., 100 Peachtree, Atlanta, GA 30303.

7. *Useful books.* The following books provide more information on using the telephone for medical self-care:

Pediatric Telephone Protocols by Julia Rosekrans, M.D., et. al.
Patient Care Publications
P.O. Box 1245
Darien, CT 06820

Telephone Medicine by Jeffrey L. Brown
C. V. Mosby Co.
11830 Westline Ind Dr.
St. Louis, MO 63142

USING THE HOME COMPUTER FOR MEDICAL SELF-CARE

COMPUTERS: WHAT THEY CAN AND CANNOT DO

Even many computer buffs are not aware of the rich variety of software programs currently available to computer users in the health field. This chapter will introduce you to some of the best of these programs—what they can do, where to get them, which machines they work on, and how much they cost.

Please keep in mind that this software cannot and should not be used for primary medical diagnosis. The programs *can*, however, educate you. They can teach you to keep your own medical records and charts, help you perform basic medical tests, give you data on different medications, provide you with illustrated anatomy and physiology lessons, advise you on the way diseases develop and how to recognize their symptoms, and furnish up-to-date information on exercise, diet, and relaxation.

With a modem, described below, you can also make contact with colossal data bases that were available only to professionals until quite recently, and that contain information extensive enough to fill entire libraries. A modem can also give you access to extracts and bibliographies on myriad medical topics and put you in direct communication with doctors, researchers, service organizations, and other laymen who share your medical interests or health problems.

The first thing you'll need, naturally, is a computer. Second, a printer is useful. Third, though not mandatory, is a modem. This handy instrument enables you to go directly on-line over your telephone and communicate with hundreds of mainframe data bases throughout the country. Finally, you will need the software itself. Home health-care programs range in price from $30 to $500. Although most stores stock only the most popular titles, they will generally special order for you; or, if you wish, you can buy directly from the manufacturer. Manufacturers' addresses are included in all entries below.

What follows is a selection of some of the most useful health-oriented software on the market today plus, for modem owners, a list of on-line data bases that feature medical information. Costs are listed along with the descriptions, although these costs are subject to change in the highly volatile computer market. Occasionally, manufacturers will send you a demonstration disk or a "sneak preview" of the more expensive programs.

Medical programs are technically considered "medical devices" and before they can be marketed they must first be checked out by the FDA's National Center for Devices and Radiological Health. This agency, however, does not test the software itself but simply screens its documentation, labeling, advertising, and related literature. Therefore, while overtly fraudulent software is usually weeded out, programming errors and faulty information sometimes slip through. Don't fall into the trap of believing that the computer is infallible, especially where matters of health are concerned.

SELF-CARE SOFTWARE PROGRAMS

General Health and Health Appraisal

Response Time. A program designed to test your reflexes and measure the speed at which you respond to an electronic stimulus (in this case a beep or buzz). Reaction time is an indication of your nerve reflex response system. This program can be used to test your level of awareness, quickness of reflexes, sobriety, and fatigue. It's also a fun parlor game. Available for the APPLE II, APPLE II+, and FRANKLIN ACE 1000; from Andent Inc., 1000 North Ave., Waukegan, IL 60085, (312) 223-5077, for $39.95.

Professional Disk. A fascinating though somewhat quirky and eclectic piece of software, *Professional Disk* contains: 1) a program to test your vulnerability to heart attack, 2) a device for embedding below-threshold-of-perception subliminal messages onto the screen, 3) an interest-calculating program to use on overdue doctors' bills, 4) an alcohol test, 5) a label-maker. Available for the APPLE II, APPLE IIE, and FRANKLIN ACE 1000; from Andent Inc. (address above), for $20.00.

Family Medical Adviser. The program asks you a number of questions concerning symptoms. You answer yes or no to all queries. The program computes the data and provides a prioritized list of possible diagnoses. Available for the APPLE II, IBM PC, and COMMODORE 64; from Navic Software, P.O. Box 14727, North Palm Beach, FL 33408, (305) 627-4132, for $38.00.

Family Medical Adviser. In a similar program, the user answers a number of yes or no questions about his or her present symptoms. The computer provides possible diagnoses based on 10,000 combinations of symptoms. Available for the APPLE II+; from Medical Software Consortium, P.O. Box 450992, Atlanta, GA 30345, for $37.50.

Total Health. This program teaches the fundamentals of a healthy life-style and how to apply them, with emphasis on nutrition and exercise. Available for the COMMODORE 64; from Practicorp, 44 Oak St., Newton Upper Falls, MA 02164, (617) 965-9870, for $29.95.

Health Risk Appraisal. An interactive program in which the user identifies his or her physical, social, and psychological patterns and the computer points out the health risks involved. Available for the APPLE II; APPLE II+; APPLE IIE; RADIO SHACK TRS-80 4, 4P, III; COMMODORE 64; IBM PC; and IBM PC jr.; from Human Relations Media, 175 Tompkins Ave., Pleasantville, NY 10570, (914) 769-6900, for $99.00.

Wellness Check. An ambitious and expensive total wellness and risk-assessment package, this program asks the user a number of multiple-choice questions concerning health habits and life-style. It then responds with a printout providing a comprehensive picture of the user's fitness level and potential health risk factors. Available for the APPLE II+; APPLE IIE; and RADIO SHACK TRS-80 12, 16; from Rhode Island Department of Health, Office of Health Promotion, 75 Davis St., Providence, RI 02908, (401) 277-6957, for $250.

Health, Age, and Longevity Profile. Based on a well-known medical study of health habits among the population of Almeda

County, California, this program isolates behavioral habits and patterns that affect longevity and matches them to the user's own habits. It then provides a projected estimate of the user's longevity. Available for the IBM PC XT; APPLE II; and RADIO SHACK TRS-80 4, 4P, III; from Medical Software (address above), for $200.

Childpace. A program designed to help track your child's social maturity, dexterity, and language development. The child (aged three months to five years) takes age-appropriate tests and the results are measured against established standards. Potential weaknesses and trouble spots, if any, are indicated. Information can be recorded on a printout. Available for the APPLE II, COMMODORE 64, IBM PC, IBM PC jr., and RADIO SHACK COLOR COMPUTER; from Computerose, 2012 East Randol Mill Rd., Ste. 223, Arlington, TX 76011, (817) 277-9153, for $39.95.

First Opinion. Users are asked a series of probing technical questions concerning the symptoms that are bothering them, then *First Opinion* lists the possible causes. A printout of the answers is provided. Available for the Hewlett-Packard 85, 86, 87; from Medical Logic International, 5 Pathfinder Dr., Sumter, SC 29150, for $295.

Personal Health. Helps the user decide when the symptoms of a particular ailment warrant a doctor's assistance. Available for the APPLE II+ and APPLE IIE; from Medical Software Consortium, P.O. Box 450992, Atlanta, GA 30345, for $49.00.

Heart Check. A comprehensive heart-assessment program. The computer gauges the health of the user's heart based on answers to questions concerning life-style, stress levels, personal habits, nutrition, weight, pulse, blood pressure, exercise, heredity, etc. A printout is provided showing the user's coronary risk profile. Available for the IBM PC XT and RADIO SHACK TRS-80 4, 4P, III; from Medical Software Consortium (address above), for $200 (Radio Shack) and $250 (IBM).

Computerized Health Appraisals. A series of fifteen programs designed to test the user's overall health and fitness level. Weight, nutrition, age, habits, heart and lungs, exercise, etc., are measured and appraised. Available for the IBM PC, APPLE II, and RADIO SHACK TRS-80 III; from Medical Software Consortium (address above), for $50.00.

Health Aide Ver 1.3. Compiles the user's complete health profile and provides suggestions for diet and exercise. Available for the APPLE II, APPLE IIE, and IBM PC; from Knossos Inc., 422 Redwood Ave., Corte Madera, CA 94925, (415) 924-8528, for $79.95.

Diet and Weight-Loss

Nutri-Bytes. An ambitious program that attempts to teach the user about nutrition from the ground up. It includes a starter nutrition test, a study of the user's eating habits, a nutrition tutorial, suggestions for diet and nutritional improvement, and a quiz on food additives. Available for the KAYPRO 2, 4, 10; APPLE II; APPLE II+; APPLE IIE; TELEVIDEO; and OSBORNE I, II; from Center for Science-Public Interest, 1755 S St., N.W., Washington, D.C. 20009, (202) 332-9110, for $39.95.

Fit and Trim. A complete weight-loss program. The user's present weight is compared with his or her ideal weight, weight-loss goals are established and printed out, diet is reviewed and suggestions for changes given, and a self-monitoring aerobic and muscle-toning exercise program is introduced. Available for the APPLE II, APPLE IIE, and FRANKLIN ACE 1000; from Andent Inc., 1000 North Ave., Waukegan, IL 60085, (312) 223-5077, for $39.00.

Weight Control and Nutrition. A program designed to help cooks prepare meals that are both nutritious *and* slimming. Available for the TI 99/4; from Texas Instruments, P.O. Box 10508, Lubbock, TX 79408, (806) 741-2000, for $39.00.

Diet Monitor V.1. The program reviews the user's eating habits and provides suggestions for more sensible dieting. Graphs and reports tailored to the user's needs are part of the package Available for the APPLE II and IBM PC; from Camrass Corporation, P.O. Box 118, Boonton, NJ 07005, (201) 328-8917, for $99.00.

Hydrostatic Body Composition. A powerful aid for serious dieters, this program measures weight, percentage of body fat, etc., through underwater weighing. Available for the IBM PC XT and RADIO SHACK TRS-80 4, 4P, III; from Medical Software Consortium, P.O. Box 450992, Atlanta, GA 30345, for $200.

Chubby Checker. Tracks calories, enters them on an easy-to-read graph, calculates ideal weight, computes how many calories you should have in each twenty-four-hour period, and helps you keep track of what you eat. Available for the Hewlett-Packard 85, 86, 87; from Health & Habitation Inc., 5 Pathfinder Dr., Sumter, SC 29150, (803) 469-9180, for $95.00.

Model Diet. A program that evaluates the user's eating habits and makes recommendations based on standard RDA requirements. The program also contains a lot of general information on nutrition. Available for the IBM PC, IBM PC jr., APPLE IIC, APPLE IIE, and COMMODORE 64; from Softsync Inc., 14 East 34th St., New York, NY 10016, (212) 685-2080, for $34.95.

Nutrition: Volumes I and II. The programs are sold separately, but together they offer a complete course in the fundmentals of nutrition. Included is a food catalog of 598 items, a nutrition report, an evaluation of the user's eating habits, a menu plan tailored to the user's nutritional needs, methods of calculating caloric intake, nutritional analysis of foods, and much more. Available for the APPLE II, APPLE II+, and APPLE IIE; from Minnesota Educational Computing Consortium, 2520 Broadway Dr., St. Paul, MN 55113, (621) 638-0600; Volume I costs $46.00, Volume II costs $45.00.

Stress Management

Ican. The user identifies stressful elements in his or her life, and the computer makes suggestions on how to reduce or eliminate them. Available for the APPLE II; from Micro Power & Light Co., 12820 Hillcrest Rd., Ste. 219, Dallas, TX 75230, (214) 239-6620, for $29.95.

Ican Stress-Management. The user chooses various words that indicate his or her stress level, and the program provides tailored advice on reducing tension. Available for the APPLE II and APPLE IIE; from Micro Learningware, P.O. Box 307, Mankato, MN 56001, (507) 625-2205, for $29.95.

Relax. An elaborate program featuring several popular stress-reduction techniques including autogenic training, phase relaxation, and biofeedback. Biofeedback equipment, workbooks, and audiocassettes come with the package. Available for the ATARI 1200 XL, 800, 800XL, 600 XL, 400; COMMODORE 64; APPLE II; APPLE II+; APPLE IIE; IBM PC; and IBM PC jr.; from Synapse Software, 5221 Central Ave., Ste. 200, Richmond, CA 94804, (415) 527-7751, for $139.95.

Stress Management. An interactive program emphasizing graphics, which is designed to help the user pinpoint and change the stressful areas in his or her life. Available for the APPLE II, APPLE II+, and APPLE IIE; from Medical Software Consortium, P.O. Box 450992, Atlanta, GA 30345, for $29.50.

Coping with Stress. Based on the principles of cognitive therapy, this program guides the user through a series of eleven response sessions designed to reveal the most negative and self-destructive elements of his or her personality. The program then offers suggestions for more productive living. Available for the IBM PC, IBM PC jr., APPLE II+, APPLE IIC, and APPLE E; from Psycomp Software, P.O. Box 994, Woodland Hills, CA 91367, (818) 992-4884, for $89.95.

Exercise and Physical Fitness

Physical Fitness. This program, based on fitness standards determined by the President's Council on Physical Fitness, helps you design an exercise regimen tailored to your needs. Available for the Ti 99/4; from Texas Instruments, P.O. Box 10508, Lubbock, TX 79408, (806) 741-2000, for $29.95.

Aerobics. This program introduces you to eighteen different aerobic routines in a series of eighty exercises (of graduated difficulty). Each workout lasts approximately twenty minutes and is designed to tone the entire body. Suggestions for appropriate music are included. Available for the ATARI 1200XL, 800XL, 800, 600XL and COMMODORE 64; from Spinnaker Software, One Kendall Sq., Cambridge, MA 02139, (617) 494-2100, for $39.00.

Runner's Historical Analysis. This program for dedicated runners logs daily mileage, times and distances, weight, calories burned, and other measurements. It can store records of daily sessions for six months. Available for the ATARI 800, 400; from Runsoft, 2512 Kirby Rd., Milton, WV 25541, for $19.95.

Personal Fitness Program. This program allows the user to plan and keep track of an exercise regime by establishing fitness goals, advising on the best methods of achieving these goals, and graphing weekly progress. Available for the ATARI 16K; from Atari Inc., 1265 Borregas, Sunnyvale, CA 94086, (408) 745-4692, for $24.95.

Keeping Medical Records

Historymaker. This ambitious and expensive program takes and records a thorough, entirely professional medical history. Available for the Hewlett-Packard 85, 86, 87; from Medical Logic International, 5 Pathfinder Dr., Sumter, SC 29150, for $495.

Medical History. A handy program that allows users to keep track of everything that takes place during a doctor's visit—examinations, shots, tests, etc. All information can be recalled instantly through a search function. Available for the RADIO SHACK TRS-80 I, III; from En-Joy Computer Projects, P.O. Box 1535, Goleta, CA 93017, for $9.95.

General Medical History Ver-1.1. A professional program that records the user's medical history down to the smallest detail. Although designed for hospitals, it can be used by the ambitious layman. Available for the APPLE II, APPLE II+, APPLE IIE, APPLE IIC, and IBM PC; from Cogitum Medical Software, Inc., 1675 Leahy St., Ste. 310, Muskegon, MI 49442, (616) 725-8322, for $450.

Medical and Health Education

Good Health Habits. Teaches children to develop proper health and hygiene habits; a game at the end adds interest. Available for the APPLE II, COMMODORE 64, and COMMODORE PET; from Right On Programs, 140 East Main St., Huntington, NY 11743, (516) 271-3177, for $18.00.

Our Bodies. A children's introduction to the workings of the body and its major organ systems; a game at the end helps make it fun. Available for the APPLE II, COMMODORE 64, and COMMODORE PET; from Right On Products (address above), for $18.00.

Meducator. A program that answers some of the most common questions about heart disease, diabetes, cancer, and high blood pressure. The program is interactive, contains a lot of graphic material, and provides users with a printout of desired information. Available for the Hewlett-Packard 85, 86, 87; from Medical Logic International, 5 Pathfinder Dr., Sumter, NC 29150, for $295.

Heart Lab. A computer simulation of heart function, the program includes animated graphics, tutorials, tests, and a feature that allows the user to test his or her own heartbeat. Although it is designed for children, it can be of use to adults as well. Available for the COMMODORE 64; from Opportunities for Learning, Inc. (must be ordered through a computer store).

Heartbeat/Heartwork/Heartflo. A graphics-oriented young person's tutorial that explains in simple terms how the heart works and what functions it performs. The program offers quizzes, a "heart saver" game, an anatomy lesson and test, a glossary of terms, and a game that lets the user diagnose and operate on an ailing human heart. Available for the APPLE II, APPLE II+, AP-

PLE IIE, and APPLE III; from J&S Software (must be ordered through a computer store).

Mental and Emotional Health

The Hypnotist. This program uses the principles of biofeedback to teach users how to induce a trance state and give themselves posthypnotic suggestions. Biofeedback equipment and thorough documentation are included. Available for the COMMODORE 64; from Psycomp Software, P.O. Box 994, Woodland Hills, CA 91367, (818) 992-4884, for $89.95.

Communicate and Win. Designed to teach techniques for successful interaction with peers and business associates. A special feature allows you to construct personality profiles of yourself and colleagues. The program is available for the APPLE; from Phoenix Software, 64 Lake Zurich Dr., Lake Zurich, IL 60047, (312) 438-4850, for $250.

Psychological Psoftware. A series of six small programs, each of which deals with a critical aspect of the psyche (intimacy, dreams, responsibility, stress, personality, and assertiveness). These programs help you assess your own emotional/psychological makeup and strengthen your weak points. Available for the APPLE II+ and APPLE IIE; from Medical Software Consortium, P.O. Box 450992, Atlanta, GA 30345, for $150.

Intimacy, the Art of Communication. A program designed to help you understand your personal relationships, locate trouble spots and danger zones, and improve your communicative skills. Available for the APPLE II, APPLE II+, and APPLE IIE; from Medical Software Consortium (address above), for $29.50.

Puppet. A program for children that emphasizes learning how to "pull your own strings," i.e., take responsibility for your behavior. Available for the APPLE II, APPLE II+, and APPLE IIE; from Medical Software Consortium (address above), for $20.00.

Personality Profile. A self-assessment program that allows you to get outside your personality and see yourself as others see you. One of the best and most popular self-help programs on the market today. Available for the APPLE II, APPLE II+, and APPLE IIE; from Medical Software Consortium (address above), for $29.50.

Dream Machine. Designed to help laymen record, analyze, and understand their dreams. Includes a 200-item dictionary of dream reference terms plus space for the user to enter descriptions of his or her dreams on permanent file. Available for the APPLE II, APPLE II+, and APPLE IIE; from Medical Software Consortium (address above), for $49.50.

Drug and Medication Use

Drug Master Provides information on over 1,200 popular drugs and medications, including how they interact. The program was designed for professional use but may be useful for the sophisticated layman. It is available for the APPLE II+, APPLE IIC, and APPLE IIE; from Medical Software Consortium (address above), for $225.

Consumer Drug Watcher. Information on actions, reactions, and interactions of 550 popular commercial drugs, many of them sold over-the-counter. This program is especially designed for the ayman. Available for the APPLE II+ and APPLE IIE; from Medical Watch Software, 1620 Ensenada Dr., Modesto, CA 95350, for $39.95.

Consumer's Guide to Prescription/Nonprescription Drugs. A program designed for the layman, which describes the action and side effects of a large number of prescription and over-the-counter drugs, including generic drugs. Available for the IBM PC; IBM PC jr; APPLE II; APPLE II+; APPLE IIE; FRANKLIN ACE 1200, 1000; HYPERION; COLUMBIA VP PORTABLE; MPC; PANASONIC SR PARTNER; PANASONIC SUPER SR PARTNER; SEEQUA CHAMELEON; COLOR CHAMELEON; CHAMELEON PLUS; COMPAQ PLUS; and COMPAQ PORTABLE; from Intellectual Software, 798 North Avenue Dr., Bridgeport, CT 06606, (203) 335-0906, for $39.95.

Drugs. A program that deals specifically with narcotic drugs: cocaine, marijuana, LSD, caffeine, alcohol, tranquilizers, opiates, etc. It assesses in detail the psycho/physical effects of these drugs, their chemical composition, legitimate medical uses, legal aspects of their use, etc. Available for the IBM PC; IBM PC jr; APPLE II; APPLE II+; APPLE IIE; FRANKLIN ACE 1200, 1000; HYPERION; COLUMBIA VP PORTABLE; MPC; PANASONIC SR PARTNER; PANASONIC SUPER SR PARTNER; SEEQUA CHAMELEON; COLOR CHAMELEON; CHAMELEON PLUS; COMPAQ PLUS; and COMPAQ PORTABLE; from Intellectual Software (address above), for $39.95.

Quitting Smoking

Why Smoke. Using a question-and-answer format, this program provides the user with a comprehensive psychological profile of why he or she smokes. A good way to get inspired to stop. Available for the RADIO SHACK TRS-80 4, 4P, III; from medical Software Consortium, P.O. Box 450992, Atlanta, GA 30345, for $50.00.

Smoker's Profile. A statistical program that projects the user's health, risk, sickness profile, life-expectancy rates, etc., according to the amount of cigarettes smoked daily. All statistics are taken from the U.S. Surgeon General's report on smoking. The program is available for the RADIO SHACK TRS-80 4, 4P, III; from Medical Software Consortium (address above), for $100.

First Aid

Med Alert!. Designed to help the user avoid accidents and be prepared for medical emergencies, the program includes space to record important phone numbers and addresses, poison antidotes, etc., along with information on dealing with specific first aid emergencies. Available for the TI 999/4, 4A; from Future Software Inc., P.O. Box 5581, Fort Worth, TX 76108, (317) 732-1687, for $34.95.

In-Depth Poisoning. Offers lessons on how to deal with poisoning emergencies, how to identify toxic materials, and how to make your home poison-safe. Available for the APPLE II, and APPLE IIE; from Medical Software Consortium, P.O. Box 450992, Atlanta, GA 30345, for $39.95.

Family Planning, Contraception, and Venereal Disease

Natural Family Planning Personal Charting Program. Helps the user chart her menstrual cycle to determine the optimum days of the month for conception. Body temperature and cervical mucus levels, along with monthly cycle patterns, are recorded and illustrated on graphs. Available for the APPLE C, APPLE E, APPLE II +, and APPLE III; from Family Life Software, 1401 South 11th Ave., St. Cloud, MN 56301, (612) 253-6032, for $39.00.

Contraception. An educational package explaining how nine different contraceptives work. Methods described include the IUD, sponge, condom, rhythm, foam, jelly, pill, diaphragm, and sterilization. Available for IBM PC; IBM PC jr; APPLE II; APPLE

II+; APPLE IIE; FRANKLIN ACE 1200, 1000; PANASONIC SR PARTNER; PANASONIC SUPER SR PARTNER; HYPERION; COLUMBIA VP PORTABLE 2116; COMPAQ PLUS; COMPAQ PORTABLE; SEEQUA CHAMELEON; COLOR CHAMELEON; CHAMELEON PLUS; and EAGLE 1600 SERIES; from Intellectual Software, 798 North Avenue Dr., Bridgeport, CT 06606, (203) 335-0906, for $34.95.

Venereal Disease. This program provides a detailed description and symptom analysis of the most prominent venereal diseases: AIDS, syphilis, herpes, and gonorrhea. Available for IBM PC; IBM PC jr; APPLE II; APPLE II+; FRANKLIN ACE 1200, 1000; PANASONIC SR PARTNER; PANASONIC SUPER SR PARTNER; HYPERION; COLUMBIA VP PORTABLE 2116; COMPAQ PLUS; COMPAQ PORTABLE; SEEQUA CHAMELEON; COLOR CHAMELEON; CHAMELEON PLUS; and EAGLE 1600 SERIES; from Intellectual Software (address above), for $34.95.

Pregnancy and Infant Care Programs

Pregnancy Package. Everything you need to know about being pregnant: diet, weight, sex, exercise, morning sickness, effects of coffee and cigarettes, potential danger signals, etc. Available for IBM PC; IBM PC jr; APPLE II; APPLE II+; APPLE IIE; FRANKLIN ACE 1200, 1000; PANASONIC SR PARTNER; PANASONIC SUPER SR PARTNER; HYPERION; COLUMBIA VP PORTABLE 2116; COMPAQ PLUS; COMPAQ PORTABLE; SEEQUA CHAMELEON; COLOR CHAMELEON; CHAMELEON PLUS; and EAGLE 1600 SERIES; from Intellectual Software (address above), for $59.95.

Pregnancy and You. Information about diet, exercise, checkups, hygiene, and nursing for the pregnant mother. Available for IBM PC; IBM PC jr; APPLE II; APPLE II+; APPLE IIE; FRANKLIN ACE 1200, 1000; PANASONIC SR PARTNER; PANASONIC SUPER SR PARTNER; HYPERION; COLUMBIA VP PORTABLE 2116; COMPAQ PLUS; COMPAQ PORTABLE; SEEQUA CHAMELEON; COLOR CHAMELEON; CHAMELEON PLUS; and EAGLE 1600 SERIES; from Intellectual Software (address above), for $44.95.

Prenatal Baby Care. A lot of good information on how to maintain optimum health while pregnant, how to spot potential problems, what to expect during labor, etc. Available for IBM

PC; IBM PC jr; APPLE II; APPLE II+; APPLE IIE; FRANKLIN ACE 1200, 1000; PANASONIC SR PARTNER; PANASONIC SUPER SR PARTNER; HYPERION; COLUMBIA VP PORTABLE 2116; COMPAQ PLUS; COMPAQ PORTABLE; SEEQUA CHAMELEON; COLOR CHAMELEON; CHAMELEON PLUS; and EAGLE 1600 SERIES; from Intellectual Software (address above), for $34.95.

New Baby Care. Covers most of what a new mother will need to know about infant care: feeding, nursing, sleeping, bathing, etc. Available for IBM PC; IBM PC jr; APPLE II; APPLE II+; APPLE IIE; FRANKLIN ACE 1200, 1000; PANASONIC SR PARTNER; PANASONIC SUPER SR PARTNER; HYPERION; COLUMBIA VP PORTABLE 2116; COMPAQ PLUS; COMPAQ PORTABLE; SEEQUA CHAMELEON; COLOR CHAMELEON; CHAMELEON PLUS; and EAGLE 1600 SERIES; from Intellectual Software (address above), for $34.95.

Rehabilitation Programs

Cogrehab Vol. 1. A clinical rehabilitation program for individuals who have suffered strokes or generalized brain damage. Seven subunits include exercises in memory rehabilitation, coordination, helping perceptual disorders, etc. Available for the APPLE II+; APPLE E; and RADIO SHACK TRS-80, 4, 4P, I, III; from Life Science Associates, 1 Fenimore Rd., Bayport, NY 11705, (516) 472-2111, for $150.

Cogrehab Vol. 2. The companion to Cogrehab Vol. 1. It runs on the same computers and costs $195.

Freerec: Free Recall. Measures the degree of damage to short- and long-term memory in stroke and brain-injured patients. Available for the IBM PC; APPLE II; APPLE III; FRANKLIN ACE 1000; and RADIO SHACK TRS-80, I, III; from Life Science Associates (address above), for $30.00.

For Modem Owners: On-Line Databases for Medical Information

AAMSI Medical Forum. A program sponsored by the American Association for Medical Systems and Informatics. Information is available on rehabilitation services, mental health, patient care services, and emergency care. The service features a computer bulletin board over which members can ask questions and confer with experts.

Access: CompuServe, 5000 Arlington Centre, P.O. Box 20212, Columbus, OH 23220

Bioethicsline. Dedicated specifically to ethical and moral questions in medicine. Articles, extracts, citations, indexes, and sub-data bases are available.

Access: National Library of Medicine (NLM), 8600 Rockville Pike, Bethesda, MD 20209, (301) 496-4193

Cancerlit. A huge data base on the subject of cancer therapy and research. Includes books, articles, journals, reports, papers, etc.

Access: National Library of Medicine (address above)

Care. Dedicated especially to self-care for laymen. Designed to help you assess and understand the symptoms of various ailments and decide whether or not a doctor's care is necessary.

Access: The Source (Source Telecomputing Corporation), 1616 Anderson Rd., McLean, VA 22102

Catline. A gigantic data base offering access to around 500,000 reprints, extracts, reports, books, monographs, technical papers, and articles on medicine.

Access: National Library of Medicine (address above)

Critical Care Medicine Library. A source for on-line books and bibliographies on medical care.

Access: BRS, 1200 Route 7, Latham, NY 12110, (518) 783-1161

FDA Newsline. The Food and Drug Administration's on-line news service features updates on FDA regulatory measures, new products passed or banned, drug approvals, etc.

Access: CompuServe (address above)

Health-Tex. Called the "lay person's version of the *Physician's Desk Reference,*" this consumer-oriented data base helps users in need of medical services to make intelligent choices about what to buy, where to buy it, when a medical situation should be treated as an emergency, how to pick the right health insurance, etc. Includes tips on gauging the need for specific medical treatments and therapies, a special service for the storage of the user's medical history, and "Health-Line Feedback," a program that tutors users in what questions to ask their doctors and pharmacists and how to get the most out of the answers.

Access: CompuServe (address above)

CHAPTER 29

MEDICAL SELF-CARE SERVICES AND RESOURCES

This appendix includes a definitive list of self-care services, resources, organizations, newsletters, books, and magazines.

SERVICES

Discount Services for the Elderly. The National Council of Senior Citizens offers its members considerable discounts on drugs, medical equipment, travel services, and much more. National Council for Senior Citizens, 1511 K St. N.W., Washington, D.C. 20005.

Mental Health Referral Service. The Mental Health Association offers referrals to legal psychiatric and mental health facilities. It also maintains a library of resource information to answer questions on mental health facilities and resources. Mental Health Association, National Headquarters, 1800 North Kent St., Arlington, VA 22209.

Self-Care for Travelers with Pacemakers. The International Association of Pacemaker Patients provides a directory of pacemaker clinics located around the country for pacemaker wearers who plan to travel. International Association of Pacemaker Patients, 610 Equitable Bldg., 100 Peachtree, Atlanta, GA 30303.

Free Talking Books for the Blind, Convalescent and Handicapped. Those who are unable to read can avail themselves of

the Library of Congress's talking book service. It is free through
local libraries, but you must apply to the Library of Congress,
National Library Service for the Blind and Physically Handicapped, Washington, D.C. 20559.

Self-Help Group for Herpes Sufferers. HELP, an organization
sponsored by the American Social Health Association, offers
members a regular newsletter, referrals to local herpes self-help
groups, and a hotline staffed by expert consultants who will answer questions concerning herpes. Membership is free. Send a
stamped, self-addressed business envelope to HELP/ASHA, P.O.
Box 100, Palo Alto, CA 94302.

Free Eyeglasses. The Lions Club will have those who are unable to afford eyeglasses tested and measured for a free pair.
Contact your local Lions Club or write to their central headquarters at Lions International, 300 22nd St., Oakbrook, IL 60521.

Home Care for Arthritis. The Arthritis Foundation offers educational programs to teach arthritis sufferers home care and home
rehabilitation techniques. Look up the local chapters of the foundation in the phone book or write to the main headquarters for
information on the society nearest you. Arthritis Foundation, 3400
Peachtree Rd., N.W., Ste. 1101, Atlanta, GA 30326.

Free Counseling Service for the Obese. The National Council
on Obesity offers free, confidential counseling on how to deal
with this difficult problem. The National Council on Obesity, P.O.
Box 35306, Los Angeles, CA 90035.

Free Counseling Service for Compulsive Eaters. Overeaters
Anonymous offers regular self-help group meetings plus a twelve-
step plan for overcoming compulsive eating. Write to Overeaters
Anonymous/World Service Office, 2190 190th St., Torrance, CA
90504, for their brochure, "Overeaters Anonymous—A Program
of Recovery for Compulsive Overeaters."

Local Referrals for People with Rare Blood Types. The National Rare Blood Club will provide a free list of men and women
in your area who have agreed to donate their rare blood to those
in need. National Rare Blood Club, 164 Fifth Ave., New York,
NY 10010.

Home-Care Programs for Brain-Damaged Children. The Institute for the Achievement of Human Potential will help evaluate
your child's rehabilitative needs and help you arrange appropriate home-care facilities. Institute for the Achievement of Human Potential, 8801 Stenton Ave., Philadelphia, PA 19118.

Home Lending Library on Food and Nutrition. The National Agricultural Library maintains a large resource library of books, tapes, audiovisual materials, and articles on the subject of diet and nutrition. For their "List of Available Publications," write to Food and Nutrition Information and Education Resources Center, National Agricultural Library, United States Department of Agriculture, Room 304, 10301 Baltimore Blvd., Beltsville, MD 20705.

Simplified Information About Health Insurance. Health insurance plans are often so complicated that it takes a specialist to understand them. The Health Insurance Institute offers a free service to help you determine which policies are best for your needs and what the policies you own really cover. You can call the Institute at (202) 862-4000 or send your written questions to Health Insurance Institute, Education and Community Services, American Council of Life Insurance, 1850 K St., N.W., Washington, D.C. 20006.

Breathing Exercise Instruction for People with Lung Problems. A program known as Easy Breathers, sponsored by the American Lung Association, teaches exercises that really help those with breathing problems. Get in touch with a local branch of the American Lung Association or write directly to American Lung Association, 1740 Broadway, New York, NY 10019.

Medical Advice for Joggers. The National Jogging Association provides information on how to avoid injuries and how to get the most out of jogging. National Jogging Association, Ste. 830, 919 18th St., N.W., Washington, D.C. 20006.

First Aid Classes. The American Red Cross offers courses in basic and advanced first aid throughout the United States. Contact your local Red Cross chapter for information on where and when the next classes near you will be held. The classes are either free or very inexpensive.

NEWSLETTERS

Medical Update. A monthly review of diagnostic and therapeutic medical advances. Benjamin Franklin Literary and Medical Society, Inc., 1100 Waterway Blvd., Indianapolis, IN 46202; $12 a year.

ADA Forecasts. Annual updates on diabetes medicine and self-care. American Diabetes Association, 2 Park Ave., 16th Floor, New York, NY 10016; free.

Health Newsletter. A consumer's newsletter on medical advances, advice, frauds, etc. Health Writers, Inc., 1127 University Ave., Madison, WI 53715; $15 a year (monthly).

Executive Fitness Newsletter. For office workers who want to maintain good health. Rodale Press, 33 East Minor St., Emmaus, PA 18049; $30 a year (quarterly).

Consuming Passions. For women with eating problems. Published monthly by Swann Mgt., P.O. Box 77, Norwood, NJ 07648; $11.95 a year (monthly).

Creative Health Newsletter. Emphasis on what's new in the holistic health field. Published bimonthly by Biokinesiology Institute, P.O. Box 1158, Shady Grove, OR 97539; $12 a year (monthly).

For You Naturally. Health and nutrition. Tele-Health, R.D. 3, Clymer Rd., Quakertown, PA 18951; $12.00 a year (monthly).

Health Maintenance Technology. Specializes in articles on early disease diagnosis. Published monthly by Health Affairs Press, P.O. Box 425, Davis, CA 95617; $20.00 a year (monthly).

Smoking and Health Newsletter. For those trying to quit. National Interagency Council on Smoking and Health, 7320 Greenville Ave., Dallas, TX 75231; free (quarterly).

Update. Reports on alcoholism and drug abuse. Alcoholism Council of Greater New York, 133 East 62nd St., New York, NY 10021; free.

Diets and Losing Weight Update. For serious dieters. Update Publicare Co., P.O. Box 570122, Houston, TX 77257; $2.00 per copy.

Voice in the Wilderness. Emphasis on natural eating and natural healing methods. Nutritional Science Association, P.O. Box 2767, Youngstown, OH 44507; $6.00 a year (bimonthly).

Medinc's. Consumer information concerning medicines, prices, diets, etc. Medical Information for Consumers, 9102 Jones Mill Rd., Chevy Chase, MD 20815; $36.00 a year (monthly).

Medical Hotline. Abstracts taken from professional medical journals and rewritten for laymen. Published by Medical News Associates, 10th Floor, 450 Park Ave. South, New York, NY 10016; $24.95 a year.

National HomeCaring Council News. Latest developments in home care. National HomeCaring Council, Inc., 67 Irving Place, New York, NY 10003; free (quarterly).

Natural Health Bulletin. Natural healing methods, preventive medicine, and the use of nutrition for medical purposes. Natural Health Bulletin, CN 5245, Princeton, NJ 08540; $31.25 a year (monthly).

Holistic Medicine. The latest in unorthodox and holistic medicine. American Holistic Medical Association, 6932 Little River Tpke., Annandale, VA 22003; $25 a year (bimonthly).

Pathway to Health. Holistic health with emphasis on the Edgar Cayce readings. A.R.E. Clinic, 4017 North 40th St., Phoenix, AZ 85018; free (quarterly).

Continuing Care. For the parents of children on home cardiopulmonary monitors. Healthdyne, Inc., 2253 Northwest Parkway, Marietta, GA 30067; free (quarterly).

Personal Fitness. Hefty monthly newsletter on all aspects of fitness, nutrition, holistic health, and preventive care Personal Fitness Consultants, Inc., 63 Vine Rd., #108, Stamford, CT 06905; $47.00 a year (monthly).

The Helper. Quarterly newsletter on research and new therapies for herpes simplex. Published by American Social Health Association, Ste. 307, 260 Sheridan Ave., Palo Alto, CA 94306; $20.00 a year (quarterly).

Diabetes Foundation Newsletter. Self-care for diabetics. Diabetes Foundation, Inc., 1330 Beacon Street, Brookline, MA 02146; free (quarterly).

Herb News. Quarterly newsletter for medical herbalists. Herb Research Foundation, P.O. Box 12602, Austin, TX 78711; $15.00 a year.

GIG. News and recipes for people allergic to gluten. Gluten Intolerance Group, P.O. Box 23053, Seattle, WA 98102; free.

In Touch for Health. For practitioners of massage, acupressure, and kinesiology. Touch for Health Foundation, 1174 North Lake Ave., Pasadena, CA 91104; $15.00 a year (monthly).

Constructive Action Newsletter. Dedicated to medical self-help and the use of exercise, nutrition, the arts, etc., as forms of therapy and disease prevention. Act-Action, 710 Lodi St., B-1104, Syracuse, NY 13203; $10 a year (monthly), $1.00 per copy.

The Home Healthcare Connection. The latest in home care. Kimberly Organization, P.O. Box 31011, St. Louis, MO 63131; $120 a year (monthly), $10.00 per copy.

Influenza. Reports on trends in influenza outbreaks, new therapies, etc. California State Department of Public Health, 2151 Berkeley Way, Berkeley, CA 94704; free.

Your Health. Preventive medicine and nutrition. International Academy of Preventive Medicine, Ste. 469, 1950 Grandview, Overland Park, KS 66210; $1.50 per copy (monthly).

Allergy Shot. Canadian newsletter about allergy diagnoses, new advances, treatment, self-care, recipes, etc. Allergy Information Association, 25 Poynter Dr., Weston, ON M9R 1K8 Canada; $15 a year (quarterly).

Health Facts. Dedicated to helping consumers make intelligent and educated decisions about health care. Center for Medical Consumers, 237 Thompson St., New York, NY 10012; $18 a year (monthly).

Cardiac Alert. Good information on techniques for preventing heart attacks. Phillips Publishing Co., 7315 Wisconsin Ave., Bethesda, MD 20814; $60 a year (monthly), $4.00 per copy.

Constructive Action for Good Health. Dedicated to putting people who are suffering from the same or similar diseases in touch with one another. Act-Action, 710 Lodi St., B-1104, Syracuse, NY 13203; $10 a year (monthly).

MEDICAL ORGANIZATIONS

National Self-Help Clearinghouse. An organization that maintains a listing of all the self-help groups in the country and provides referrals. An extremely helpful and timely resource. National Self-Help Clearinghouse, Graduate School University Center, City University of New York, 33 West 42nd St., New York, NY 10036.

Self-Help Institute. An organization that performs a service similar to that of the National Self-Help Clearinghouse. Self-Help Institute, Center for Urban Affairs, Northwestern University, Evanston, IL.

Medic-Alert Foundation International. People suffering from serious, potentially dangerous ailments such as insect sting allergies, epilepsy, or heart problems register with the Medic-Alert main office and receive identification tags. In case of emergency, a physician can identify the ailment from the tag and call the Medic-Alert office, open twenty-four hours a day, where all pertinent medical information on the patient is kept on permanent record. Medic-Alert Foundation International, 1000 North Palm, Turlock, CA.

American Allergy Association. Dedicated to helping seriously allergic people cope with their symptoms. Provides information on eliminating household allergens, devising an allergy-free diet, locating hypoallergenic products, etc. American Allergy Association, P.O. Box 7273, Menlo Park, CA 94025.

The Phoenix Society. Provides posthospital aid and counseling to badly burned and scarred patients. The Phoenix Society, Inc., 11 Rust Hill Rd., Levittown, PA 19056.

Emphysema Anonymous, Inc. A nonprofit, volunteer-staffed organization designed to help emphysema victims deal with (and know more about) their disease. Emphysema Anonymous, Inc., P.O. Box 66, 1364 Palmetto Ave., Ft. Meyers, FL 33902.

The People's Medical Society. An organization maintained by the Rodale Press that offers membership by mail. Benefits include a newsletter, self-care literature, updates on medical consumer items, evaluations of hospitals and physicians, etc. For a free kit listing membership benefits, write to The People's Medical Society, 14 East Minor St., Emmaus, PA 18049.

National Psoriasis Foundation. A volunteer organization that sponsors self-help groups for psoriasis sufferers and provides other services as well. National Psoriasis Foundation, Ste. 200, 6415 Southwest Canyon Court, Portland, OR 97221.

National Amputation Foundation. A self-help organization designed to help amputees accustom themselves to the physical and emotional changes that result from a major amputation. National Amputation Foundation, 12-45 150th St., Whitestone, NY 11357.

Sex Information and Education Council of the United States. Provides information, literature, and referrals for people suffering from any type of sexual problem. Sex Information and Education Council of the United States, Ste. 407, 84 Fifth Ave., New York, NY 10011.

Anorexia Nervosa and Associated Disorders. A self-help society furnishing referrals and counseling for teenagers suffering from anorexia. Anorexia Nervosa and Associated Disorders, Ste. 2020, 550 Frontage Rd., Northfield, IL 60093.

La Leche League International, Inc. Offers instruction, counseling, and breast self-care advice for mothers who wish to breastfeed their infants. La Leche League International, Inc., 9616 Minneapolis, Franklin Park, IL 60131.

Epilepsy Concern. Designed to aid and counsel epileptics on a person-to-person basis. Epilepsy Concern also helps interested parties establish local chapters. Epilepsy Concern, 1282 Wynnewood Dr., West Palm Beach, FL 33409.

Healthright. Provides education and counseling on women's

health-care issues. Healthright, Room 1319, 175 Fifth Ave., New York, NY 10010.

United Stroke Program. A nonprofit organization that offers free self-rehabilitation programs for stroke victims. United Stroke Program, Inc., Ste. 101, 522 South Sepulveda Blvd., Los Angeles, CA 90040.

Home-Oriented Maternity Experience (HOME). Provides information, advice, counseling, and support for couples who want to experience childbirth at home. Home-Oriented Maternity Experience, 511 New York Ave., Tacoma Park, Washington, D.C. 20012.

Take Off Pounds Sensibly Club, Inc. (TOPS). A self-help group organized along the lines of Alcoholics Anonymous and dedicated to helping overweight members reduce in a sensible, realistic, and supportive atmosphere. Take Off Pounds Sensibly Club, Inc., P.O. Box 07489, Milwaukee, WI 53207.

Western Center for Health Planning. An organization that offers medical information to consumers and trains medical consumer groups. Western Center for Health Planning, Ste. 535, 703 Market St., San Francisco, CA 94103.

Neurotics Anonymous. A self-help group organized similarly to Alcoholics Anonymous. A series of small weekly meetings are designed to help members come to terms with mental and emotional problems that interfere with their well-being. Neurotics Anonymous, International Liaison, Inc., 1341 G St., N.W., Washington, D.C.

TERRAP. Designed to help members confront and deal with their phobias, especially agoraphobia (fear of the outdoors). TERRAP, Inc., 1010 Doyle St., Menlo Park, CA 94025.

International Association for Medical Assistance to Travelers. Helps travelers locate English-speaking doctors in 120 countries. Members receive an annual directory listing physicians who can be contacted twenty-four hours a day. International Association for Medical Assistance to Travelers, Empire State Bldg., Ste. 5620, 350 Fifth Avenue, New York, NY 10001.

The Center for Medical Consumers and Health-Care Information, Inc. Provides consumers with accurate, reliable, and up-to-date information on the best health-care alternatives for their particular situation. The Center features a large (and free) lending library of books on medical subjects, maintains a counseling service, and publishes a newsletter called *Health Facts*. The Center for Medical Consumers and Health Care Information, 237 Thompson St., New York, NY 10012, (212) 674-7105.

United Ostomy Association. A self-help group for patients who have undergone ostomy surgery, the Association seeks to teach them methods of self-management and to help them return to normal lives as quickly as possible after surgery. United Ostomy Association, 1111 Wilshire Blvd., Los Angeles, CA 90017.

National Association of Councils of Stutterers. An organization that specializes in forming self-help groups for chronic stutterers. National Association of Stutterers, c/o Speech & Hearing Clinic, The Catholic University of America, Washington, D.C. 20064.

SOURCES FOR SELF-CARE AIDS AND EQUIPMENT

Spenco Catalog. Medical equipment with an emphasis on sports medicine and home health care. Spenco Medical Corporation, P.O. Box 2501, Waco, TX 76702-2501, (800) 433-3334.

Cleo, Inc. Catalog specializes in home aids for the sick and convalescent: wheelchairs, exercise equipment, and aids for sleeping, lifting, standing, driving, reading, dressing, eating, bathing, etc. Cleo, Inc., 3957 Mayfield Rd., Cleveland, OH 44121, (800) 321-0595 (in Ohio call [800] 222-CLEO).

Sears Home Health-Care Catalog. Sears's typical large selection. The emphasis is on beds, incontinent supplies, self-testing and self-diagnostic equipment, bath safety devices, mastectomy needs, and fashion care clothing. The catalog features a helpful list of organizations for the disabled, self-care information and referral associations, rehabilitative services, etc. Sears Home Health Care, Department 742 BSC, 18-38, P.O. Box 5544, Chicago, IL 60680, (800) 323-3274.

3M Products for Health Care. An exhaustive and highly technical listing of professional medical equipment, this interesting catalog contains a few home health products scattered throughout. 3M, Medical-Surgical Division, St. Paul, MN 55144-1000.

Health Supplies of America. The most complete and reasonably priced of the consumer-oriented home health-care suppliers. This company offers a broad line of self-care equipment ranging from respiratory supplies to urological equipment. A best bet. Health Supplies of America, P.O. Box 288, Farmville, NC 27828, (800) 334-1187 (in North Carolina, call [800] 672-4214).

Medical Self-Care Catalog. Associated with *Medical Self-Care Magazine,* this company is one of the few in the United States that caters exclusively to consumers interested in preventive medicine. Their selection has grown considerably throughout the years and their current issues are models of interesting and useful self-care offerings. Highly recommended. *The Medical Self-Care Catalog,* P.O. Box 999, Pt. Reyes, CA 94956, (415) 663-8462.

Fred Sammons, Inc. A comprehensive catalog of medical self-help aids. The only catch is that all articles must be ordered through a physician or health-care professional. There are, however, many items here that are not offered by consumer-oriented companies. Fred Sammons, Inc., P.O. Box 32, Brookfield, IL 60513-0032, (800) 323-5574 (in Illinois call [800] 942-2129).

Abbey Medical Catalog. Although this is one of the largest and most complete medical equipment catalogs in the United States, all equipment must be ordered through a health-care professional. Abbey Medical Catalog Sales Department, 13782 Crenshaw Blvd., Gardena, CA 90249, (800) 421-5156 (in California, call [800] 262-1294).

GENERAL SELF-CARE SERVICES, AIDS, AND RESOURCES

Directory of Health-Care Professionals Who Support Medical Self-Care. Many issues of the magazine *Medical Self-Care* include a comprehensive state-by-state listing of physicians, nurses, therapists, natural healers, chiropractors, etc., who encourage self-care and will cooperate fully in a program of preventive and/or therapeutic self-maintenance. Issue numbers 6, 8, 29, 30, and 32 have included these listings. Back issues of *Medical Self Care* can be purchased for $2.50 each. *Medical Self Care,* P.O. Box 1000, Pt. Reyes, CA 94956.

Directory of Medical Self-Care Classes. Early issues of *Medical Self-Care* (issues 1, 2, 3, 4, 8) include information on medical self-care classes around the country. See entry above for information on ordering back issues.

The Strength in Us: Self-Help Groups in the Modern World. This book by Alfred Katz and Eugene Bender, published by New Viewpoints/Franklin Watts, 387 Park Ave. South, New York, NY 10016, is an excellent source of information on self-help groups in America: how and why they work, how to use them, how to start one yourself.

The Family Circle Guide to Self-Help. A book on self-help that includes a long list of self-help organizations throughout the country. It can be ordered in paperback from Ballantine Books, 400 Hahn Rd., Westminster, MD 21157 (301) 848-1900.

Medical Passport. A booklet designed for travelers, especially those suffering from chronic ailments such as diabetes or heart disease that require special medication. You record all your pertinent medical data in the booklet (immunization, current medications, allergies, drug intolerances, etc.) and keep it on your person while traveling. The "passport" will help the doctor help you in case of a medical emergency. It costs $4.00 from The Medical Passport Foundation, P.O. Box 820, Deland, FL 32720.

Medical Self-Care Tapes. New Dimensions Tapes, 267 States St., San Francisco, CA 94114, carries a large and interesting line of self-care audiocassettes including interviews with Moshe Feldenkrais, Linus Pauling, Frederick Leboyer, Michio Kushi, and many others.

BOOKS

The Activated Patient: A Course Guide, Keith Sehnert, M.D., and Joseph Nocerino. A course guide used in a sixteen-session workshop on medical self-care given by the authors. Information on ordering can be obtained from Center for Continuing Health Education, Georgetown University, P.O. Box 7268, Arlington, VA 22207.

Advanced First Aid & Emergency Care, prepared by the American National Red Cross for the Instruction of Advanced First Aid Classes, New York: Doubleday & Company, 1973 (and updates). Still the best of all first aid manuals.

Alive and Well: Decisions in Health, Arlene and Howard Eisenberg, New York: McGraw Hill Book Company, 1979. Some useful self-care information.

The Allergy Self-Help Book, Sharon Faelten and the Editors of *Prevention* Magazine, Emmaus, Pennsylvania: Rodale Press, 1983. Self-care for allergy sufferers.

Cancer: How to Prevent It and How to Help Your Doctor Fight It, George E. Berkley, Ph.D., Englewood Cliffs: Prentice-Hall, 1978. Emphasizes nutrition.

The Complete Book of Medical Tests, Mark A. Moskowitz and Michael E. Osband, New York: W. W. Norton, 1984. Good general work.

A Doctor's Guide to Home Medical Care, Trevor Weston, M.D., Chicago: Contemporary Books, Inc., 1982. Includes a limited amount of self-care material, but the title is misleading: The book's main purpose is to identify symptoms and advise the reader when these symptoms are serious enough to warrant a doctor's visit.

Do-It-Yourself Medical Testing: Over 165 Tests You Can Do At Home, Cathey Pinckney and Edward R. Pinckney, M.D., New York: Facts On File Publications, 1983. Remarkably complete, although some of these tests should probably be done under the supervision of a health-care professional.

The Essential Guide to Nonprescription Drugs, David R. Zimmerman, New York: Harper & Row, 1983. A comprehensive and well-written guide to over-the-counter medications.

The Family Doctor's Health Tips, Keith W. Sehnert, M.D., Deephaven, Minnesota: Meadowbrook Press, 1981. Very brief, but contains some useful information on self-care.

Getting Well Again, O. Carl Simonton, M.D., Los Angeles: J. P. Tarcher, 1978. A lot of useful information both on conventional therapies for cancer and on self-care techniques (such as visualization and relaxation techniques).

Healing at Home, Mary Howell, M.D., Boston: Beacon Press, 1979. Emphasizes home medical and emotional care for children.

Health Hazards Manual for Artists, Michael McCann, Ph.D. A booklet advising painters, sculptors, potters, etc., on the potential dangers of various art materials. It costs $3.50 from The Foundation for the Community of Artists, Ste. 412, 280 Broadway, New York, NY 10007.

Healthwise Handbook, Toni Roberts Beard, Kathleen McIntosh Tinker, Donald W. Kemper, Boise, Idaho: Healthwise, Inc., 1980.

Help Yourself to Health, Art Ulene, M.D. (with Sandy Feldman, M.D.), New York: Perigee Books, 1980. Interesting.

The Home Alternative to Hospitals and Nursing Homes, Mara Brand Covell, New York: Rawson Associates, 1983. The emphasis is on actual methods and techniques for home care, e.g., nursing skills, cooking and feeding of home-care patients, taking the vital signs, changing beds, identifying problems, etc.

The Home Health Care Solution, Janet Zhun Nassif, New York: Harper & Row, 1985. Loaded with solid facts and useful information—an excellent introduction to the administrative mechanics of home care.

How to Be Your Own Doctor (Sometimes), Keith W. Sehnert, M.D., New York: Grosset and Dunlap, 1981. One of the early books on medical self-care and still one of the best.

How to Practice Prospective Medicine, Lewis Robbins, Jack Hall. A manual of preventive medicine that lists fourteen causes of death, matches them up to your age, sex, and race, explains how to figure the risk factor in each category, then tells you what you can do to improve the odds. The book costs $12.50 from Health Hazard Appraisal, Methodist Hospital of Indiana, 1604 North Capitol Ave., Indianapolis, IN 46202.

The Johnson & Johnson First Aid Book, Stephen N. Rosenberg, M.D., New York: Warner Books, 1985. Another solid first aid guide.

A Manual of Laboratory Diagnostic Tests, Frances Fischback, Philadelphia: J. B. Lippincott, 1984. Highly technical, but useful for those ambitious enough to wrestle with it.

Medical and Dental X-Rays: A Consumer's Guide to Avoiding Unnecessary Radiation Exposure, Priscilla W. Laws, Washington: Health Research Group, 1974. (Order from Health Research Group, 2000 P St., N.W., Washington, D.C. 20036.)

Medical Self-Care: Access to Health Tools, Tom Ferguson, M.D., New York: Summit Books, 1980. An excellent collection of the best articles from the magazine *Medical Self-Care.*

Medical Self-Care and Assessment, Brent Q. Hafen, Ph.D., with Molly J. Brog, Ph.D., Kathryn J. Frandsen, Ed.D., Englewood, Colorado: Morton Publishing Company, 1983. Generally interesting and informative.

Medical Self-Care: Women's Health and *Medical Self-Care: Men's Health.* Both books are compiled from articles in *Medical Self-Care* and are available for $7.95 (women's) and $5.95 (men's) plus $1.00 postage from Medical Self Care, P.O. Box 717, Inverness, CA 94937.

Medical Symptoms and Treatments, by the editors of *Consumer Guide* with Jeffrey W. Ellis, M.D., New York: Beekman House, 1982. Helps readers match symptoms with diseases.

The Medicine Show, by the editors of *Consumer Reports,* New York: Pantheon Books, 1974. Another valuable insider's look at drugs.

Non-Prescription Drugs and Their Side Effects, Robert J. Benowicz, New York: Berkley Books, 1983. Especially useful for cold drugs, gastrointestinal drugs, and skin medications.

The People's Book of Medical Tests, David Sobel, M.D., Tom Ferguson, M.D., New York: Summit Books, 1985. Covers the field thoroughly, with an especially helpful section on medical self-testing.

The People's Handbook of Medical Care, Arthur Frank, M.D. and Stuart Frank, M.D., New York: Random House, 1972.

The People's Pharmacy—3, Joe Graedon, New York: Bantam Books, 1985. Inside information on which drugs really work and which drugs don't. An update of a classic—earlier editions included *The People's Pharmacy* and *The People's Pharmacy—2.*

A Physician's Complete Guide to Medical Self-Care, Timothy Rumsey and O. Otteson, New York: Rutledge Press, 1981. Good overall survey, with some information on performing medical tests at home.

The Runner's Complete Medical Guide, Richard Mangi, M.D., Peter Jokl, M.D., O. William Dayton, New York: Summit Books, 1979. One of the best self-help resources for runners.

Take Care of Yourself: A Consumer's Guide to Medical Care, Donald M. Vickery, M.D., James F. Fries, M.D., Massachusetts: Addison-Wesley Publishing Company, 1977. Contains a lot of useful information but tends to send people to the doctor a little too quickly.

Your Child: A Medical Guide, by the editors of *Consumer Guide* with Ira J. Chasnoff, M.D., New York: Beekman House, 1983. A lot of helpful and sensible advice for treating children.

Your Health Care and How to Manage It, Lawrence L. Weed, M.D. Solid instruction on how to keep your own medical records. It costs $3.80 from PROMIS Laboratory, University of Vermont, Burlington, VT 05401.

MAGAZINES

American Health—A solid health magazine containing some self-care information. $11.95 a year from American Health, P.O. Box 10034, Des Moines, IA 50347 (monthly).

Health—A popular fitness magazine that occasionally carries self-help articles, usually with a women's slant. $9.97 from Health, P.O. Box 6013, Palm Coast, FL 32037 (monthly).

Medical Self Care—By far the best and most comprehensive periodical in this country on preventive medicine and self-help. The articles and interviews cover a wide range of self-care situations from women's diseases to improving health standards on the job. Joe Graedon, author of *The People's Pharmacy,* has a regular column, and the list of self-help resources in each issue is alone worth the price of a subscription. On sale at most newsstands or by subscription. $11.97 a year from Medical Self Care, P.O. Box 1000, Pt. Reyes, CA 94956.

Nutrition Action—A magazine on food and nutrition featuring regular updates and warnings about food additives. $10.00 a year from Center for Science in the Public Interest, 1755 South St., N.W., Washington, D.C. 20009 (monthly).

Prevention—Emphasizes preventive self-help techniques, vitamins, and diet. $11.97 a year from *Prevention,* Emmaus, PA 18098-0007 (monthly).

Women's Health—A new magazine filled with thoughtful articles, columns, resource listings, etc. Although geared to women, men will find much of value here, too. Published semiannually by Rodale Press, Inc., Emmaus, PA 18049. Rodale also publishes a newsletter known as *Women's Health,* which costs $24.00 a year.

LISTS, PAMPHLETS, BIBLIOGRAPHIES, AND OTHER LITERATURE

Academic Medical Center—Affiliated Programs Participating in or Interested in Provider-Assisted Patient Self-Care—Dr. James I. Hudson has compiled a list of doctors and medical professors at universities throughout the country who are involved in self-care projects. Free from James I. Hudson, M.D., Director, Department of Health Services Association of American Medical Colleges, Ste. 200, One Dupont Circle, N.W., Washington, D.C. 20036.

Blue Cross booklets—Blue Cross publishes a large number of free pamphlets on self-care. For their list, write Blue Cross, 840 North Lakeshore Dr., Chicago, IL 60611.

Bibliography of Medical Books for the Layperson, Marilyn McLean Philbrook—An annotated bibliography of nontechnical books on medicine and health care. $2.50 from Publication Sales Office, Boston Public Library, P.O. Box 286, Boston, MA 02117.

Booklets on self-care—HEALTHWISE, 1612 N. 13th, Boise, Idaho 83702, is a small medical clinic that specializes in classes in self-care, training for self-care instructors, and production of self-care audiovisual materials. It also publishes a line of useful booklets, including *The Healthwise Handbook, Healthwise Instructors' Guide,* and *Self-Care Education: Impact on HMO Costs.* Inquire about their line of self-care videotapes.

Directory of health-oriented software—Lists software programs, many of them for laymen, in most fields of medicine. $50.00 from Moore Data Management, 1660 South Hwy. 100, Minneapolis, MN 55416.

Health Activities Project Activity Folios—The University of California will send you a free list of teaching materials used to instruct children in concepts of how the body works and how to take care of it. H.A.P./Lawrence Hall of Science, University of California, Berkeley, CA 94720.

Health Research Group—This excellent consumer organization, affiliated with Ralph Nader, will send you a free list of pamphlets that deal with controversial health concerns. Some examples are "Taking the Pain Out of Finding a Good Dentist," "Trimming the Fat Off Health Care Costs: A Consumer's Guide to Taking Over Health Planning," "Getting Yours: A Consumer's Guide to Obtaining Your Medical Records." Health Research Group, Department P, 2000 P St., N.W., Ste. 708, Washington, D.C. 20036.

Lending library books on cancer—A full line of books for cancer patients and their families. Free from Cancer Lending Library, P.O. Box 466, Sebastopol, CA 95472.

List of Resources on Medical Alternatives and Holistic Health—The list costs $1.00 from Phyllis Ochs, Schenectady County Public Library, Liberty and Clinton Sts., Schenectady, NY 12305.

Patient Brochure and Self-Help Manual—Walt Stoll, M.D., has compiled a booklet on self-care that he hands out to his patients. For $1.00 (postage and handling), he will send you a copy as well. Walt Stoll, M.D., 1412 North Broadway, Lexington, KY 40505.

Patient Information Library—Provides booklets and posters on many aspects of healing and disease. Patient Information Library, P.O. Box 50490, Palo Alto, CA 94303.

Report on Blood Pressure Cuffs—An article for comparison shoppers, first published in *Consumer Reports,* March 1979. Dated, but a good place to start your research if you're thinking of buying a cuff. Reprints cost $1.00 from Consumers Union, 256 Washington St., Mt. Vernon, NY 10550.

Self-health publications—The Health Education Center, 200 Ross St., Pittsburgh, PA 15219-2067, will send you a free copy of their unusual list of self-care books, which includes a health profile for teenagers and a bibliography of literature on health fairs.

Textbook for self-care courses—A 500-page textbook written for a college-level course on disease prevention and medical self-care, *An Invitation to Health: Your Personal Responsibility,* contains flow charts and clinical algorithms designed to help readers make informed self-care decisions. By Barbara J. Coombs, Dianne R. Hales, and Brian K. Williams, it costs $13.95 from The Benjamin/Cummings Publishing Company, 2727 Sand Hill Rd., Menlo Park, CA 94025.

INDEX